Obesity and Respiratory Disease

Guest Editors

CHARLES S. DELA CRUZ, MD, PhD
DAVID A. BEUTHER, MD, FCCP
RICHARD A. MATTHAY, MD

CLINICS IN CHEST MEDICINE

www.chestmed.theclinics.com

September 2009 • Volume 30 • Number 3

SAUNDERS an imprint of ELSEVIER, Inc.

W.B. SAUNDERS COMPANY
A Division of Elsevier Inc.

1600 John F. Kennedy Boulevard • Suite 1800 • Philadelphia, Pennsylvania 19103

http://www.theclinics.com

CLINICS IN CHEST MEDICINE Volume 30, Number 3
September 2009 ISSN 0272-5231, ISBN-13: 978-1-4377-1201-8, ISBN-10: 1-4377-1201-0

Editor: Sarah E. Barth
Developmental Editor: Donald Mumford

Clinics in Chest Medicine (ISSN 0272-5231) is published quarterly by Elsevier Inc., 360 Park Avenue South, New York, NY 10010-1710. Months of issue are March, June, September, and December. Periodicals postage paid at New York, NY and additional mailing offices. Subscription prices are $251.00 per year (domestic individuals), $400.00 per year (domestic institutions), $122.00 per year (domestic students/residents), $275.00 per year (Canadian individuals), $491.00 per year (Canadian institutions), $342.00 per year (international individuals), $491.00 per year (international institutions), and $171.00 per year (international and Canadian students/residents). International air speed delivery is included in all Clinics subscription prices. All prices are subject to change without notice. **POSTMASTER:** Send address changes to *Clinics in Chest Medicine,* Elsevier Health Sciences Division, Subscription Customer Service, 3251 Riverport Lane, Maryland Heights, MO 63043. **Customer Service: Telephone: 1-800-654-2452** (U.S. and Canada); **1-314-447-8871** (outside U.S. and Canada). **Fax: 1-314-447-8029.** E-mail: **journalscustomerservice-usa@elsevier.com** (for print support); **journalsonlinesupport-usa@elsevier.com** (for online support).

Reprints. For copies of 100 or more of articles in this publication, please contact the Commercial Reprints Department, Elsevier Inc., 360 Park Avenue South, New York, NY 10010-1710. Tel.: 212-633-3812; Fax: 212-462-1935; E-mail: reprints@elsevier.com.

Clinics in Chest Medicine is covered in *MEDLINE/PubMed (Index Medicus), Current Contents/Clinical Medicine, EMBASE/ Excerpta Medica, Science Citation Index,* and *ISI/BIOMED.*

Printed and bound in the United Kingdom

Transferred to Digital Print 2011

Contributors

GUEST EDITORS

CHARLES S. DELA CRUZ, MD, PhD
Instructor, Section of Pulmonary and Critical Care Medicine, Department of Internal Medicine, Yale University School of Medicine, New Haven, Connecticut

RICHARD A. MATTHAY, MD
Professor of Medicine, Section of Pulmonary and Critical Care Medicine, Department of Internal Medicine, Yale University School of Medicine, New Haven, Connecticut

DAVID A. BEUTHER, MD, FCCP
Assistant Professor, National Jewish Health and Department of Pulmonary and Critical Care Medicine, University of Colorado at Denver Health Sciences Programs, Denver, Colorado

AUTHORS

ERIC J. ADKINS, MD
Fellow, Pulmonary and Critical Care Medicine, Division of Pulmonary, Allergy, Critical Care and Sleep Medicine, Center for Critical Care, The Ohio State University Medical Center, Columbus, Ohio

DAVID A. BEUTHER, MD, FCCP
Assistant Professor, National Jewish Health and Department of Pulmonary and Critical Care Medicine, University of Colorado at Denver Health Sciences Programs, Denver, Colorado

GEORGE A. BRAY, MD
Boyd Professor, Pennington Biomedical Research Center, Baton Rouge, Louisiana

LEE J. BROOKS, MD
Clinical Professor of Pediatrics, University of Pennsylvania School of Medicine; and Attending Physician, Division of Pulmonary Medicine and Sleep Center, The Children's Hospital of Pennsylvania, University of Pennsylvania, Philadelphia, Pennsylvania

VICTORIA A. CATENACCI, MD
Assistant Professor of Medicine, Division of Endocrinology, Diabetes and Metabolism, Department of Medicine, University of Colorado at Denver, Denver, Colorado

CHARLES S. DELA CRUZ, MD, PhD
Instructor, Section of Pulmonary and Critical Care Medicine, Department of Internal Medicine, Yale University School of Medicine, New Haven, Connecticut

ERIC J. DEMARIA, MD
Professor of Surgery, Vice Chair, and Chief, Network General Surgery; and Director, EndoSurgery/Bariatric Surgery, Department of Surgery, Duke University Medical Center, Durham, North Carolina

ALI A. EL SOLH, MD, MPH
Associate Professor of Medicine and Social and Preventive Medicine, Veterans Affairs Western New York Healthcare System; Department of Medicine, The Western New York Respiratory Research Center, School of Medicine and Biomedical Sciences; Department of Social and Preventive Medicine; and School of Public Health, State University of New York at Buffalo, Buffalo, New York

ELIZABETH K. FIORINO, MD
Fellow, Division of Pulmonary Medicine and Sleep Center, The Children's Hospital of Philadelphia, University of Pennsylvania School of Medicine, Philadelphia, Pennsylvania

MOATAZ M. GADDOR, MD
Postdoctoral Research Associate, Department of Surgery, Duke University Medical Center, Durham, North Carolina

JOSE GOLDMAN, MD, PhD
Department of Internal Medicine, Michigan State University, East Lansing, Michigan

JOHN HARRINGTON, MD, MPH
Assistant Professor, Department of Internal Medicine, Division of Sleep Medicine, National Jewish Health, Denver, Colorado

JAMES O. HILL, PhD
Professor, Department of Pediatrics; Professor, Department of Medicine; and Director, Center for Human Nutrition, University of Colorado at Denver, Denver, Colorado

SHYOKO HONIDEN, MS, MD
Assistant Professor of Medicine, Department of Medicine, Section of Pulmonary and Critical Care Medicine, Yale University School of Medicine, New Haven, Connecticut

TEOFILO LEE-CHIONG, MD
Professor, Department of Internal Medicine, Division of Sleep Medicine, National Jewish Health, Denver, Colorado

STEPHEN W. LITTLETON, MD
Fellow in Sleep Medicine, Section of Pulmonary and Critical Care Medicine, University of Chicago, Chicago, Illinois

RICHARD A. MATTHAY, MD
Professor of Medicine, Section of Pulmonary and Critical Care Medicine, Department of Internal Medicine, Yale University School of Medicine, New Haven, Connecticut

JOHN R. MCARDLE, MD
Associate Professor of Medicine, Department of Medicine, Section of Pulmonary and Critical Care Medicine, Yale University School of Medicine, New Haven, Connecticut

JENNIFER W. MCCALLISTER, MD
Assistant Professor, Division of Pulmonary, Allergy, Critical Care and Sleep Medicine, Center for Critical Care, The Ohio State University Medical Center, Columbus, Ohio

BABAK MOKHLESI, MD, MSc
Associate Professor, Department of Medicine; Director, Sleep Medicine Fellowship Program; and Director, Sleep Disorders Center, Section of Pulmonary and Critical Care Medicine, University of Chicago, Chicago, Illinois

JAMES M. O'BRIEN, Jr, MD, MSc
Associate Professor, Division of Pulmonary, Allergy, Critical Care and Sleep Medicine, Center for Critical Care, The Ohio State University Medical Center, Columbus, Ohio

ANTHONY N. PASSANNANTE, MD
Professor of Anesthesiology, and Vice-Chair for Clinical Operations, Department of Anesthesiology, University of North Carolina Hospitals, Chapel Hill, North Carolina

FRANCOISE ROUX, MD, PhD
Assistant Professor, Department of Medicine, Section of Pulmonary and Critical Care Medicine, Yale Center for Sleep Medicine, Yale University School of Medicine, New Haven, Connecticut

NEOMI SHAH, MD, MPH
Assistant Professor, Department of Medicine, Section of Pulmonary, Montefiore Medical Center, Albert Einstein College of Medicine, Bronx, New York

AKSHAY SOOD, MD, MPH
Associate Professor of Medicine, Department of Medicine, University of New Mexico School of Medicine, Albuquerque, New Mexico

PAUL D. STEIN, MD
Director of Research Education, St. Joseph
Mercy Oakland Hospital, Pontiac; and
Department of Internal Medicine, College of
Osteopathic Medicine, Michigan State
University, DMC Campus, Detroit, Michigan

MICHAEL TIELBORG, MD
Assistant Professor of Anesthesiology,
Department of Anesthesiology, University
of North Carolina Hospitals, Chapel Hill,
North Carolina

HOLLY R. WYATT, MD
Associate Professor of Medicine,
Division of Endocrinology, Diabetes and
Metabolism, Department of Medicine,
University of Colorado at Denver, Denver,
Colorado

BASIL M. YURCISIN, MD
Minimally Invasive Surgery Fellow,
Department of Surgery, Duke University
Medical Center, Durham, North
Carolina

Contributors

PAUL D. STEIN, MD
Director of Research Education, St. Joseph Mercy Oakland Hospital, Pontiac; and Department of Internal Medicine, College of Osteopathic Medicine, Michigan State University, DMC Campus, Detroit, Michigan

MICHAEL TIELBORG, MD
Assistant Professor of Anesthesiology, Department of Anesthesiology, University of North Carolina Hospitals, Chapel Hill, North Carolina

HOLLY R. WYATT, MD
Associate Professor of Medicine, Division of Endocrinology, Diabetes and Metabolism, Department of Medicine, University of Colorado at Denver, Denver, Colorado

BASIL M. YURCISIN, MD
Minimally Invasive Surgery Fellow, Department of Surgery, Duke University Medical Center, Durham, North Carolina

Contents

Victoria A. Catenacci, James O. Hill, and Holly R. Wyatt

Obesity has reached epidemic proportions in the United States, with 35.1% of adults being classified as obese. Obesity affects every segment of the US population and continues to increase steadily, especially in children. Obesity increases the risk for many other chronic diseases, including diabetes mellitus, cardiovascular disease, and nonalcoholic fatty liver disease, and decreases overall quality of life. The current US generation may have a shorter life expectancy than their parents if the obesity epidemic is not controlled, and there is no indication that the prevalence of obesity is decreasing. Because of the complexity of obesity, it is likely to be one of the most difficult public health issues our society has faced.

Akshay Sood

Obesity, particularly severe obesity, affects resting and exercise-related respiratory physiology. Severe obesity classically produces a restrictive ventilatory abnormality characterized by reduced expiratory reserve volume. Obstructive ventilatory abnormality may also be associated with abdominal obesity. Decreased peak work rates are usually seen among obese subjects in a setting of normal or decreased ventilatory reserve and normal cardiovascular response to exercise. Weight loss may reverse many adverse physiologic consequences of severe obesity on the respiratory system.

Neomi Shah and Francoise Roux

Obstructive sleep apnea is a common disorder, and obesity is a known risk factor for its development. The prevalence of obesity is increasing worldwide, and a corresponding increase in the prevalence of obstructive sleep apnea and its cardiovascular and noncardiovascular consequences is likely. This article reviews the established evidence supporting obesity as a risk factor for obstructive sleep apnea and discusses the evidence suggesting that obesity is also a consequence of obstructive sleep apnea. There is evidence that treating obesity reduces the severity of obstructive sleep apnea and that treating obstructive sleep apnea decreases obesity. However, the evidence does not support a sustained correlation between weight loss and improvement in sleep-disordered breathing.

Stephen W. Littleton and Babak Mokhlesi

Obesity-hypoventilation syndrome (OHS), also historically described as the Pickwickian syndrome, consists of the triad of obesity, sleep disordered breathing, and chronic hypercapnia during wakefulness in the absence of other known causes of hypercapnia. Its exact prevalence is unknown, but it has been estimated that

10% to 20% of obese patients with obstructive sleep apnea have hypercapnia. OHS often remains undiagnosed until late in the course of the disease. Early recognition is important because these patients have significant morbidity and mortality. Effective treatment can lead to significant improvement in patient outcomes, underscoring the importance of early diagnosis. The authors review the definition and epidemiology of OHS, in addition to the current multifaceted understanding of the pathophysiology, and provide useful clinical approaches to diagnosis and treatment.

Population-based studies have defined a significant, bidirectional, dose-dependent association between obesity and asthma. Obesity does not cause airflow obstruction, but can result in pulmonary restriction and a reduction in airway diameter, and that could contribute to airway hyper-responsiveness. Mouse models of asthma have demonstrated that obesity and adipokines can enhance airway hyper-responsiveness, airway inflammation, and allergic responses, but it is unclear whether obesity-associated inflammatory mechanisms are relevant in human asthma. Shared environmental and genetic factors are incompletely understood, but very likely to be relevant. Obese asthma appears to be a distinct and novel phenotype of asthma, associated with a reduction in lung volumes, lack of eosinophilic inflammation, altered response to asthma controller therapy, glucocorticoid resistance, and poor asthma control.

Various abnormalities of hemostasis have been described in obesity, mainly concerning increased levels of plasminogen activator inhibitor-1, but other abnormalities of coagulation and platelet activation have been reported as well. Circulating microparticles have also been observed in obese patients. These suggest that obesity would be a risk factor for venous thromboembolism (VTE). Analysis of the database of the National Hospital Discharge Survey showed compelling evidence that obesity is, in fact, a risk factor for VTE. Obesity is also a risk factor for recurrent VTE. A synergistic effect of oral contraceptives with obesity has been shown.

Acute lung injury (ALI) and the acute respiratory distress syndrome (ARDS) are common indications for ICU admission and mechanical ventilation. ALI/ARDS also consumes significant health care resources and is a common cause of death in ICU patients. Obesity produces changes in respiratory system physiology that could affect outcomes for ALI/ARDS patients and their response to treatment. Additionally, the biochemical alterations seen in obese patients, such as increased inflammation and altered metabolism, could affect the risk of developing ALI/ARDS in patients with another risk factor (eg, sepsis). The few studies that have examined the influence of obesity on the outcomes from ALI/ARDS are inconclusive. Furthermore, observed results could be biased by disparities in provided care.

Obesity is becoming a worldwide problem of epidemic proportions, and its effect on the heart is increasingly being recognized. Obesity is often associated with an increased risk for heart failure. In this article, the authors review the evidence for obesity-related cardiomyopathy. The importance of metabolic disturbances in the development of cardiomyopathy in obese patients is highlighted. The authors also briefly explore whether obesity plays a role in the development of pulmonary hypertension. Better recognition and understanding of both obesity cardiomyopathy and pulmonary hypertension are needed in the obese patient population.

Medications can significantly increase weight loss compared with placebo in most trials. In general, patients can expect a weight loss of 8% to 10% from baseline provided they adhere to the weight-loss program and take medications regularly. All medications have side effects that need to be considered before initiating treatment, however. For sibutramine, there is an increase in blood pressure and heart rate that may require discontinuation of the drug in a small percentage of patients. For orlistat, the principal side effect is gastrointestinal in origin resulting from the increased activity of the lower bowel. Cannabinoid receptor antagonists, once a promising target, are no longer under study. Other medications are in clinical trials and on their way.

Laparoscopic Roux-en-Y gastric bypass and laparoscopic adjustable gastric banding are the most commonly performed weight reduction operations in the United States. Preoperative assessment and selection should be performed by a multidisciplinary team to obtain optimal results. The most devastating complication of bariatric surgery is leak, which can carry a high risk of mortality if not detected and treated expediently. New nationwide databases have been developed to monitor outcomes and facilitate better understanding of the mechanisms of bariatric surgery. New horizons for the advancement of bariatric surgery are in the realm of surgery in adolescent and geriatric populations, the use of weight-loss surgery in lower body mass index (<35 kg/m^2) populations, and the use of surgery to cure the comorbidities of obesity.

Airway management is a major factor underlying morbidity and mortality in the obese population. The validity of anthropomorphic prediction model in assessing a difficult airway is less accurate compared with lean subjects. Preoperative evaluation and anticipation of potential complications are critical for safe and successful intubation. Application of noninvasive positive airway pressure can prevent atelectasis and improve oxygenation during the anesthetic induction as well during the postoperative period and after liberation from mechanical ventilation. When performed by trained operators, bedside percutaneous dilatation tracheostomy in obese patients has a safety profile comparable to surgical tracheostomy but provides advantages including ease of performance and lesser cost, and obviates transporting a critically ill patient outside the intensive care unit.

> The global obesity epidemic presents anesthesia providers with unique and complex challenges as an increasing number of patients with elevated body mass index present for medical care. Pharmacokinetics, respiratory and cardiac physiology, positioning, regional anesthetic techniques, monitoring, and postoperative care are all profoundly affected by increased body mass. In recent years, the occult impact of undiagnosed obstructive sleep apnea on perioperative morbidity and mortality has marshaled increased attention from both patients and practitioners. A summary and discussion of the Practice Guidelines developed by the American Society of Anesthesiologists regarding the care of patients with obstructive sleep apnea is provided.

> The exact prevalence of obesity among critically ill patients is not known, but some evidence suggests that in the United States one in four patients in the intensive care unit is obese. The authors review the physiologic alterations in obesity that are relevant in critical illness and highlight some common diseases associated with obesity. Various practical challenges in the care of the critically ill obese patient, including drug dosing, are also reviewed.

> The prevalence of childhood obesity has more than tripled over the past five decades. Obesity results in low lung volumes, likely through increased loading of the chest wall and abdomen. The prevalence of asthma in children has paralleled the rise in obesity; obesity may increase the severity of asthma, but a direct link has been difficult to establish. Obesity is a risk factor for obstructive sleep apnea (OSA) in children as well as adults. Obese children may be at increased risk for persistent OSA following adenotonsillectomy treatment for OSA. Severe obesity and OSA may lead to the obesity-hypoventilation syndrome, with hypoxia, hypercapnia, and reduced ventilatory drive. Obesity can increase a child's risk for complications of anesthesia and recovery from surgery.

> In this article, the combined effects of aging and obesity on the respiratory system are examined. Following a concise epidemiologic overview of the prevalence of obesity among older adults, the occurrence of prospective, often variable, health consequences related to this trend are considered as well as the observed effects of the association of both aging and obesity on respiratory anatomy, physiology, and diseases. Last, findings of research related to weight loss on respiratory function in obese older adults are summarized.

Clinics in Chest Medicine

THE CLINICS ARE NOW AVAILABLE ONLINE!

Access your subscription at:
www.theclinics.com

Preface

Obesity has become a worldwide epidemic, with more than 1 billion overweight adults (body mass index [BMI] 25 to 29.9) and at least 300 million obese adults (BMI >30). Obesity is now a major health concern, contributing significantly to increased morbidity and mortality; obese persons have a 50% to 100% greater risk of death from any cause than normal-weight persons.

This edition of the *Clinics in Chest Medicine* comprehensively reviews the effects of obesity on pulmonary disease and critical care medicine in 15 articles written by authors from 14 academic medical centers. The opening article by Catenacci, Hill, and Wyatt reviews the remarkable epidemiology of obesity, with a discussion of the genesis of the obesity epidemic and how it has become one of the most difficult public health issues currently and for future generations. Next, the effect of obesity on resting and exercise respiratory physiology is discussed in detail in the article by Sood.

We include two articles on the role of obesity in obstructive sleep apnea (OSA) and the obesity hypoventilation syndrome (OHS). Shah and Roux discuss the well-established causative role of obesity in OSA and review the less well-known data that suggest obesity may also be a consequence of OSA. Littleton and Mokhlesi review the current understanding of OHS, a syndrome consisting of obesity, sleep-disordered breathing, and chronic hypercapnia.

The ensuing four articles explore the association of obesity with various cardiopulmonary diseases. Beuther examines the role of obesity in asthma and other obstructive lung diseases. Stein and Goldman review the importance of obesity as a risk factor for venous thromboembolic disease. McCallister, Adkins, and O'Brien explore the influence of obesity on the outcomes of acute lung injury and the acute respiratory distress syndrome. Dela Cruz and Matthay highlight the potential importance of obesity in the pathogenesis of cardiomyopathy and pulmonary hypertension.

Five articles are devoted to the treatment of obesity. Bray extensively reviews the medical therapy for obesity, whereas Yurcisin, Gaddor, and DeMaria discuss advances in bariatric surgery for weight reduction in obese patients. El Solh focuses on the multiple issues related to airway management of obese patients and emphasizes the importance of technically skilled practitioners. Passannante and Tielborg discuss the issues related to anesthesia in obese patients, and Honiden and McArdle review the important issue of obesity in the intensive care unit, reviewing the physiologic alterations in obesity and the practical challenges in the care of critically ill obese patients.

The final two articles in this issue focus on obese patients at the extremes of age. Fiorino and Brooks discuss obesity in children, including the increased prevalence of obesity and obesity-related diseases in the young. Harrington and Lee-Chiong discuss the combined effects of aging and obesity on the respiratory system.

We thank Sarah Barth, Publisher, Elsevier, for her invaluable assistance in the preparation of this issue of *Clinics in Chest Medicine*.

Charles S. Dela Cruz, MD, PhD
Section of Pulmonary and Critical Care Medicine
Department of Internal Medicine
Yale University School of Medicine
333 Cedar Street
New Haven, CT 06520, USA

David A. Beuther, MD, FCCP
National Jewish Health
Department of Pulmonary and Critical Care medicine
University of Colorado at Denver Health
Sciences Programs
Denver, CO 80045, USA

Richard A. Matthay, MD
Section of Pulmonary and Critical Care Medicine
Department of Internal Medicine
Yale University School of Medicine
333 Cedar Street
New Haven, CT 06520, USA

Clin Chest Med 30 (2009) xiii
doi:10.1016/j.ccm.2009.06.002
0272-5231/09/$ – see front matter © 2009 Elsevier Inc. All rights reserved.

The Obesity Epidemic

Victoria A. Catenacci, MD[a,c], James O. Hill, PhD[a,b,c],
Holly R. Wyatt, MD[a,c],*

KEYWORDS
- Etiology • Definition • Prevalence • Susceptibility
- Health Risk • Co-morbidities

RAPID RISE OF AN EPIDEMIC

Many public health officials and organizations have tried to alert the public about the dangers of obesity.[1] Reports estimate that obesity was responsible for approximately 365,000 preventable deaths in 2000.[1,2] This number was second only to that attributable to tobacco smoking. More recent reports indicate that obesity lessens life expectancy markedly, especially among younger adults.[3] Despite this knowledge and the increased media coverage about the health, social, psychologic, and economic consequences of excess body fat, the prevalence of obesity has reached epidemic proportions and continues to escalate. Between 1980 and 2004, the prevalence of obesity more than doubled from 15% to 33% in adults and the prevalence of overweight more than tripled from 5.5% to 17% in children.[4] It is not going to be possible to meet the objectives set for "Healthy People 2010" of reducing obesity prevalence in adults to 15% and in children to 5%.[5] Recent projections based on the National Health and Nutrition Examination Surveys (NHANES) predict that if the current trends continue, more than half (51.1%) of US adults are likely to be obese and 86.3% are likely to be overweight or obese by 2030.[6] In children, at the current rate, the prevalence of overweight is likely to nearly double by 2030.[6]

DEFINITIONS OF OVERWEIGHT AND OBESITY

Overweight and obesity are currently defined based on body mass index (BMI), which is determined as weight (kilograms) divided by height (square meters). **Table 1** shows the categories of BMI. A healthy BMI range is 18.5 to 24.9 kg/m^2. Overweight is defined as a BMI from 25 to 29.9 kg/m^2, and obesity is defined as a BMI of 30 kg/m^2 or greater.[7] Obesity can further be subdivided based on subclasses of BMI, as shown in **Table 1**. Extreme obesity is defined as a BMI greater than 40 kg/m^2. Waist circumference can also be used in combination with a BMI value to evaluate health risk for individuals. In children (2–19 years of age), at risk for becoming overweight is defined as a BMI-for-age greater than or equal to the 85th percentile and less than the 95th percentile on the Centers for Disease Control and Prevention (CDC) growth charts. Overweight is defined as a BMI-for-age greater than or equal to the 95th percentile on the CDC growth charts.[8]

PREVALENCE OF OVERWEIGHT AND OBESITY

The strongest data on obesity prevalence rates over time in the United States come from the results of the NHANES. The NHANES periodically collect measured heights and weights in representative samples of the population for adults,

This work was supported by grant K23 DK078913-02 from the National Institutes of Health.
Portions of this article were adapted from Hill JO, Catenacci V, Wyatt HR. Obesity: overview of an epidemic. Psychiatr Clin N Am 2005;28:1–23.
a Division of Endocrinology, Diabetes, and Metabolism, Department of Medicine, University of Colorado Denver, 4455 East 12th Avenue, Denver, CO 80220, USA
b Department of Pediatrics, University of Colorado Denver, 4455 East 12th Avenue, Denver, CO 80220, USA
c Center for Human Nutrition, University of Colorado Denver, 4455 East 12th Avenue, Denver, CO 80220, USA
* Corresponding author.
E-mail address: holly.wyatt@ucdenver.edu (H.R. Wyatt).

Clin Chest Med 30 (2009) 415–444
doi:10.1016/j.ccm.2009.05.001

Table 1
Categories of BMI and disease risk[a] relative to normal weight and waist circumference

	BMI kg/m²	Obesity Class	Men ≤ 102cm (≤ 40 in) Women ≤ 88 cm (≤ 35 in)	>102 cm (<40 in) >88 cm (>35 in)
Underweight	<18.5		—	—
Normal[b]	18.5–24.9		—	—
Overweight	25.0–29.9		Increased	High
Obesity	30.0–34.9	I	High	Very high
	35.0–39.9	II	Very high	Very high
Extreme obesity	≥40	III	Extremely high	Extremely high

[a] Disease risk for type 2 diabetes, hypertension, and CVD.
[b] Increased waist circumference can also be a marker for increased risk even in persons of normal weight.
  Data from National Heart, Lung, and Blood Institute Obesity Education Initiative Expert Panel. Clinical guidelines on the identification, evaluation, and treatment of overweight and obesity in adults: the evidence report. Obes Res 1998;6(Suppl 2):51s–210s.

adolescents, and children in the United States. The most recently reported NHANES data were collected during the period 1999 through 2006.[9,10] As shown in **Fig. 1**, obesity rates in adults (20–74 years of age) have been gradually increasing over the past 3 or more decades, with the latest statistics showing that in 2005 to 2006, approximately 67.3% of the US population was overweight or obese and approximately 35.1% was obese.[10] **Fig. 2** shows the trends since 1960 for overweight, obesity, and extreme obesity in adults.[10] Because the surveys before 1988 only include individuals up through 74 years of age, trends are shown for adults 20 to 74 years of age. Although obesity rates have doubled, the

prevalence of overweight at approximately 32% to 34% has remained stable over that same period. It seems in **Fig. 2** that the increases noted in overweight or obese prevalence rates over time have been fueled by significant increases in the obese category and not by increases in the overweight category. NHANES data from 2005 through 2006 represented the first time that the prevalence of obesity (35.1%) exceeded the prevalence of overweight (32.2%) reported in the survey.

It further seems that increasing BMI and increasing obesity prevalence rates are affecting the entire adult population, with no group being completely immune. We are experiencing increases in obesity rates among men and women

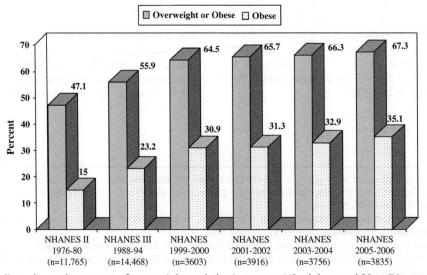

Fig. 1. Age-adjusted prevalence rates of overweight and obesity among US adults, aged 20 to 74 years, over time. (*Data from* National Center for Health Statistics Web site, December 2008). Available at: http://www.cdc.gov/nchs/products/pubs/pubd/hestats/overweight/overweight_adult.htm. Accessed January 16, 2009.

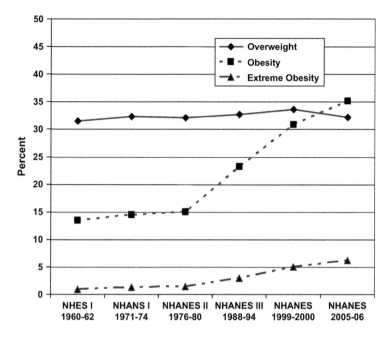

Fig. 2. Trends in overweight, obesity, and extreme obesity among US adults, aged 20–74 years, over time. (*Data from* National Center for Health Statistics Web site, December 2008). Available at: http://www.cdc.gov/nchs/products/pubs/pubd/hestats/overweight/overweight_adult.htm. Accessed January 16, 2009.

of all ethnic groups, of all ages, and of all educational and socioeconomic levels.[4,9,11,12] Although the entire population seems to be getting heavier, there is evidence that obesity affects some subgroups in the population to a greater extent than others. For example, African-America and Hispanic women have had a higher prevalence of obesity (BMI >30) than white women or men of any ethnic background (**Fig. 3**). Note that obesity prevalence rates increased over time in all gender-ethnic groups (**Figs. 4** and **5**). Further, obesity rates have consistently been higher in those with a low socioeconomic status (SES) and in those with a lower education level.[13,14] As shown in **Figs. 6** and **7**, however, similar weight gain seems to be occurring in all income and education levels.[15]

The fact that minority and low-SES individuals are disproportionally affected by obesity may not be surprising because our least expensive foods are those containing high levels of fat and sugar.[16] This means that the way to get the most calories for the least money is to eat a diet that is high in fat and sugar. This illustrates the interaction of biology and economics in supporting the obesity epidemic. Those foods for which we have a high biologic preference (foods high in sugar and high in energy density) and which contribute to overeating are currently the least expensive and most accessible.[16,17] Further, minority and low-SES individuals may engage in less physical activity than those in other sectors of the population. In low-SES populations, there are often issues of neighborhood safety, such that children are not

allowed to go outside and play. People who have more financial resources combat these circumstances more easily and, consequently, are more physically active and less obese than those with fewer resources.

Those individuals who are already overweight or obese may also be gaining weight at a more rapid

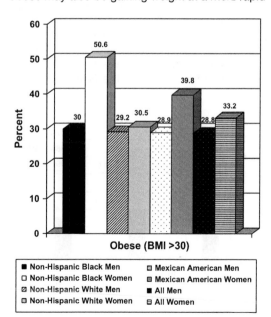

Fig. 3. Prevalence of obesity among adults aged 20 years and older by race and ethnicity for men and women in the United States: 1999 through 2004. (*Data from* Ogden CL, Yanovski SZ, Carroll MD, et al. The epidemiology of obesity. Gastroenterology 2007;132:2087–102).

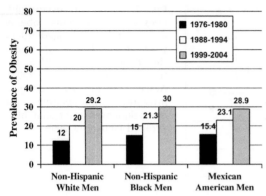

Fig. 4. Prevalence rates of obesity in men by race and ethnicity over time. (*Data from* Flegal KM, Carroll MD, Kuczmarski RJ, et al. Overweight and obesity in the United States: prevalence and trends, 1960–1994. Int J Obes 1998;22:39–47; and Ogden CL, Yanovski SZ, Carroll MD, et al. The epidemiology of obesity. Gastroenterology 2007;132:2087–102).

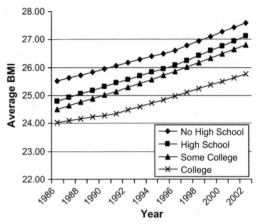

Fig. 6. Weight gain by education level over time. (*Data from* Centers for Disease Control and Prevention. Behavioral Risk Factor Surveillance System Survey data. Atlanta (GA): US Department of Health and Human Services, Centers for Disease Control and Prevention; 1998–2002).

pace than those who are not. For example, data from the Behavioral Risk Factor Surveillance System (a random-digit telephone survey of the household population of the United States) shows that it is not just that more Americans are becoming obese but that it is the most severe obesity that is increasing the most in relative terms. From 2000 through 2005, the prevalence of obesity (self-reported) increased by 24%, the prevalence of a self-reported BMI greater than 40 increased by 50%, and the prevalence of a BMI greater than 50 increased by 75% (**Fig. 8**). The greatest relative increase has been in the proportion of individuals with a BMI greater than

50 kg/m^2.[18,19] The most recent NHANES data also confirm this trend: the percentage of the population with a BMI greater than 40 has increased from 0.9% in the 1960s to approximately 6% at the current time.[10]

Obesity rates are high in most age groups. **Fig. 9** shows obesity prevalence rates for different age groups for men and women (from the NHANES 1999–2004). Obesity rates, in general, increase with age until approximately 75 years of age, when rates decline. This could be attributable to increasing mortality from obesity-related conditions.

Children have not been immune from the obesity epidemic. **Figs. 10** and **11** show the prevalence

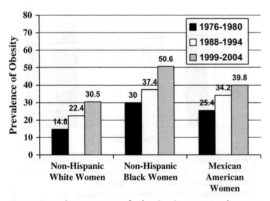

Fig. 5. Prevalence rates of obesity in women by race and ethnicity over time. (*Data from* Flegal KM, Carroll MD, Kuczmarski RJ, et al. Overweight and obesity in the United States: prevalence and trends, 1960–1994. Int J Obes 1998;22:39–47; and Ogden CL, Yanovski SZ, Carroll MD, et al. The epidemiology of obesity. Gastroenterology 2007;132:2087–102).

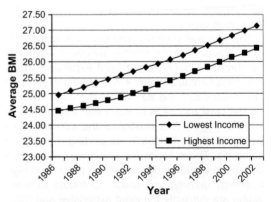

Fig. 7. Weight gain by income level over time. (*Data from* Centers for Disease Control and Prevention. Behavioral Risk Factor Surveillance System Survey data. Atlanta (GA): US Department of Health and Human Services, Centers for Disease Control and Prevention; 1998–2002).

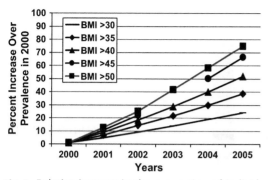

Fig. 8. Relative increase in the proportion of individuals with a BMI greater than 30 kg/m^2. (*Data from* Sturm R. Increases in morbid obesity in the USA: 2000–2005. Public Health 2007;121:492–6).

over time of overweight in children and adolescents. In this figure, based on NHANES data,[9,20] overweight is defined from age- and gender-specific growth charts developed by Cole and colleagues.[21] In 2003 through 2006, at least 16% of US children were overweight and 32% were higher than the 85th percentile; just as with adults, the prevalence of overweight has increased over time.[9,22] The prevalence of overweight in Mexican-American boys 6 to 11 years of age and 12 to 19 years of age is significantly greater than in non-Hispanic white boys. Non-Hispanic black girls have a significantly greater prevalence of overweight than non-Hispanic white girls based on NHANES 1999 through 2004 data.[4] Further, just as with adults, overweight seems to be increasing more rapidly in minority children than in white children of all ages (**Figs. 12** and **13**). A report from the Foundation for Child Development[23] has found that when considering overall

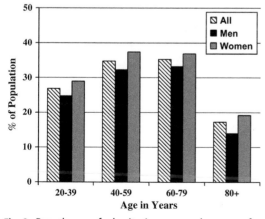

Fig. 9. Prevalence of obesity in men and women for different age groups for 1999 through 2004. (*Data from* Ogden CL, Yanovski SZ, Carroll MD, et al. The Epidemiology of Obesity. Gastroenterology 2007;132:2087–102; with permission.)

health, children are faring only slightly better today than they did 30 years ago. Increasing childhood obesity was suggested as a major reason for such slight progress.

GRADUAL FATTENING OF AMERICANS

Hill and colleagues[24] examined the trends in the increase of obesity in the United States. Their analysis suggests that the obesity epidemic arose from gradual yearly weight gain in the population produced from a slight consistent degree of positive energy balance (ie, energy intake exceeding energy expenditure). Using longitudinal and cross-sectional data sets, they found that the average adult in the United States has gained an average of 1 to 2 lb/y for the past 2 to 3 decades. **Fig. 14**, from NHANES data, shows how the BMI distribution has moved to the right over the past several years. This figure also shows the projected BMI distribution in 2008 if weight gain continues at its current rate. In **Fig. 14**, the authors show the distribution of weight gain over an 8-year period, using data from the Coronary Artery Risk Development in Young Adults (CARDIA)[12] and NHANES[20] studies. In the lower panel, they show this distribution in excess energy stored per day, assuming that an excess of 3500 kcal produces 1 lb of weight gain. Finally, the authors assumed that excess energy was stored with an efficiency of 50% (a conservative assumption). They concluded that weight gain in 90% of the adult population is attributable to a positive energy balance of 100 kcal/d or less (**Fig. 15**). Thus, it seems that the obesity epidemic arose gradually over a long period because of a slight but consistent degree of positive energy balance.

HEALTH RISKS ASSOCIATED WITH OBESITY

Obesity is linked to the most prevalent and costly medical problems seen in our country, including type 2 diabetes, hypertension, coronary artery disease (CAD), and many forms of cancer. **Box 1** lists the complications and diseases that are directly or indirectly related to obesity.

Type 2 Diabetes and Impaired Glucose Tolerance

BMI, abdominal fat distribution, and weight gain are important risk factors for the development of type 2 diabetes. It is estimated that 90% of individuals with type 2 diabetes are obese.[25] Data from the NHANES III found that almost 70% of adult men and women in the United States with type 2 diabetes have a BMI of 27 or greater and that the risk for diabetes increases linearly with BMI.[26]

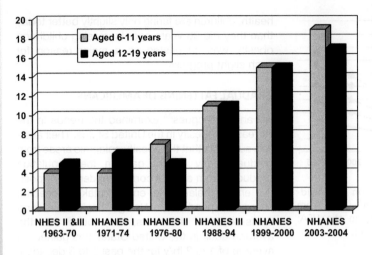

Fig. 10. Prevalence of overweight in children and adolescents over time. (*Data from* Ogden CL, Flegal KM, Carroll MD, et al. Prevalence and trends in overweight among US children and adolescents, 1999–2000. JAMA 2002;288:1728–32; and Ogden CL, Yanovski SZ, Carroll MD, et al. The epidemiology of obesity. Gastroenterology 2007;132:2087–102).

Data from 8 years of follow-up of a cohort of more than 113,000 US women aged 30 to 55 years in the Nurses Health Study found that among women with a BMI of 23 to 23.9 kg/m², the relative risk for diabetes was 3.6 times that of women having a BMI less than 22 kg/m².[27] A recent analysis indicated that the prevalence of impaired fasting glucose was 13.1% among adolescents in 2005 to 2006.[28] Overweight adolescents had a nearly a twofold higher prevalence of impaired fasting glucose than did those with a normal body weight.[28]

Dyslipidemia

Visceral obesity is associated with elevated triglycerides, low high-density lipoprotein (HDL) cholesterol, and increased small dense low-density lipoprotein particles.[29] Data from the NHANES III suggest that the prevalence of hypercholesterolemia (total cholesterol >240 mg/dL) increased progressively with BMI in men. In women, the prevalence was highest at a BMI of 25 to 27 and did not increase further with increasing BMI.[30]

Metabolic Syndrome

It is clear that obesity is often associated with a cluster of metabolic disorders that increase the risk for cardiovascular disease and diabetes. These metabolic disorders include insulin resistance, glucose intolerance, hypertension, hyperlipidemia, and markers of increased

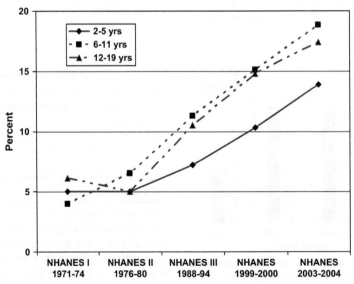

Fig. 11. Trends in child and adolescent overweight. (*Data from* National Center for Health Statistics Web site, April 2006.) Available at: http://www.cdc.gov/nchs/products/pubs/pubd/hestats/overweight/overweight_child_03.htm. Accessed January 16, 2009.

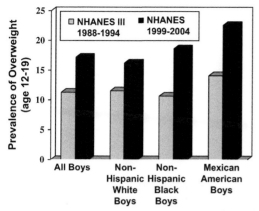

Fig. 12. Overweight prevalence by race and ethnicity for adolescent boys aged 12 to 19 years. (*Data from* Ogden CL, Flegal KM, Carroll MD, et al. Prevalence and trends in overweight among US children and adolescents, 1999–2000. JAMA 2002;288:1728–32; and Ogden CL, Yanovski SZ, Carroll MD, et al. The epidemiology of obesity. Gastroenterology 2007;132:2087–102).

inflammation. This condition is often referred to as the metabolic syndrome, formerly known as syndrome X. Formal diagnostic criteria for the metabolic syndrome for clinical use have been proposed by numerous groups and professional organizations. Diagnostic criteria set forth by the National Heart, Lung, and Blood Institute and the

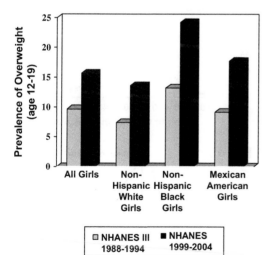

Fig. 13. Overweight prevalence by race and ethnicity for adolescent girls aged 12 to 19 years. (*Data from* Ogden CL, Flegal KM, Carroll MD, et al. Prevalence and trends in overweight among US children and adolescents, 1999–2000. JAMA 2002;288:1728–32; and Ogden CL, Carroll MD, Curtin LR, et al. Prevalence of overweight and obesity in the United States, 1999–2004. JAMA 2006;295:1549–55).

American Heart Association have set the following criteria for defining metabolic syndrome: (1) abdominal obesity (waist circumference ≥ 40 in men and ≥ 35 in women), (2) hypertension (systolic or diastolic $\geq 130/85$), (3) high triglycerides (≥ 150 mg/dL), (4) low HDL cholesterol (<40 mg/dL in men and <50 mg/dL in women), and (5) impaired glucose tolerance (≥ 100 mg/dL).[31] A person must have three of the five criteria to meet the diagnosis of metabolic syndrome. If a person is on a medication to treat one of these conditions, he or she is considered to have that condition. In a controversial paper, the American Diabetes Association took a position that there is currently not enough information to define metabolic syndrome and that this designation should not be used in clinical practice.[32] That organization thought it was not clear if the syndrome had any greater risk than the sum of the individual parts. Although the opposing view has caused some confusion for clinicians, many obesity experts believe that continuing to use the outlined criteria as a screening strategy is reasonable, and this screening strategy likely represents the mainstream of clinical care at the current time.[33]

Coronary Artery Disease

Obese persons, particularly those with abdominal fat distribution, are at increased risk for CAD. The risk for CAD begins to increase at a BMI of 23 for men and 22 for women.[34] It was previously thought that most of the increased risk was mediated by obesity-related increases in risk factors, particularly hypertension, dyslipidemia, impaired glucose tolerance or diabetes, and the metabolic syndrome. Several long-term epidemiologic studies, including the Nurses Health Study and the Framingham Study, have shown that overweight and obesity increased the risk for CAD even after correction for other known risk factors, however.[35,36] The American Heart Association added obesity to its list of major risk factors for CAD.[37]

Sleep Apnea

Obese men and women are also at high risk for sleep apnea, in which partial or complete upper airway obstruction during sleep leads to episodes of apnea or hypopnea. The interruption in nighttime sleep and repeated episodes of hypoxemia lead to daytime somnolence, morning headache, and systemic hypertension and can eventually result in pulmonary hypertension and right heart failure. In a study of 200 obese women and 50 obese men (mean BMI of 45.3) and 128 controls matched for age and gender, 40% of obese men

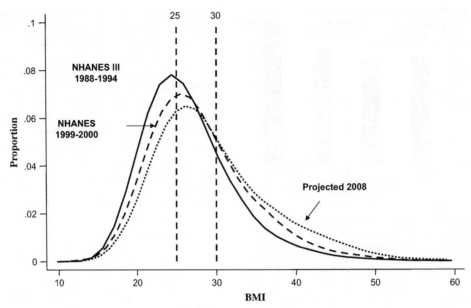

Fig. 14. BMI distribution over time. (*Adapted from* Hill JO, Wyatt HR, Reed GW, et al. Obesity and the environment: where do we go from here? Science 2003;299:853–5; with permission).

and 3% of obese women demonstrated sleep apnea warranting therapeutic intervention. Another 8% of men and 5.5% of women showed sleep apneic activity that warranted recommendation for evaluation in the sleep laboratory. In contrast, none of the 128 controls demonstrated sleep apneic activity severe enough for therapeutic intervention.[38]

Nonalcoholic Fatty Liver Disease

Obesity is associated with a spectrum of liver disease known as nonalcoholic fatty liver disease (NAFLD) or nonalcoholic steatohepatitis. Manifestations of this disorder include hepatomegaly; abnormal liver function test results; and abnormal liver histologic findings, including macrovesicular steatosis, steatohepatitis, fibrosis, and cirrhosis.[39,40] The exact prevalence of this disorder in obese patients is not fully known; however, data from autopsy studies suggest that steatohepatitis occurs in approximately 20% of obese patients.[41] NAFLD progresses to cirrhosis in approximately 10% of patients; however, the high prevalence of obesity and obesity-related liver disease makes NAFLD an important cause of cirrhosis.

Cancer

Overweight and obesity are associated with increased risk for esophageal, pancreatic, renal cell, postmenopausal breast, endometrial, cervical, and prostate cancers.[42–46] Several studies have also found a direct link between

BMI and colon cancer in men and women.[47,48] A recent prospective study of more than 900,000 adults in the United States found that increased body weight and obesity were associated with increases in death rates for all cancers combined.[49]

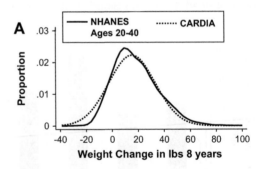

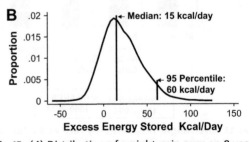

Fig. 15. (*A*) Distribution of weight gain over an 8-year period using data from the NHANES and CARDIA studies. (*B*) Distribution of excess energy stored per day accounting for predicted weight gain. (*Adapted from* Hill JO, Wyatt HR, Reed GW, et al. Obesity and the environment: where do we go from here? Science 2003;299:853–5; with permission).

Box 1
Comorbidities and complications of obesity

Cardiovascular
  Atherosclerotic cardiovascular disease
  Dyslipidemia
  Hypertension
  Congestive heart failure
  Varicose veins
  DVT/ Pulmonary embolism
Pulmonary
  Obstructive sleep apnea
  Hypoventilation syndrome
  Asthma
  Pulmonary hypertension
  Dyspnea
Psychological
  Depression
  Poor self-image
  Poor quality of life
  Eating disorders
Gastrointestinal
  Gallbladder disease/Cholelithiasis
  Gastroesophageal reflux disease
  Nonalcoholic fatty liver disease
  Hernias
Dermatologic
  Acanthosis nigricans
  Striae distensae
  Hirsuitism
  Venous stasis
  Cellulitits
  Acrochordon
  Intertrigo

Neurologic
  Stroke
  Idiopathic intracranial hypertension
  Dementia
Musculoskeletal
  Degenerative osteoarthritis
  Restrictive mobility
  Low back pain
Genitourinary
  Polycystic ovary syndrome
  Menstrual abnormalities
  Infertility
  Urinary stress incontinence
  End stage renal disease
  Hypogonadism/ Impotence
  Obesity-related glomerulopathy
Metabolic
  Type 2 diabetes
  Impaired glucose tolerance
  Hyperuricemia/ Gout
  Insulin resistance
  Metabolic syndrome
  Vitamin D deficiency
Cancer
  Breast
  Colon
  Prostate
  Uterine

It was estimated that overweight and obesity could account for approximately 14% of all deaths attributable to cancer in men and 20% of all deaths attributable to cancer in women.

Health Risks for Obesity in Children and Adolescents

It is not just adults whose health is being affected by obesity. As more and more children and adolescents are becoming obese, they are beginning to develop chronic diseases usually seen much later in life. For example, a larger number of obese children and adolescents are now being diagnosed with type 2 diabetes,[50] a disease that was virtually nonexistent in this population a few generations ago. Similarly, there is evidence that obesity in children and adolescents facilitates progression of cardiovascular disease.[51]

Quality of Life and Function

Obesity has been associated with impaired quality of life. A 1998 study measured the impact of obesity on functional health status and subjective well-being. Health-related quality of life, as measured by the Medical Outcomes Study Short Form-36 Health Survey, of more than 300 obese persons seeking treatment for obesity at a university-based weight management center was compared with that of the general population and with that of other patients with chronic medical conditions. Obese participants (mean BMI of 38.1) reported significantly lower scores (more impairment) on all eight quality-of-life domains, especially bodily pain and vitality. The morbidly obese (mean BMI of 48.7) reported significantly worse physical, social, and role functioning; worse perceived general health; and greater bodily pain than did the mildly obese (mean BMI of 29.2) or moderately to severely obese (mean BMI of 34.5). The obese participants also reported significantly greater disability attributable to bodily pain than did participants with other chronic medical conditions.[52]

Bias and discrimination against the obese have been clearly documented.[53,54] Discrimination has been shown in employment, education, and health care.[53] Social stigmatization of obese children is present[54] and could represent one of the most serious consequences of obesity in children.

HOW DID THE EPIDEMIC ARISE?
Obesity is a Disorder of Energy Regulation

The size of the body fat mass is the result of the balance between energy intake and energy expenditure. If energy intake is sustained at a level that is too high for a given level of energy expenditure or if energy expenditure is sustained at a level that is too low for a given level of energy intake, obesity develops.[55] Such a simple statement fails to reflect the complex nature of obesity and the numerous biologic and environmental factors that have an impact on energy balance (**Fig. 16**). We know, for example, that genes can influence each component of energy balance and can explain differences among individuals in body weight and body composition.[56] Although we can conclude that our genes are permissive for weight gain, the gradual weight gain of the population over the past 4 to 5 decades has occurred too quickly to be primarily attributable to genetic factors. Dr. Kelly Brownell was among the first to point out the potential role that environmental factors play in facilitating food intake and discouraging physical activity. Our current food environment is marked by an overabundance of inexpensive energy-rich foods.[24] Similarly, we have created a physical activity environment with only a rare need for physical activity to secure food and shelter and for transportation.[24] These

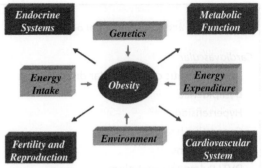

Fig.16. Pathogenesis and consequences of obesity. The size of body fat mass is the result of the balance between energy intake and energy expenditure. If intake is too high for a given expenditure or if expenditure is too low for a given intake, obesity develops over the long term. An imbalance between energy intake and expenditure can be caused by genetic or environmental factors. In most cases, genetic and environmental factors act together in the pathogenesis of overweight and obesity. Adipose tissue is not only an important energy depot but an active endocrine organ, which has an influence on cardiovascular and metabolic function, fertility, and endocrine systems. It is therefore understandable that obesity is associated with various cardiovascular, metabolic, and endocrine diseases. (*From* Hofbauer KG. Molecular pathways to obesity. Int J Obes Relat Metab Disord 2002;26(Suppl 2):S19; with permission).

environmental influences serve to reduce physical activity (which reduces energy intake) and to increase energy intake. In this "obesogenic environment," the prevalence of obesity has increased to unthinkable levels, with the age-adjusted prevalence of obesity exceeding 30%.[9] Obesity also has multiple health implications, and it has recently been hypothesized that babies born at the beginning of the twenty-first century may have shorter life expectancies than their parents.[57]

Most Americans seem to be in a state of positive energy balance over time, producing gradual weight gain and obesity. It is important to emphasize that a minor imbalance between energy intake and energy expenditure may lead to severe obesity: if energy intake exceeds energy expenditure by 5% each day, this results in a gain of 5 kg of fat mass over 1 year. A gain of 5 kg of fat mass per year leads to morbid obesity over several years.[58] There is considerable debate as to whether and to what extent, the body has physiologic processes that serve to maintain energy balance. It does seem that there is some physiologic regulation of energy balance because changes on one side (ie, energy intake, energy expenditure) of the energy balance equation do produce changes on the other side. For example, chronic changes in the amount of food consumed lead to changes in metabolism that serve to oppose a change in body weight.[59] Similarly, chronic changes in physical activity seem to have some impact on food intake.[60,61] It is clear that such compensatory physiologic changes are not sufficient to prevent changes in body weight in the face of positive or negative energy balance completely,[60,61] however, suggesting a relatively weak physiologic regulation of energy balance. Further, the physiologic system may be biased to protect more against body weight loss than against body weight gain. This makes some sense in that for most of mankind's history, starvation was a much more serious problem than obesity.[62]

The extent to which the body's physiologic regulatory mechanisms serve to maintain a healthy weight may depend on the level of "energy flux." Energy flux refers to the absolute level of energy intake and energy expenditure under conditions of energy balance.[63–65] There are several lines of evidence to suggest that a high level of physical activity improves the precision of control of food intake and that energy balance is better regulated at a higher level of energy flux.[66–69] For example, the same individual could achieve energy balance by ingesting and expending 1700 kcal/d (lower flux) or by ingesting and expending 2500 kcal/d (higher flux). A high level of energy expenditure (high flux) may create an environment in which our body weight regulation systems function optimally (under more accurate physiologic control mechanisms). In an environment in which high levels of physical activity are necessary for securing food and shelter and for transportation and in which food is inconsistently available, the body's physiologic regulatory mechanisms work well and serve to help facilitate sufficient food intake to avoid loss of body mass. As the environment has gradually changed to one in which high levels of physical activity are not required in daily life and in which food is abundant, inexpensive, and served in large portions, however, the physiologic regulation of body weight seems to be insufficient to oppose weight gain and obesity (**Fig. 17**).

As such, the obesity epidemic seems to be the result of individual susceptibility to obesity within a permissive environment. Susceptibility to obesity seems to be a polygenic trait and not the consequence of a single metabolic defect in most people.[70,71] As long as access to food is limited and energy expenditure is high, the body weight of susceptible individuals barely differs from normal. Under conditions of high energy intake or reduced energy expenditure, however, body weight in a susceptible population increases more (**Fig. 18**).[55] Our biology developed to work

best in a different environment, one in which food was inconsistent and high levels of physical activity were required to secure food and shelter and for transportation. In previous environments, this biology was adequate to allow most people to maintain a healthy weight without conscious effort. Body weight regulation was achieved for most with simple physiologic control. **Fig. 19** illustrates how the situation is different in today's environment. Securing food and shelter and moving around in our environment do not require the high levels of physical activity needed in the past.[24] Technology has made it possible to be productive while being largely sedentary. Under such conditions, weight gain can only be prevented with conscious efforts to eat less or to be physically active. Successful energy balance and avoiding weight gain in our current environment thus depend more on cognitive (not physiologic) control to keep intake equal to energy expenditure.

Individual Susceptibility to Obesity

Genetic factors

Most people regulate their body weight within a defined range that is likely determined by genetic factors. Some have described regulation of body weight as a "set point" model, in which each individual has a preferred level of body weight to defend. The gradual weight gain over time of the population suggests that this may not be the best description, however. A better model may be a "settling point." This model would predict that an individual within a constant environment with constant genetic factors would defend a specific body weight level. If genes or the environment changes, however, the level of body weight defended would change. This model is a better fit with data suggesting that as the environment has changed over the past few decades, the chronic body weight of the population has increased. There are several lines of evidence to show strong genetic influences on body weight.

Family studies Within any given environment, there is a certain degree of variation in body weight among individuals. It is estimated that up to 40% of variation in BMI can be explained by genetic factors.[72] BMI is correlated among first-degree family members,[73] and parental overweight is the most potent risk factor for childhood overweight.[74,75] In these nuclear family studies that examine sibling-sibling and sibling-parent correlations, however, it is difficult to separate genetic factors from the effect of the environment. Adoption studies provide another approach for

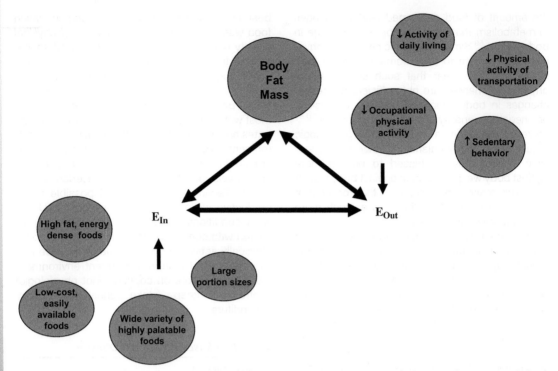

Fig. 17. Environmental factors provide a constant pressure toward positive energy balance and an increase in body fat mass. (*Adapted from* Hill JO, Wyatt HR, Melanson EL. Genetic and environmental contributions to obesity. Med Clin N Am 2000;84:333–46; with permission).

estimating heritability based on the similarity of adoptive children's body weight to that of their adoptive and biologic parents. These studies suggest a stronger role for genetics than for environment in predicting future weight. The BMI of the biologic parents is much more strongly correlated with the adult weight of the adoptive child than is the BMI of the adoptive parents.[76] Twin studies have been an integral part of the research into the genetics of obesity and provide even stronger support for the effect of genetic factors on BMI. Twin studies suggest that genetic differences between individuals clearly play important role in determining body weight. Maes and colleagues[77] summarized data on approximately 29 twin studies and found that heritability estimates were generally in the range of 50% to 90% for BMI, with the strongest correlation in monozygotic twin pairs. The observation holds true whether twins were reared separately or apart.[78]

Monogenic obesity Although several single genes causing obesity have been identified in rodents,[79] only a few monogenic causes of obesity have been described in humans. The gene whose contribution is thought to be most prevalent is the melaocortin-4 receptor (MC4R) gene.[80] MC4R mutations have been suggested as the most frequent single gene cause of obesity and are estimated to be present in approximately 4% of patients with severe obesity.[81] Melaocortin-3 receptor and MC4R are involved in suppression of food intake by α-melanocyte–stimulating hormone (MSH), and deficiency of MC4R leads to massive obesity in humans. A much rarer form of obesity has been described with mutations in pro-opiomelanocortin (POMC),[82] the precursor for the peptides that act on MC4R. Perhaps the best known single-gene mutation involves the recently isolated hormone leptin. Leptin is a 167-amino acid protein produced by fat cells and is thought to be critical in the regulation of body fat and body weight. Leptin signals the brain through leptin receptors about the size of adipose stores. Mutations in genes for leptin[83] and the leptin receptor have also been associated with obesity.[84] Few individuals with these defects have been identified, however. Treatment of leptin-deficient (but not leptin receptor-deficient) children leads to weight loss. The peroxisome proliferator activator receptor-γ (PPARγ)[85] is important in the control of fat cell differentiation and proliferation. Defects in the PPARγ receptor have been reported to cause modest obesity that begins later in life. Another defect described is in the prohormone convertase-1 (PC-1).[86] In one

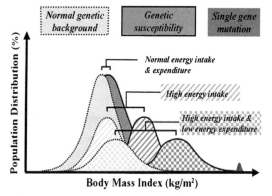

Fig. 18. Genetic susceptibility to obesity. Under conditions of normal energy intake and expenditure, subpopulations with a normal genetic background or with a genetic susceptibility to obesity have comparable BMIs (expressed as mass in kilograms divided by squared height in meters). When energy intake is high, the BMI distribution curve shifts to the right. This shift is more pronounced in a subpopulation with genetic susceptibility for obesity. An additional reduction in energy expenditure results in a further increase in BMI and a wider separation of the subpopulations. Patients with rare monogenic forms of obesity show a marked increase in BMI irrespective of the environmental conditions. (*From* Hofbauer KG. Molecular pathways to obesity. Int J Obes Relat Metab Disord 2002;26(Suppl 2): S19; with permission).

family, defects in this gene and in a second gene were associated with obesity. Members of the family with only the PC-1 defect were not obese, suggesting that it was the interaction of the two

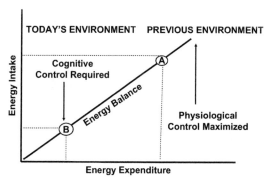

Fig. 19. Energy balance in different environments. (A) Past environment required high levels of activity and allowed energy balance and a stable body weight to be achieved under physiologic control. Activity was the "driver" and "pulled along" food intake. (B) Current environment has created a different situation in which little physical activity is required for daily activities. Energy balance is achieved through conscious efforts to eat less to match the low levels of expenditure. (*From* Hill JO, Catenacci V, Wyatt HR. Obesity: overview of an epidemic. Psychiatr Clin N Am 2005;28:17; with permission).

genes that led to obesity. These genes illustrate the potentially powerful effect that specific genes can have on obesity; however, these disorders are extraordinarily rare at the present time.

Common obesity susceptibility It is likely that obesity is a highly polygenic and complex disorder, resulting from the input of multiple genes that influence food intake and energy expenditure, with additional interactions between genes and environment. An additional 250 genes, markers, and chromosomal regions have been linked to obesity, but the clinical importance of each association is not yet known.[72] Several approaches are now being used to identify these genes, and 25 genome sites have been identified as possible links in the development of obesity. These susceptibility genes likely code for differences in genes that code for metabolic and hormonal factors, such as regulation of aspects of energy intake and energy expenditure.

Regulation of food intake

Humans regulate their food intake in a complex way that is incompletely understood. Many hormones and peptides seem to be involved in the food intake regulatory system. Gastrointestinal peptides play an important role in mediation of hunger and satiety. Ghrelin, produced by the stomach, is a potent stimulus for food intake and may be involved in meal initiation. Cholecystokinin, gastrin-releasing peptide, and neuromedin B all have been implicated in reducing food intake. Pancreatic peptides also modulate feeding: glucagon and glucagon-like peptide-1 (GLP-1) reduce food intake. Plasma nutrient levels may also be important afferent satiety signals. For example, a small drop in circulating glucose levels has been found to precede the onset of eating. Longer range signals of satiety may be related to body energy stores (eg, body fat, glycogen). Leptin is a hormone secreted into the circulation from adipocytes as fat cell size increases and may serve as a signal within the brain to decrease food intake and increase energy expenditure.[81]

Signals from the periphery, including the gastrointestinal tract and adipose tissue, are monitored by a sophisticated neural system within the brain that interprets and integrates a continuous stream of information from the internal and external environment. Monoamine systems, such as serotonin and norepinephrine, and amino acids and neuropeptides, such as neuropeptide Y (NPY), agouti-related peptide (AGRP), POMC, MSH, cocaine and amphetamine-related transcript (CART), melanin-concentrating hormone (MCH), and corticotrophin-releasing hormone (CRH), are known to influence eating behavior.[87] Leptin is transported across the blood-brain barrier and has an impact on receptors in the central nervous system, inhibiting the production of several orexigenic neuropeptides (NPY, AGRP, and MCH) while enhancing the production of hormones known to inhibit food intake (MSH [which acts on MC4R], CART, and CRH).[58,88] Genetic variations in these complex pathways involved in the regulation of energy intake may play a large role in individual differences in food intake and food-related behaviors. Genetic among individuals in levels or activity of these peptides and hormones or their receptors could potentially affect energy intake and body weight. Genes may also influence preference for certain foods or for certain macronutrients. Regulation of daily food intake probably plays a greater role in maintaining energy balance than the small changes in metabolic rates that occur during overfeeding or underfeeding in determining body weight.[58]

Regulation of energy expenditure

Total energy expenditure (TEE) is the sum of resting energy expenditure (REE) and thermic effect of food and energy expended in physical activity (PAEE). The components of TEE and a comparison of TEE in sedentary and active individuals are shown in **Fig. 20**. It has been argued that slight differences in REE are important for the development of obesity.[89] Individual differences in REE on the order of 5% to 10% have

been identified in certain populations and have been found to predict weight gain over time.[90] As pointed out by Bessard and colleagues,[91] however, the concept of "a low metabolic rate at the origin of weight gain" does not take into account the fact that the gain in body weight caused by a low resting metabolic rate should result in an increase in REE over time, which would essentially normalize the low metabolic rate. Even if a low resting metabolic rate plays a role in weight gain in some people, a weight gain of approximately 5 to 10 kg is sufficient to normalize the metabolic rate. Thus, a low resting metabolic rate could only explain up to 10 kg of weight gain. Greater increases in body weight, and therefore the development of obesity, must involve excessive caloric intake, low levels of physical activity, or other metabolic factors.

Individual differences in PAEE clearly have a significant impact on body weight. PAEE is the most variable component of energy expenditure and can easily range from 10% of TEE in sedentary individuals to 40% of TEE in highly active individuals. Physical activity provides the greatest source of flexibility in the energy expenditure system and is the component through which large differences in energy expenditure can be achieved. For example, the US Pima Indians, who live a typical North American lifestyle, have a high prevalence of obesity and type 2 diabetes. In contrast, Mexican Pima Indians, who still live a traditional lifestyle in the Sierra Madre Mountains, are quite lean when compared with their American counterparts (average BMI: 24.9 versus 33.4) despite an estimated separation of these populations 700 to 1000 years ago.[92] Esparza and colleagues[93] compared the physical activity level of 40 Mexican Pima Indians from a remote mountainous area of northwest Mexico with that of 40 age- and gender-matched Pima Indians from the Gila River Indian Community in Arizona. They found that physical activity was significantly greater in Mexican Pima Indians when compared with US Pima Indians (TEE adjusted for resting metabolic rate: 3289 ± 454 versus 2671 ± 454 kcal/d; $P < .0001$). These results emphasize the importance of physical activity in the prevention of obesity in genetically susceptible populations.

PAEE can be separated into two components: exercise activity thermogenesis and nonexercise activity thermogenesis (NEAT). NEAT has an enormous variety of constituents, including the energy expenditure of occupation, leisure, sitting, standing, ambulation, talking, and fidgeting. Recent evidence suggests that NEAT may be biologically determined and plays an important role in body weight regulation.[94,95] Levine and

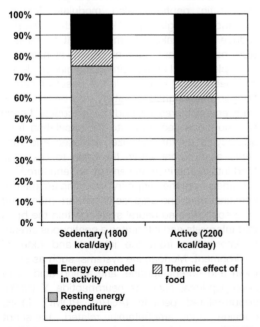

Fig. 20. Components of TEE in sedentary and active individuals.

colleagues[95] measured changes in energy storage and energy expenditure in 16 nonobese volunteers who were fed 1000 kcal/d in excess of weight maintenance requirements for 8 weeks. Volitional activity was kept at constant low levels, and compliance was confirmed through questionnaires and accelerometer-derived measurements of physical activity. Changes in NEAT were found to account for the 10-fold differences in fat storage and directly predicted resistance to fat gain with overfeeding ($r = 0.77$, $P<.001$). These results suggest that as humans overeat, activation of NEAT dissipates excess energy to preserve leanness and that failure to activate NEAT may result in ready fat gain. In a subsequent study, Levine and Kotz[96] reported that obese individuals were seated, on average, 2 hours longer per day than lean individuals and that this did not change when the obese individuals lost weight or when lean individuals gained weight, suggesting that NEAT is biologically determined. This is supported by additional work from Levine's laboratory demonstrating a biologic basis for NEAT's role in body weight regulation in rodents.[97] Presently, the genetic basis of NEAT remains undefined, but NEAT may be extremely important in determining the response to the environmental factors that lead to obesity.

Until quite recently, brown adipose tissue (BAT) has been thought to be primarily important in small mammals and infants to maintain body temperature. It has been generally thought that BAT is rapidly lost after birth and that humans do not possess more than vestigial amounts of BAT later in life. As such, any significant function in the adult human physiology and metabolism was dismissed because of low numbers of brown adipocytes.[98] Recent observations made as a result of the use of fluorodeoxyglucose positron emission tomography (FDG PET) to trace tumor metastasis may change the prior thinking about the role of brown fat in humans, however. Nedergaard and colleagues[99] reported symmetric areas of increased tracer uptake in the upper parts of the human body on FDG PET scans corresponding to BAT deposits. These investigators conclude that a substantial fraction of adult humans possess active BAT and that this tissue has potential to be of metabolic significance for normal human physiology. For example, it is possible that BAT could be activated in times of caloric excess and could be "protective" against the development of obesity in this way. A few retrospective attempts have been made to examine whether there is a correlation between the possession of active BAT and low body weight (BMI). Some of these studies claim such a relation;[100] others claim that

such correlations do not exist.[101,102] Further research is needed to confirm the presence and determine the metabolic significance of these deposits of brown fat in humans. Nevertheless, this finding implies that there may be aspects of individual regulation of energy expenditure and susceptibility to obesity that are not fully understood.

Environmental Promoters of Obesity

Dietary factors

Many dietary factors can directly and indirectly change the balance between energy intake and expenditure and influence body weight. Dietary factors that have been implicated in the development of obesity include dietary fat, energy density, calcium intake, sugar-sweetened beverages, portion size, dietary variety, and economic factors related to convenience and cost.

Dietary fat Diets high in fat have been suggested to increase the risk for obesity. In experimental studies, sedentary animals given ad libitum high-fat diets gain weight and become obese as compared with those given a low-fat diet. In humans, however, the relation between dietary fat and the development of obesity is somewhat controversial. Ingestion of excess calories is clearly central in the development of obesity. Because subjects tend to eat a constant weight of food on high- and low-fat diets, high-fat diets seem to increase the risk for overeating and excessive caloric intake. The epidemiologic literature on the relation between fat intake and body weight was critically reviewed by Lissner and Heitmann.[103] Although the data are not entirely consistent, these researchers concluded that the greater the amount of dietary fat that humans consume is, the greater is their body weight. In addition, it seems that a reduction in dietary fat without intentional restriction of energy intake causes weight loss.[104]

Energy density Increasing energy density of foods may be another major contributor to the obesity epidemic. Energy density is defined as "the amount of energy in a given weight of food (kcal/g or kJ/g)".[105] Water content is a major determinant of energy density because the amount of water added to a food increases food weight but not energy. Thus, soups, milk, and beverages typically have a low energy density, as do natural fruits and vegetables. Processed foods high in fat and sugar are energy dense and often highly palatable, which may lead to overeating.[106] Several short-term feeding studies have shown a positive relation between the energy density of foods and energy intake.[105,107] Studies have also shown that energy intake increases as energy density increases even when the dietary fat content is maintained at a constant level.[68]

Dietary calcium intake The potential impact of calcium in the development of obesity has recently attracted a great deal of attention. Calcium plays an important role in regulating lipogenesis, and it has been postulated that a higher calcium intake could have an "antiobesity effect".[108,109] Population studies have shown that the level of calcium intake is inversely related to the obesity rate.[110,111] Epidemiologic studies have also reported an association between higher dietary calcium levels and reduced BMI.[111] In a 24-week randomized controlled trial of 32 obese adults maintained on a 500-kcal/d deficit diet, Zemel and colleagues[112] found that weight loss was enhanced in men and women assigned to high-calcium and high-dairy diets. These results have not been confirmed by several larger trials,[113–115] however, and most prospective studies have not found beneficial effects of calcium or dairy products on weight gain.[116–119]

Sugar-sweetened beverages The time trend data over the past several decades have suggested that the increase in obesity rates has been closely paralleled by an increase in consumption of sugar-sweetened beverages. Malik and colleagues[120] recently conducted a systematic review of 30 studies on this topic, with greater weight given to data from large prospective studies and randomized clinical trials. They found that most (but not all) studies reported a significant positive association between the intake of sugar-sweetened beverages and increases in overweight or obesity in children. Ludwig and colleagues[121] found that for each additional serving of sugar-sweetened drink per day, BMI increased by 0.24 units and the odds of obesity increased by 60%. Several prospective studies have examined the relation between sugar-sweetened beverage consumption and obesity in adults. In the largest study, Schulze and colleagues[122] found that women who increased consumption of sugar-sweetened beverages gained the most weight, whereas women who decreased their consumption gained the least weight over a 4-year follow-up period. Finally, a recent cohort study of more than 7000 Spanish men and women found a positive association between higher consumption of sugar-sweetened beverages and risk for weight gain.[123] Thus, the weight of evidence indicates that greater consumption of sugar-sweetened beverages is associated with weight gain and obesity in children

and adults. It has been suggested that one reason for this association may be that sugars consumed in liquid form rather than in solid form are less likely to be compensated for during the day.[124,125] Thus, it has been hypothesized that sugars, when consumed in drinks, contribute to excess energy intake by "bypassing" regulatory systems;[121,124,126,127] however, this is still controversial.

High-fructose corn syrup Sucrose consumption has declined from 80% of total caloric sweeteners in 1970 to 40% in 1997 because high-fructose corn syrup (HFCS) has primarily been used to substitute for sucrose as a caloric sweetener in the United States. The increase in the consumption of high-fructose corn sweeteners has occurred over the same period as the epidemic of obesity, prompting recent concerns about HFCS as a cause of the obesity epidemic.[128] The digestion, absorption, and metabolism of fructose differ from those of glucose.[128] Unlike glucose, fructose does not stimulate insulin secretion[129] or enhance leptin production.[128] Once inside the cell, fructose can enter the pathways that provide the glycerol backbone for triglyceride synthesis more efficiently than glucose.[87] Thus, there is concern that high fructose consumption, as is occurring with the increasing consumption of soft drinks and the use of high-fructose corn sweeteners, may be a "fat equivalent".[87] A recent study reported by Soenen and Westerterp-Platenga[125] investigated the effects of HFCS, sucrose, or milk drinks, however, and the results suggest that "all beverages may be created equal." Caloric compensation for the beverages tested (the reduction of food intake at the test meal 50 minutes later as a percentage of calories in the preload beverage) was incomplete, averaging less than 40% for women and 60% for men. There was no difference between beverages in caloric compensation; visual analog scale ratings of satiety; or postprandial blood concentrations of glucose, insulin, GLP-1, or ghrelin. In an interesting editorial accompanying that article, Dr. G. Harvey Anderson stated that although a food solution to obesity remains elusive, "a reductionist approach that focuses on one food or one component of the food supply, in the presence of too much, is unlikely to succeed."[130]

Portion size Over the past several decades, portion sizes have increased markedly,[131] with the advent of supersizing and ever larger baked goods and candy bars. Americans associate quantity with quality; thus, restaurants and food manufacturers are providing larger and larger quantities as evidence of value. Young and Nestle[132] determined marketplace portion sizes, identified changes in these sizes with time, and compared these marketplace portions with federal standards as defined by the US Department of Agriculture (USDA) and the Food and Drug Administration (FDA). They found that most marketplace portions exceed standard serving sizes by at least a factor of 2 and sometimes by eight fold. Short-term experimental studies have demonstrated that adults provided with large portions of food have significant higher energy intake.[133,134] The greater energy content of larger food portions could be contributing to the increasing prevalence of overweight and obesity.

Dietary variety Before this century, refined sugars and flours were luxury items used only on special occasions. Our current diet consists of numerous highly palatable snacks and deserts produced from fats, refined sugars, and starches. The aggressive and sophisticated marketing of the food industry targets children and adolescents with appealing images of sweetened cereals, candies, cookies, and high-caloric beverages. Studies have suggested that a large variety of sweets, snacks, condiments, entrees, and carbohydrates, coupled with a small variety of vegetables, promotes long-term increases in energy intake and body fatness. McCrory and colleagues[135] evaluated 71 healthy men and women who provided accurate reports of dietary intake and completed a body composition assessment. These researchers found that dietary variety was positively associated with energy intake within each of 10 food groups. In multiple regression analysis with age and gender controlled for, dietary variety of sweets, snacks, condiments, entrees, and carbohydrates (as a group) was positively associated with body fatness, whereas variety from vegetables was negatively associated with body fatness.

Economic factors influencing diet The average American spends only approximately 10.7%[136] of his or her net income on food. Food with high levels of fat and sugar is particularly inexpensive. Drewnowski and Specter[16] explored the relation between fat and sugar consumption, energy density of food, and energy costs of food and came to the following conclusions. First, the rates of obesity in the United States follow a socioeconomic gradient, such that the highest obesity rates are associated with the lowest incomes and low levels of education. Second, there is an inverse relation between energy density of food and energy cost of food, such that energy-dense foods composed of fats and sugars are lower in cost. Third, the high energy density and palatability of sweets and fats are associated with higher energy intakes. Fourth, poverty and food insecurity are associated with lower food expenditures and lower quality diets. This economic approach suggests that food choices and diet are influenced by economic resources and food costs. Low-cost energy-dense diets are likely to be highly palatable, contain added sugars and fats, and promote the development of obesity and overweight.

Declining levels of physical activity
A low level of physical activity decreases TEE and causes weight gain unless matched by a decrease in energy intake. In 2005, only approximately half of US adults reported engaging in the levels of leisure time physical activity (LTPA) recommended by the CDC (30 minutes of moderate activity at least five times a week or 20 minutes of vigorous activity at least three times a week) and 25% of US adults reported engaging in no LTPA.[137] LTPA accounts for only a small proportion of total physical activity energy expenditure; thus, it is perhaps even more important to examine trends in other types of physical activity, including occupational, transportation, and household activities.

Brownson and colleagues[138] conducted a comprehensive review of trends in physical activity in the United States over the past 50 years. This study showed that LTPA has been relatively stable or slightly increasing over time. Nevertheless, although LTPA has not decreased, and may have even increased moderately, this increase has not compensated for substantial decreases in activities related to work, transportation, and household chores. Improvements in technology over the past several decades have significantly reduced energy expenditure required for daily living. Use of automated equipment in the household (ie, central heat, washing machines, dishwashers) has decreased the energy required in preparing food and maintaining a comfortable home. Physical activity in the workplace has also been reduced. Estimates based on data from the US census bureau show that in the past 50 years, the percentage of the labor force in high-activity occupations (farm workers, waiters and waitresses, construction laborers, and cleaning service workers) has declined from approximately 30% in 1950 to 23% in 2000, whereas the percentage of laborers in low-activity occupations has increased from 23% in 1950 to 42% in 2000.[139] This shift in job categories, combined with increased automation and computer use, has led to a substantial decline in occupational physical activity. Another major contributor to the decline in overall physical activity is the dramatic increase in the use of cars for transportation, a trend that has been accompanied by a decline in walking and public transportation. Furthermore, increased concern about crime limits walking and playing outside in some areas. In contrast, sedentary behaviors have increased dramatically.[138] Television, video games, and the Internet have replaced active forms of entertainment and leisure time activities in many adults and children. According to the 1998 Nielsen Report on Television (A.C. Nielsen Co., Media Research Division, Northbrook, Illinois), the average US male adult watches 29 hours of television a week and the average female adult watches 34 hours of television a week.

In contrast, a recent article published by Westerterp and Speakman[140] examined trends over the past 20 years in measurements of the energy expenditure of physical activity directly measured with doubly labeled water in subjects from The Netherlands (n = 366) and North America (n = 393). Because doubly labeled water has only been used to measure free living energy expenditure in human population studies since 1982, this is the earliest period for which direct measures of human energy expenditure are available. These researchers found that energy expenditure of physical activity has not declined significantly since the 1980s to the present, a period of time over which obesity rates have increased. On the basis of this analysis, they concluded that reduced energy expenditure attributable to lowered physical activity energy expenditure is unlikely to have fueled the obesity epidemic. As these investigators themselves point out, however, it is possible that none of these measurements of energy expenditure were made early enough to capture the change in energy expenditure that is predisposing our society to weight gain. An alternative explanation may also lie in the impact of increasing body size on physical activity energy expenditure. It is possible that the lack of difference in physical activity energy expenditure over this period was a result of an increase in body weight over time in the populations studied. As body weight increases, there is a consequent increase in physical activity energy expenditure attributable to an increase in the energetic cost of moving a larger body mass. Thus, it is possible that although we, as a population, may move less, this does not necessarily translate to a lower energy expenditure of activity because of our increased body size. In effect, we achieve energy balance at a higher level of energy flux (and at a higher level of energy intake) because of the increased physical activity energy expenditure associated with a greater body mass.

Comparisons of the level of physical activity in obese and lean individuals have provided conflicting results and are confounded by the fact that an individual's level of activity may decline as he or she gains weight. Data from the UK population indicate that decreased physical activity preceded the increase in the prevalence of obesity in that population, however.[141] In addition, more than 30 prospective cohort studies have examined the association between physical activity and weight change over time. For example, cross-sectional analysis of baseline and follow-up data from the NHANES I revealed that recreational physical activity was inversely related to body weight. The estimated relative risk for major weight gain for those in the low-activity level at the follow-up survey compared with those in the high-activity level was 3.1 (95% confidence interval [CI]: 1.6–6.0) in men and 3.8 (95% CI: 2.3–6.5) in women. In addition, the relative risk for persons whose activity level was low at the baseline and follow-up surveys was 2.3 (95% CI: 0.9–5.8) in men and 7.1 (95% CI: 2.2–23.3) in women.[142] Schmitz and colleagues[143] examined the longitudinal relationship between changes in physical activity and weight gain during 10 years of follow up among a cohort of 5115 black and white men and women aged 18 to 30 years at baseline in the CARDIA Study. Over the 10 year follow up period, change in physical activity was inversely associated with weight change within all four race and sex subgroups ($P<.05$). As with studies of dietary factors and obesity, many methodologic issues may complicate epidemiologic studies of physical activity and obesity, including inaccurate and imprecise measurements of physical activity, reverse causation, and confounding by diet and other lifestyle factors. Nevertheless, cumulative evidence from prospective studies and randomized clinical trials indicates that physical activity plays an important role in weight control, probably mediated through multiple pathways, including increasing TEE, reducing fat mass, and maintaining lean body mass and resting metabolic rate among others.

Novel hypotheses about environmental promoters of obesity

Although most attention has traditionally focused on high caloric diet and sedentary lifestyle as the root causes of the obesity epidemic, there is a growing recognition that the roles of additional environmental factors should not be ignored.

Prenatal and early postnatal environment The environment encountered during fetal and early postnatal life may affect adult body weight. The "fetal origins" hypothesis, first proposed by Barker and colleagues[144,145] and elaborated by several groups over the past 15 years to be termed the *developmental origins of adult health and disease*, provides an alternative explanation for the increasing rates of obesity. This hypothesis states that exposure to an unfavorable environment during development (in utero or in the early post-natal period) programs changes in fetal or neonatal development, such that the individual is then at greater risk for developing adulthood disease, including obesity.[146,147] Several studies have found that adult men and women born small for gestational age were more likely to have a higher BMI, a higher waist-to-hip circumference ratio, the metabolic syndrome, and CAD than those who were normal size at birth.[148–151] More than a dozen studies now confirm that maternal smoking is associated with offspring obesity. In a meta-analysis of 14 studies, Oken and colleagues[152] estimated that maternal smoking during pregnancy increased the odds that the offspring would be obese (defined by BMI cut points) between the ages of 3 and 33 years by 50%. Adjustment for factors related to social and economic position did not markedly change these estimates; however, residual confounding is still possible. Higher maternal BMI at the onset of pregnancy and greater amount of weight gain during pregnancy have been shown to have an impact on body weight of offspring. Oken and colleagues[153] also showed that excess weight gain during pregnancy was associated with a higher risk for obesity in the offspring at the age of 3 years. Maternal diabetes also increases the risk for being overweight as children and adults.[154]

A body of evidence also suggests that breast-feeding could be protective against obesity.[155–162] A US survey of more than 15,000 children aged 9 to 14 years and their mothers found that among subjects who had been only or mostly fed breast milk compared with those only or mostly fed formula, the odds ratio for being overweight was 0.78 (95% CI: 0.66–0.91) after adjustment for age, gender, sexual maturity, energy intake, time watching television, physical activity, and mother's BMI, in addition to other variables reflecting social, economic, and lifestyle factors.[162] A meta-analysis of duration of breastfeeding estimated a 4% decreased risk for obesity for each additional month of breastfeeding.[157] Other recent cohort studies[163,164] have found no significant effect, however. The reasons for these contradictory findings are unclear but may be related to differences in the methods used for ascertaining individuals' exposure to breast milk, differences in the methods used for measuring and adjusting

for confounders, the selection of disparate end points for the measurement of obesity, and the statistical power of the studies.[165] According to Clifford, "the possibility remains that even if the effect of breast feeding on future obesity is small the public health impact can be tremendous."[165] Although confounding still may be an issue (eg, mothers who breastfeed may be more vigilant regarding other aspects of the environment that could affect weight gain), the best evidence to date suggests that having been breastfed lowers the risk for future obesity. In fact, the recent Endocrine Society clinical practice guideline for prevention and treatment of pediatric obesity recommends breastfeeding infants for at least 6 months for the prevention of obesity.[166]

The reason why breastfeeding might reduce the risk for obesity later in life is unclear. Observations using a rat model provide support for the theory that mother's milk is the ideal diet for newborns and that an increased carbohydrate intake during infancy—even in the form of carbohydrate-enriched milk formula—could program for chronic hyperinsulinemia, hyperphagia, obesity, and related disorders.[167] Recent studies have also suggested that leptin may be the specific compound responsible for some of the beneficial effects of breastfeeding. Leptin is present in breast milk but is not present in infant formula, and when it is ingested during the suckling period, it can be absorbed by the immature stomach, exerting biologic effects.[168]

Viral infections In recent years, viral infections have been recognized as a possible cause of obesity. Although several viruses have been reported to induce obesity (infecto-obesity) in animal models, until recently, the viral etiology of human obesity has not received much attention because the virus studies were not able to infect humans. In a series of articles over the past 10 years, however, Dhurandhar and colleagues have demonstrated that a human adenovirus, adenovirus-36 (Ad-36), is capable of inducing adiposity in experimentally infected chickens, mice, and nonhuman primates (marmosets).[169–171] Animals inoculated with Ad-36 show a higher fat percentage combined with low levels of serum cholesterol and triglycerides.[170] Ad-36 is known to increase the replication, differentiation, lipid accumulation, and insulin sensitivity in fat cells and reduces those cells' leptin secretion and expression.[172] Recent studies have shown that, in the United States, antibodies to Ad-36 were more prevalent in obese subjects (30%) than in nonobese subjects (11%).[173] In addition, in twins discordant for infection with Ad-36, the infected twins were heavier and fatter than their cotwins.[173] It has recently been postulated that Ad-36 may be a contributing factor to the worldwide increasing problem of obesity.[172,174]

Environmental toxins Growing scientific evidence supports the hypothesis that numerous environmental chemicals with hormone-like activity can interfere with complex endocrine signaling pathways and cause adverse health effects.[175-179] Environmental estrogens (ie, chemicals with estrogenic potential) have been reported to alter adipogenesis using in vitro model systems, but other classes of endocrine-disrupting chemicals (EDCs) are now coming under scrutiny as well. Concern regarding these compounds initially focused only on potential reproductive and carcinogenic effects. More recently, however, obesity has been proposed to be yet another adverse health effect of exposure to EDCs during critical stages of development.[180-185] These recent findings highlight the possible involvement of "environmental obesogens," chemicals that can disrupt the normal controls of adipogenesis and energy balance, in the worldwide increase in obesity rates.

Examples of these compounds include bisphenol A (BPA), organotins, and phytoestrogens. BPA, an endocrine disruptor, is detectable at nanomolar levels in human serum worldwide. BPA is widely found in polycarbonate plastic used to make a variety of common products, including baby and water bottles. Concerns about the use of BPA in consumer products grabbed headlines in 2008 when several governments issued reports questioning its safety and some retailers pulled products made from it off their shelves. Subsequently, the first study of BPA's effects on humans was published in September 2008 by Lang and colleagues.[186] The cross-sectional study of almost 1500 people assessed exposure to BPA by looking at levels of the chemical in urine. These researchers found that high BPA levels were significantly associated with heart disease, diabetes, and abnormally high levels of certain liver enzymes. An editorial in the same issue notes that "while this preliminary study needs to be confirmed and cannot prove causality, there is precedent for analogous effects in animal studies, which add[s] biological plausibility to the results reported by Lang et al."[187] Recent studies have also suggested a mechanism for a link between BPA and obesity. A study by Hugo and colleagues[188] reported that BPA at environmentally relevant doses inhibits the release of adiponectin, a hormone made by fat cells, which may protect against the metabolic syndrome. The mechanism by which BPA suppresses adiponectin has not been determined. These investigators concluded that "given the endurance of BPA in the environment, its presence in serum from humans worldwide, and the suppression of adiponectin release at nanomolar concentrations, BPA may indeed be the bona fide endocrine disruptor that adversely affects metabolic homeostasis and its manifestations."[188] As such, BPA has been at the center of the debate over potential adverse effects of man-made chemicals, and there are substantial disagreements over interpretation of studies and differences of opinion regarding the potential toxicity of BPA. Although the FDA has reassured consumers that BPA is safe, it has convened an outside panel of experts to review this issue. In contrast, in September of 2008, the US National Toxicology Program issued a report in which it expressed "some concern" that infants were at risk from exposure to the chemical, and the Canadian government has formally declared BPA a hazardous substance as of October 2008.

Phytoestrogens, contained in various food and food supplements (particularly in soy products), are another class of chemicals receiving attention. Genestein is one of the most abundant phytoestrogens in the human diet, and in mouse models, it has been found to induce adipose deposition in male mice.[189] Use of soy-based infant formula containing genestein has also been associated with obesity later in life.[190] Organotins represent a class of widespread persistent organic pollutants with potent endocrine-disrupting properties in invertebrates and vertebrates. New data identify tributyltin chloride and triphenyltin chloride as nanomolar agonist ligands for retinoid X receptor (RXRα, RXRβ, and RXRγ) and PPARγ, nuclear receptors that play important roles in lipid homeostasis and adipogenesis.[191] Clearly, many uncertainties remain about the full extent of health consequences that may follow exposure to EDCs. Whether the results of these agents in experimental and animal models can be extrapolated to health hazards in humans also remains to be determined. This is an area that merits further research, however.

Sleep deprivation Over the past several years, there has been increasing evidence for the role of sleep deprivation in the development of obesity. The increasing epidemic of obesity has been paralleled by a similar epidemic of sleep deprivation. The development of electricity and indoor lighting initiated a steady reduction in human durations, which has been advanced by widespread use of television and computers, and adult sleep duration has decreased significantly since the turn of the century. Overall, research in adults suggests that short sleepers are heavier than those who sleep 7 to 8 hours, with supportive findings from most cross-sectional analyses, in addition to three prospective studies.[192–195] Postulated mechanisms for the relation between sleep deprivation and obesity include altered thermoregulation (a drop in core body temperature decreases energy expenditure), increased fatigue (leading to decreased TEE), increased hunger (attributable to elevations in ghrelin and decreases in leptin levels), and increased time to eat (attributable to less time asleep).[193] Clearly, there is the issue of reverse causation (obesity is a known risk factor for obstructive sleep apnea) and other confounders, such as coexisting chronic medical and psychiatric conditions, medication use, differences in SES, and shared genetic mechanisms that may regulate sleep and body weight. Because of the increasing prevalence of sleep deprivation in our society, however, any association between reduced sleep and obesity has substantial importance from a public health standpoint and merits further research.

DEALING WITH THE COMPLEXITY OF OBESITY

The more we understand about the etiology of obesity, the more complex it seems. Obesity involves interaction between our biology, our behavior, and the environment in which we live. We have efforts underway in our scientific community to focus on each of the major issues but few, if any, efforts to integrate among areas. Focusing only on one of these major areas is likely to be incomplete. We need to understand the underlying biology of obesity, but only in rare cases is obesity the result of a single biologic "defect." Similarly, we need to understand better how to change behavior, but to do this, we have to appreciate our biology and the environment in which we live.

Figuring out how to change the environment to make a difference in obesity also requires appreciation of biology and behavior. Finally, obesity even involves the ways we constructed our society, our shared collective world view, and the material base of this world view. For example, a recent analysis of economics and lifestyle[17,196,197] suggests the need to understand better the complex economic factors that are supporting our current diet and physical activity patterns and to think about how these could be changed to support a more healthy lifestyle. We must begin to examine ways in which we can replace those aspects of society that support obesity with those that support healthier lifestyles. We need to begin to construct a vision of what our society would look like if it supported maintenance of a healthy body weight and produced obesity prevalence rates that were acceptable.

STRATEGIES FOR GETTING OUT OF THE OBESITY EPIDEMIC

It is important that we begin to craft strategies that could get us out of the obesity epidemic. **Fig. 21**, adopted from the work of Dr. Stephan Rossner, illustrates some possibilities. If we do nothing, the weight of the population is likely to continue to increase until a time when all those who are not genetically protected are overweight or obese. How might we reduce obesity prevalence rates to acceptable levels over time?

One possibility is to reduce weight in many of those people who are already overweight or obese. The problem is that our ability to produce and maintain substantial weight loss is not good.[198–200] Most people who lose large amounts of weight regain this weight completely within a few years.[198–200] Rarely does anyone go permanently from the obese category to the healthy

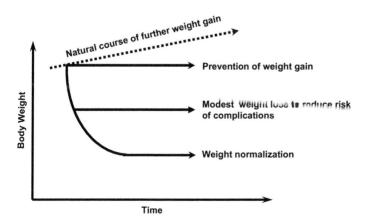

Fig. 21. Possible outcomes of obesity treatments. (*Adapted from* Rossner S. Factors determining the long-term outcome of obesity treatment. In: Bjorntorp P, Brodoff BN, editors. Obesity. Philadelphia: JB Lippincott; 1992. p. 712–9; with permission).

weight category. A recent large-scale clinical trial comparing weight-loss diets of different macronutrient compositions illustrates these challenges.[201] In this 2-year study, 811 overweight adults were randomly assigned to one of four diets of different macronutrient composition designed to produce an energy deficit of 750 kcal/d from baseline. The targeted percentages of energy derived from protein, carbohydrate, and fat of the four dietary arms were 20%, 15%, and 65%; 20%, 25%, and 55%; 40%, 15%, and 45%; and 40%, 25% and 35%, respectively. Participants received extensive group and individual behavioral counseling in addition to access to a Web-based self-monitoring tool. Weight loss across the four diet types did not vary, as found in previous randomized controlled trials comparing different diet types.[202] Although average weight loss across groups at 6 months was approximately 6 kg (7% of initial weight), at 2 years, the average weight loss was 4 kg. Although weight loss did vary among subjects, at 2 years, only approximately a third of subjects had lost at least 5% of their initial body weight. In regard to more substantial weight loss, only 14% to 15% of participants had lost greater than 10% of their initial body weight and only 2% to 4% had lost greater than 20 kg. In an accompanying editorial, Martijn Katan makes several important observations about this study.[203] He notes that weight loss at 6 months fits reasonably with the planned dietary energy deficit of 750 kcal/d. After 12 months, however, subjects started to regain weight, which suggests that they were eating more than planned. Katan[203] believes that weight regain during the second year, although slow, suggests that, in the end, many participants might have eventually regained their original weight even if treatment had continued. Katan[203] also highlights the facts that this study was led by experienced investigators and performed in highly motivated and carefully selected subjects who were offered 59 group and 13 individual training sessions over the course of 2 years. Despite all these measures, the average BMI of study subjects after 2 years of participation was around 31 to 32 and was trending upward. The inability of the subjects in this study to achieve and maintain significant weight loss raises significant concerns about the effectiveness of individual treatment to address obesity within our current environment.

Another possible way to reverse the obesity epidemic is through prevention. This could begin with stopping the gradual weight gain in the adult population and identifying and stopping excessive weight gain in children. We have previously demonstrated that weight gain in most adults can be prevented with small changes in energy balance of 100 kcal/d or less.[204] Preventing further weight gain in the population could have significant positive impacts on health and health care costs of the population because increasing BMI is associated with increasing risk for chronic disease and increasing health care costs.[19] The extent of changes in energy balance required for children and adolescents has not been quantified but is certainly going to be less than that required for significant weight loss. By using a strategy of stopping excessive weight gain, the prevalence of obesity would decrease with each successive generation. The impact of a community-based intervention to address weight regain has been studied in a 12-year school- and community-based effort to prevent overweight in school-aged children in two small towns in France.[205] Almost everyone in these towns in northern France, including the local government, teachers, physicians, business owners, and media, was recruited to join in an effort to encourage children to eat better and increase their activity. The towns built additional infrastructure to support physical activity (eg, recreational facilities, playgrounds), mapped out walking paths, and offered workshops and individual counseling to families to improve dietary behaviors. Although this was not a randomized trial, the results were impressive. In the 2004 school year, the prevalence of overweight in children in the intervention towns had dropped to 8.8% in contrast to 17.8% in the neighboring comparison towns. The study investigators conclude that their results suggest that interventions targeting a variety of population groups can have synergistic effects on overweight prevalence over a long period.

The bottom line is that, currently, we do not have a good ability to produce and maintain significant amounts of weight in large numbers of overweight and obese individuals. Although we can certainly improve our obesity treatment strategies over time, we cannot, at present, rely on this strategy alone to reverse the obesity epidemic. The success of this small study in France suggests a new strategy for preventing and treating obesity that involves a comprehensive and community-based transformation of the food and activity environment. Although it may take decades to reverse the obesity epidemic using this strategy, this study gives hope that we may actually be able to produce and maintain the behavior changes that would be required to reverse trends toward increasing rates of overweight and obesity by actions at a community level. This can be done through a combination of focusing on specific behavior change and modifying the environment in ways to support and sustain the desired behavior changes.

SUMMARY

In pursuing "the good life," we have created an environment and a society that unintentionally promote weight gain and obesity, given our genetic and biologic make-up. The consequences of the obesity epidemic are severe, affecting the health, quality of life, and economics of our nation. Dealing with the epidemic of obesity is likely to be one of the greatest challenges our society has faced. To reverse the obesity epidemic, we must develop specific strategies that recognize the complexity of the issue. Obesity involves biology, behavior, and the environment. We must re-examine the ways in which our society currently promotes obesity and determine what things can be changed. We must re-examine the ways in which we build our communities, the ways in which we produce and market our foods, and the ways in which we inadvertently promote sedentary behavior.

There is a growing realization that it is time to get serious about public health efforts to reverse the obesity epidemic. Although obesity prevalence rates have been increasing since the 1980s, it is only within the past 5 years that the issue has become a high priority for the public health community and policy makers. Thus, it is not surprising that we do not yet have any large-scale national initiatives to deal with the problem. The need to develop such initiatives is apparent, but, at present, there is no clear strategy for doing so.

There is some reason to be optimistic about dealing with obesity. We have successfully addressed many previous threats to public health. It was probably inconceivable in the 1950s to think that major public health initiatives could have such a dramatic effect on reducing the prevalence of smoking in the United States. Yet, this serious problem was addressed by a combination of strategies involving public health, economics, political advocacy, behavior change, and environmental change. Similarly, Americans have been persuaded to use seat belts and to recycle, addressing two other challenges to public health.[206]

Nevertheless, there is also reason to be pessimistic. Certainly, we can learn from our previous efforts for social change, but we must realize that our challenge with obesity may be greater. In the other examples cited previously, we had clear goals in mind. Our goals were to stop smoking, increase the use of seat belts, and increase recycling. The difficulty of achieving these goals should not be minimized, but they were clear and simple goals. With obesity, there is no clear agreement about goals. There is no agreement among experts as to which strategies should be implemented on a widespread basis to achieve the behavioral changes in the population needed to reverse the high prevalence rates of obesity. We need a success model that helps us to understand what to do to address obesity. Although we need success models, there is a great deal of urgency in responding to the obesity epidemic. Once we get serious about addressing obesity, it is likely to take decades to reverse obesity rates to levels seen 30 years ago. Meanwhile, the prevalence of overweight and obesity increases yearly, and we are rapidly losing the opportunity to prevent obesity in most people.

REFERENCES

1. Mokdad AH, Marks JS, Stroup DF, et al. Actual causes of death in the United States, 2000. JAMA 2004;291(10):1238–45.
2. Mokdad AH, Marks JS, Stroup DF, et al. Correction: actual causes of death in the United States, 2000. JAMA 2005;293(3):293–4.
3. Fontaine KR, Redden DT, Wang C, et al. Years of life lost due to obesity. JAMA 2003;289(2):187–93.
4. Ogden CL, Yanovski SZ, Carroll MD, et al. The epidemiology of obesity. Gastroenterology 2007; 132(6):2087–102.
5. USDHHS USDoHaHS. Healthy people 2010. Available at: http://www.healthypeople.gov/. Accessed January 16, 2009.
6. Wang Y, Beydoun MA, Liang L, et al. Will all Americans become overweight or obese? Estimating the progression and cost of the US obesity epidemic. Obesity (Silver Spring) 2008;16(10):2323–30.
7. Clinical guidelines on the identification, evaluation, and treatment of overweight and obesity in adults—the evidence report. National Institutes of Health. Obes Res 1998;6(Suppl 2):51S–209S.
8. Flegal KM, Tabak CJ, Ogden CL. Overweight in children: definitions and interpretation. Health Educ Res 2006;21(6):755–60.
9. Ogden CL, Carroll MD, Curtin LR, et al. Prevalence of overweight and obesity in the United States, 1999–2004. JAMA 2006;295(13):1549–55.
10. Prevalence of overweight, obesity and extreme obesity among adults: United States, trends 1976–80 through 2005–2006. Available at: http://www.cdc.gov/nchs/products/pubs/pubd/hestats/overweight/overweight_adult.htm. Accessed January 16, 2009.
11. Hedley AA, Ogden CL, Johnson CL, et al. Prevalence of overweight and obesity among US children, adolescents, and adults, 1999–2002. JAMA 2004;291(23):2847–50.
12. Lewis CE, Jacobs DR Jr, McCreath H, et al. Weight gain continues in the 1990s: 10-year trends in weight and overweight from the CARDIA study.

Coronary Artery Risk Development in Young Adults. Am J Epidemiol 2000;151(12):1172–81.

13. Molarius A, Seidell JC, Sans S, et al. Educational level, relative body weight, and changes in their association over 10 years: an international perspective from the WHO MONICA Project. Am J Public Health 2000;90(8):1260–8.

14. Sobal J, Stunkard AJ. Socioeconomic status and obesity: a review of the literature. Psychol Bull 1989;105(2):260–75.

15. Truong K, Sturm R. Weight gain trends across socio-demographic groups in the United States. Am J Public Health 2005;95(9):1602–6.

16. Drewnowski A, Specter SE. Poverty and obesity: the role of energy density and energy costs. Am J Clin Nutr 2004;79(1):6–16.

17. Cawley J. An economic framework for understanding physical activity and eating behaviors. Am J Prev Med 2004;27(Suppl 3):117–25.

18. Sturm R. Increases in morbid obesity in the USA: 2000–2005. Public Health 2007;121(7):492–6.

19. Sturm R, Ringel JS, Andreyeva T. Increasing obesity rates and disability trends. Health Aff (Millwood) 2004;23(2):199–205.

20. Flegal KM, Carroll MD, Ogden CL, et al. Prevalence and trends in obesity among US adults, 1999–2000. JAMA 2002;288(14):1723–7.

21. Cole TJ, Bellizzi MC, Flegal KM, et al. Establishing a standard definition for child overweight and obesity worldwide: international survey. BMJ 2000;320(7244):1240–3.

22. Ogden CL, Carroll MD, Flegal KM. High body mass index for age among US children and adolescents, 2003–2006. JAMA 2008;299(20):2401–5.

23. Land K. The Foundation for Child Development index of child well-being (CWI), 1975–2002, with projections for 2003. Durham (NC): Duke University; 2004.

24. Hill JO, Wyatt HR, Reed GW, et al. Obesity and the environment: where do we go from here? Science 2003;299(5608):853–5.

25. Allison DB, Saunders SE. Obesity in North America. An overview. Med Clin North Am 2000; 84(2):305–32.

26. Overweight, obesity, and health risk. National Task Force on the Prevention and Treatment of Obesity. Arch Intern Med 2000;160(7):898–904.

27. Colditz GA, Willett WC, Stampfer MJ, et al. Weight as a risk factor for clinical diabetes in women. Am J Epidemiol 1990;132(3):501–13.

28. Li C, Ford ES, Zhao G, et al. Prevalence of pre-diabetes and its association with clustering of cardiometabolic risk factors and hyperinsulinemia among U.S. adolescents: National Health and Nutrition Examination Survey 2005–2006. Diabetes Care 2009;32(2):342–7.

29. Terry RB, Wood PD, Haskell WL, et al. Regional adiposity patterns in relation to lipids, lipoprotein cholesterol, and lipoprotein subfraction mass in men. J Clin Endocrinol Metab 1989;68(1):191–9.

30. Brown CD, Higgins M, Donato KA, et al. Body mass index and the prevalence of hypertension and dyslipidemia. Obes Res 2000;8(9):605–19.

31. Grundy SM, Cleeman JI, Daniels SR, et al. Diagnosis and management of the metabolic syndrome. An American Heart Association/National Heart, Lung, and Blood Institute Scientific Statement. Executive summary. Cardiol Rev 2005;13(6):322–7.

32. Kahn R, Buse J, Ferrannini E, et al. The metabolic syndrome: time for a critical appraisal: joint statement from the American Diabetes Association and the European Association for the Study of Diabetes. Diabetes Care 2005;28(9):2289–304.

33. Bessesen DH. Treatment of the obese patient. Assessment of the obese patient. Totowa (NJ): Humana Press, Inc; 2007. p. 195–218.

34. Stamler J, Wentworth D, Neaton JD. Is relationship between serum cholesterol and risk of premature death from coronary heart disease continuous and graded? Findings in 356,222 primary screenees of the Multiple Risk Factor Intervention Trial (MRFIT). JAMA 1986;256(20):2823–8.

35. Hubert HB, Feinleib M, McNamara PM, et al. Obesity as an independent risk factor for cardiovascular disease: a 26-year follow-up of participants in the Framingham Heart Study. Circulation 1983;67(5):968–77.

36. Manson JE, Willett WC, Stampfer MJ, et al. Body weight and mortality among women. N Engl J Med 1995;333(11):677–85.

37. Eckel RH, Krauss RM. American Heart Association call to action: obesity as a major risk factor for coronary heart disease. AHA Nutrition Committee. Circulation 1998;97(21):2099–100.

38. Vgontzas AN, Tan TL, Bixler EO, et al. Sleep apnea and sleep disruption in obese patients. Arch Intern Med 1994;154(15):1705–11.

39. Adler M, Schaffner F. Fatty liver hepatitis and cirrhosis in obese patients. Am J Med 1979;67(5):811–6.

40. Matteoni CA, Younossi ZM, Gramlich T, et al. Nonalcoholic fatty liver disease: a spectrum of clinical and pathological severity. Gastroenterology 1999; 116(6):1413–9.

41. Wanless IR, Lentz JS. Fatty liver hepatitis (steatohepatitis) and obesity: an autopsy study with analysis of risk factors. Hepatology 1990;12(5):1106–10.

42. Chow WH, Gridley G, Fraumeni JF Jr, et al. Obesity, hypertension, and the risk of kidney cancer in men. N Engl J Med 2000;343(18):1305–11.

43. Huang Z, Hankinson SE, Colditz GA, et al. Dual effects of weight and weight gain on breast cancer risk. JAMA 1997;278(17):1407–11.

44. Michaud DS, Giovannucci E, Willett WC, et al. Physical activity, obesity, height, and the risk of pancreatic cancer. JAMA 2001;286(8):921–9.

45. Romero Y, Cameron AJ, Locke GR 3rd, et al. Familial aggregation of gastroesophageal reflux in patients with Barrett's esophagus and esophageal adenocarcinoma. Gastroenterology 1997;113(5):1449–56.

46. Schottenfeld D, Fraumeni JF. Cancer epidemiology and prevention. New York: Oxford Press; 1996.

47. Giovannucci E, Ascherio A, Rimm EB, et al. Physical activity, obesity, and risk for colon cancer and adenoma in men. Ann Intern Med 1995;122(5):327–34.

48. Giovannucci E, Colditz GA, Stampfer MJ, et al. Physical activity, obesity, and risk of colorectal adenoma in women (United States). Cancer Causes Control 1996;7(2):253–63.

49. Calle EE, Rodriguez C, Walker-Thurmond K, et al. Overweight, obesity, and mortality from cancer in a prospectively studied cohort of U.S. adults. N Engl J Med 2003;348(17):1625–38.

50. Fagot-Campagna A, Pettitt DJ, Engelgau MM, et al. Type 2 diabetes among North American children and adolescents: an epidemiologic review and a public health perspective. J Pediatr 2000;136(5):664–72.

51. Freedman DS, Dietz WH, Srinivasan SR, et al. The relation of overweight to cardiovascular risk factors among children and adolescents: the Bogalusa Heart Study. Pediatrics 1999;103(6 Pt 1):1175–82.

52. Burton WN, Chen CY, Schultz AB, et al. The economic costs associated with body mass index in a workplace. J Occup Environ Med 1998;40(9):786–92.

53. Puhl R, Brownell K. Bias, discrimination, and obesity. Obes Res 2001;9:788–805.

54. Schwartz MB, Puhl R. Childhood obesity: a societal problem to solve. Obes Rev 2003;4(1):57–71.

55. Hofbauer KG. Molecular pathways to obesity. Int J Obes Relat Metab Disord 2002;26(Suppl 2):S18–27.

56. Allison DB, Pietrobelli A, Faith MS, et al. Genetic influences on obesity. In: Eckel RH, editor. Obesity: mechanisms and clinical management. Philadelphia: Lippencott Williams and Wilkins; 2003. p. 31–74.

57. Olshansky SJ, Passaro DJ, Hershow RC, et al. A potential decline in life expectancy in the United States in the 21st century. N Engl J Med 2005;352(11):1138–45.

58. Jequier E. Leptin signaling, adiposity, and energy balance. Ann N Y Acad Sci 2002;967:379–88.

59. Horton TJ, Drougas H, Brachey A, et al. Fat and carbohydrate overfeeding in humans: different effects on energy storage. Am J Clin Nutr 1995;62(1):19–29.

60. Blundell JE, Stubbs RJ, Hughes DA, et al. Cross talk between physical activity and appetite control: does physical activity stimulate appetite? Proc Nutr Soc 2003;62(3):651–61.

61. Epstein LH, Paluch RA, Consalvi A, et al. Effects of manipulating sedentary behavior on physical activity and food intake. J Pediatr 2002;140(3):334–9.

62. Am P. Fires of life: the struggles of an ancient metabolism in a modern world. BNF Nutr Bull 2001;26:13–27.

63. Bullough RC, Gillette CA, Harris MA, et al. Interaction of acute changes in exercise energy expenditure and energy intake on resting metabolic rate. Am J Clin Nutr 1995;61(3):473–81.

64. Goran MI, Calles-Escandon J, Poehlman ET, et al. Effects of increased energy intake and/or physical activity on energy expenditure in young healthy men. J Appl Physiol 1994;77(1):366–72.

65. van Aggel-Leijssen DP, van Baak MA, Tenenbaum R, et al. Regulation of average 24h human plasma leptin level; the influence of exercise and physiological changes in energy balance. Int J Obes Relat Metab Disord 1999;23(2):151–8.

66. Mayer J, Roy P, Mitra KP. Relation between caloric intake, body weight, and physical work: studies in an industrial male population in West Bengal. Am J Clin Nutr 1956;4(2):169–75.

67. Mayer J, Marshall NB, Vitale JJ, et al. Exercise, food intake and body weight in normal rats and genetically obese adult mice. Am J Physiol 1954;177(3):544–8.

68. Stubbs RJ, Harbron CG, Murgatroyd PR, et al. Covert manipulation of dietary fat and energy density: effect on substrate flux and food intake in men eating ad libitum. Am J Clin Nutr 1995;62(2):316–29.

69. Stubbs RJ, Ritz P, Coward WA, et al. Covert manipulation of the ratio of dietary fat to carbohydrate and energy density: effect on food intake and energy balance in free-living men eating ad libitum. Am J Clin Nutr 1995;62(2):330–7.

70. Boutin P, Froguel P. Genetics of human obesity. Best Pract Res Clin Endocrinol Metab 2001;15(3):391–404.

71. Barsh GS, Farooqi IS, O'Rahilly S. Genetics of body-weight regulation. Nature 2000;404(6778):644–51.

72. Bouchard C, Perusse L. Genetics of obesity. Annu Rev Nutr 1993;13:337–54.

73. Bouchard C, Perusse L, Leblanc C, et al. Inheritance of the amount and distribution of human body fat. Int J Obes 1988;12(3):205–15.

74. Agras WS, Hammer LD, McNicholas F, et al. Risk factors for childhood overweight: a prospective study from birth to 9.5 years. J Pediatr 2004;145(1):20–5.

75. Agras WS, Mascola AJ. Risk factors for childhood overweight. Curr Opin Pediatr 2005;17(5):648–52.

76. Price RA, Cadoret RJ, Stunkard AJ, et al. Genetic contributions to human fatness: an adoption study. Am J Psychiatry 1987;144(8):1003–8.

77. Maes HH, Neale MC, Eaves LJ. Genetic and environmental factors in relative body weight and human adiposity. Behav Genet 1997;27(4):325–51.

78. Stunkard AJ, Harris JR, Pedersen NL, et al. The body-mass index of twins who have been reared apart. N Engl J Med 1990;322(21):1483–7.

79. Comuzzie AG, Allison DB. The search for human obesity genes. Science 1998;280(5368):1374–7.

80. Farooqi IS, Yeo GS, Keogh JM, et al. Dominant and recessive inheritance of morbid obesity associated with melanocortin 4 receptor deficiency. J Clin Invest 2000;106(2):271–9.

81. Eckel RH. Obesity: a disease or a physiologic adaptation. In: Eckel RH, editor. Obesity: mechanisms and clinical management. Philadelphia: Lippencott Williams and Wilkins; 2003. p. 3–30.

82. Krude H, Biebermann H, Luck W, et al. Severe early-onset obesity, adrenal insufficiency and red hair pigmentation caused by POMC mutations in humans. Nat Genet 1998;19(2):155–7.

83. Montague CT, Farooqi IS, Whitehead JP, et al. Congenital leptin deficiency is associated with severe early-onset obesity in humans. Nature 1997;387(6636):903–8.

84. Clement K, Vaisse C, Lahlou N, et al. A mutation in the human leptin receptor gene causes obesity and pituitary dysfunction. Nature 1998;392(6674):398–401.

85. Ristow M, Muller-Wieland D, Pfeiffer A, et al. Obesity associated with a mutation in a genetic regulator of adipocyte differentiation. N Engl J Med 1998;339(14):953–9.

86. Jackson RS, Creemers JW, Ohagi S, et al. Obesity and impaired prohormone processing associated with mutations in the human prohormone convertase 1 gene. Nat Genet 1997;16(3):303–6.

87. Bray GA. How do we get fat? An epidemiologic and metabolic approach. Clin Dermatol 2004;22(4):281–8.

88. Cowley MA, Pronchuk N, Fan W, et al. Integration of NPY, AGRP, and melanocortin signals in the hypothalamic paraventricular nucleus: evidence of a cellular basis for the adipostat. Neuron 1999;24(1):155–63.

89. Ravussin E, Lillioja S, Knowler WC, et al. Reduced rate of energy expenditure as a risk factor for body-weight gain. N Engl J Med 1988;318(8):467–72.

90. Tataranni PA, Harper IT, Snitker S, et al. Body weight gain in free-living Pima Indians: effect of energy intake vs expenditure. Int J Obes Relat Metab Disord 2003;27(12):1578–83.

91. Bessard T, Schutz Y, Jequier E. Energy expenditure and postprandial thermogenesis in obese women before and after weight loss. Am J Clin Nutr 1983;38(5):680–93.

92. Ravussin E, Valencia ME, Esparza J, et al. Effects of a traditional lifestyle on obesity in Pima Indians. Diabetes Care 1994;17(9):1067–74.

93. Esparza J, Fox C, Harper IT, et al. Daily energy expenditure in Mexican and USA Pima Indians: low physical activity as a possible cause of obesity. Int J Obes Relat Metab Disord 2000;24(1):55–9.

94. Levine JA, Lanningham-Foster LM, McCrady SK, et al. Interindividual variation in posture allocation: possible role in human obesity. Science 2005;307(5709):584–6.

95. Levine JA, Eberhardt NL, Jensen MD. Role of non-exercise activity thermogenesis in resistance to fat gain in humans. Science 1999;283(5399):212–4.

96. Levine JA, Kotz CM. NEAT—non-exercise activity thermogenesis—egocentric and geocentric environmental factors vs. biological regulation. Acta Physiol Scand 2005;184(4):309–18.

97. Novak CM, Kotz CM, Levine JA. Central orexin sensitivity, physical activity, and obesity in diet-induced obese and diet-resistant rats. Am J Physiol Endocrinol Metab 2006;290(2):E396–403.

98. Astrup A, Bulow J, Madsen J, et al. Contribution of BAT and skeletal muscle to thermogenesis induced by ephedrine in man. Am J Physiol 1985;248(5 Pt 1):E507–15.

99. Nedergaard J, Bengtsson T, Cannon B. Unexpected evidence for active brown adipose tissue in adult humans. Am J Physiol Endocrinol Metab 2007;293(2):E444–52.

100. Rousseau C, Bourbouloux E, Campion L, et al. Brown fat in breast cancer patients: analysis of serial (18)F-FDG PET/CT scans. Eur J Nucl Med Mol Imaging 2006;33(7):785–91.

101. Sturkenboom MG, Franssen EJ, Berkhof J, et al. Physiological uptake of [18F]fluorodeoxyglucose in the neck and upper chest region: are there predictive characteristics? Nucl Med Commun 2004;25(11):1109–11.

102. Cohade C, Mourtzikos KA, Wahl RL. "USA-Fat": prevalence is related to ambient outdoor temperature—evaluation with 18F-FDG PET/CT. J Nucl Med 2003;44(8):1267–70.

103. Lissner L, Heitmann BL. Dietary fat and obesity: evidence from epidemiology. Eur J Clin Nutr 1995;49(2):79–90.

104. Astrup A, Grunwald GK, Melanson EL, et al. The role of low-fat diets in body weight control: a meta-analysis of ad libitum dietary intervention studies. Int J Obes Relat Metab Disord 2000;24(12):1545–52.

105. Ello-Martin JA, Ledikwe JH, Rolls BJ. The influence of food portion size and energy density on energy intake: implications for weight management. Am J Clin Nutr 2005;82(Suppl 1):236S–41S.

106. Drewnowski A. Energy density, palatability, and satiety: implications for weight control. Nutr Rev 1998;56(12):347–53.

107. Rolls BJ, Roe LS, Meengs JS. Reductions in portion size and energy density of foods are additive and

lead to sustained decreases in energy intake. Am J Clin Nutr 2006;83(1):11–7.

108. Zemel MB. The role of dairy foods in weight management. J Am Coll Nutr 2005;24(Suppl 6):537S–46S.

109. Zemel MB, Shi H, Greer B, et al. Regulation of adiposity by dietary calcium. FASEB J 2000; 14(9):1132–8.

110. Davies KM, Heaney RP, Recker RR, et al. Calcium intake and body weight. J Clin Endocrinol Metab 2000;85(12):4635–8.

111. Pereira MA, Jacobs DR Jr, Van Horn L, et al. Dairy consumption, obesity, and the insulin resistance syndrome in young adults: the CARDIA study. JAMA 2002;287(16):2081–9.

112. Zemel MB, Thompson W, Milstead A, et al. Calcium and dairy acceleration of weight and fat loss during energy restriction in obese adults. Obes Res 2004; 12(4):582–90.

113. Shapses SA, Heshka S, Heymsfield SB. Effect of calcium supplementation on weight and fat loss in women. J Clin Endocrinol Metab 2004;89(2):632–7.

114. Lorenzen JK, Molgaard C, Michaelsen KF, et al. Calcium supplementation for 1 y does not reduce body weight or fat mass in young girls. Am J Clin Nutr 2006;83(1):18–23.

115. Gunther CW, Legowski PA, Lyle RM, et al. Dairy products do not lead to alterations in body weight or fat mass in young women in a 1-y intervention. Am J Clin Nutr 2005;81(4):751–6.

116. Rajpathak SN, Rimm EB, Rosner B, et al. Calcium and dairy intakes in relation to long-term weight gain in US men. Am J Clin Nutr 2006;83(3):559–66.

117. Berkey CS, Rockett HR, Willett WC, et al. Milk, dairy fat, dietary calcium, and weight gain: a longitudinal study of adolescents. Arch Pediatr Adolesc Med 2005;159(6):543–50.

118. Gonzalez AJ, White E, Kristal A, et al. Calcium intake and 10-year weight change in middle-aged adults. J Am Diet Assoc 2006;106(7):1066–73 [quiz 1082].

119. Macdonald HM, New SA, Campbell MK, et al. Longitudinal changes in weight in perimenopausal and early postmenopausal women: effects of dietary energy intake, energy expenditure, dietary calcium intake and hormone replacement therapy. Int J Obes Relat Metab Disord 2003;27(6):669–76.

120. Malik VS, Schulze MB, Hu FB. Intake of sugar-sweetened beverages and weight gain: a systematic review. Am J Clin Nutr 2006;84(2):274–88.

121. Ludwig DS, Peterson KE, Gortmaker SL. Relation between consumption of sugar-sweetened drinks and childhood obesity: a prospective, observational analysis. Lancet 2001;357(9255):505–8.

122. Schulze MB, Manson JE, Ludwig DS, et al. Sugar-sweetened beverages, weight gain, and incidence of type 2 diabetes in young and middle-aged women. JAMA 2004;292(8):927–34.

123. Bes-Rastrollo M, Sanchez-Villegas A, Gomez-Gracia E, et al. Predictors of weight gain in a Mediterranean cohort: the Seguimiento Universidad de Navarra Study 1. Am J Clin Nutr 2006;83(2): 362–70 [quiz 394–65].

124. DiMeglio DP, Mattes RD. Liquid versus solid carbohydrate: effects on food intake and body weight. Int J Obes Relat Metab Disord 2000;24(6): 794–800.

125. Soenen S, Westerterp-Plantenga MS. No differences in satiety or energy intake after high-fructose corn syrup, sucrose, or milk preloads. Am J Clin Nutr 2007;86(6):1586–94.

126. Canty DJ, Chan MM. Effects of consumption of caloric vs noncaloric sweet drinks on indices of hunger and food consumption in normal adults. Am J Clin Nutr 1991;53(5):1159–64.

127. Ludwig DS, Majzoub JA, Al-Zahrani A, et al. High glycemic index foods, overeating, and obesity. Pediatrics 1999;103(3):E26.

128. Bray GA, Nielsen SJ, Popkin BM. Consumption of high-fructose corn syrup in beverages may play a role in the epidemic of obesity. Am J Clin Nutr 2004;79(4):537–43.

129. Curry DL. Effects of mannose and fructose on the synthesis and secretion of insulin. Pancreas 1989; 4(1):2–9.

130. Anderson GH. Much ado about high-fructose corn syrup in beverages: the meat of the matter. Am J Clin Nutr 2007;86(6):1577–8.

131. Nielsen SJ, Popkin BM. Patterns and trends in food portion sizes, 1977–1998. JAMA 2003;289(4):450–3.

132. Young LR, Nestle M. Expanding portion sizes in the US marketplace: implications for nutrition counseling. J Am Diet Assoc 2003;103(2):231–4.

133. Rolls BJ, Morris EL, Roe LS. Portion size of food affects energy intake in normal-weight and overweight men and women. Am J Clin Nutr 2002; 76(6):1207–13.

134. Diliberti N, Bordi PL, Conklin MT, et al. Increased portion size leads to increased energy intake in a restaurant meal. Obes Res 2004;12(3):562–8.

135. McCrory MA, Fuss PJ, McCallum JE, et al. Dietary variety within food groups: association with energy intake and body fatness in men and women. Am J Clin Nutr 1999;69(3):440–7.

136. Putnam JA, Allshouse JE. Food consumption, prices and expenditures, 1970–1997. Washington, DC: Food and Rural Economic Division, US Department of Agriculture; 1999.

137. Kruger J. Prevalence of regular physical activity among adults—United States, 2001 and 2005. MMWR Morb Mortal Wkly Rep 2007;56(46):1209–12.

138. Brownson RC, Boehmer TK, Luke DA. Declining rates of physical activity in the United States: what are the contributors? Annu Rev Public Health 2005;26:421–43.

139. King GA, Fitzhugh EC, Bassett DR Jr, et al. Relationship of leisure-time physical activity and occupational activity to the prevalence of obesity. Int J Obes Relat Metab Disord 2001;25(5):606–12.

140. Westerterp KR, Speakman JR. Physical activity energy expenditure has not declined since the 1980s and matches energy expenditures of wild mammals. Int J Obes (Lond) 2008;32(8):1256–63.

141. Prentice AM, Jebb SA. Obesity in Britain: gluttony or sloth? BMJ 1995;311(7002):437–9.

142. Williamson DF, Madans J, Anda RF, et al. Recreational physical activity and ten-year weight change in a US national cohort. Int J Obes Relat Metab Disord 1993;17(5):279–86.

143. Schmitz KH, Jacobs DRJ, Leon AS, et al. Physical activity and body weight: associations over ten years in the CARDIA study. Coronary Artery Risk Development in Young Adults. Int J Obes Relat Metab Disord 2000;24:1475–87.

144. Barker DJP. Fetal and infant origins of adult disease. London: BMJ Publishing Group; 1992.

145. Barker DJP. Mothers, babies, and disease in later life. London: BMJ Publishing Group; 1994.

146. Gluckman PD, Hanson MA. Developmental origins of disease paradigm: a mechanistic and evolutionary perspective. Pediatr Res 2004;56(3):311–7.

147. Hanson M, Gluckman P, Bier D, et al. Report on the 2nd World Congress on Fetal Origins of Adult Disease, Brighton, U.K., June 7–10, 2003. Pediatr Res 2004;55(5):894–7.

148. Barker DJ, Winter PD, Osmond C, et al. Weight in infancy and death from ischaemic heart disease. Lancet 1989;2(8663):577–80.

149. Phillips DI, Barker DJ, Hales CN, et al. Thinness at birth and insulin resistance in adult life. Diabetologia 1994;37(2):150–4.

150. Valdez R, Athens MA, Thompson GH, et al. Birthweight and adult health outcomes in a biethnic population in the USA. Diabetologia 1994;37(6):624–31.

151. Barker DJ, Hales CN, Fall CH, et al. Type 2 (non-insulin-dependent) diabetes mellitus, hypertension and hyperlipidaemia (syndrome X): relation to reduced fetal growth. Diabetologia 1993;36(1):62–7.

152. Oken E, Levitan EB, Gillman MW. Maternal smoking during pregnancy and child overweight: systematic review and meta-analysis. Int J Obes (Lond) 2008;32(2):201–10.

153. Oken E, Taveras EM, Kleinman KP, et al. Gestational weight gain and child adiposity at age 3 years. Am J Obstet Gynecol 2007;196(4):322.e1–8.

154. Dabelea D, Hanson RL, Lindsay RS, et al. Intrauterine exposure to diabetes conveys risks for type 2 diabetes and obesity: a study of discordant sibships. Diabetes 2000;49(12):2208–11.

155. von Kries R, Koletzko B, Sauerwald T, et al. Does breast-feeding protect against childhood obesity? Adv Exp Med Biol 2000;478:29–39.

156. Bergmann KE, Bergmann RL, Von Kries R, et al. Early determinants of childhood overweight and adiposity in a birth cohort study: role of breast-feeding. Int J Obes Relat Metab Disord 2003;27(2):162–72.

157. Harder T, Bergmann R, Kallischnigg G, et al. Duration of breastfeeding and risk of overweight: a meta-analysis. Am J Epidemiol 2005;162(5):397–403.

158. Toschke AM, Vignerova J, Lhotska L, et al. Overweight and obesity in 6- to 14-year-old Czech children in 1991: protective effect of breast-feeding. J Pediatr 2002;141(6):764–9.

159. Taveras EM, Rifas-Shiman SL, Scanlon KS, et al. To what extent is the protective effect of breastfeeding on future overweight explained by decreased maternal feeding restriction? Pediatrics 2006;118(6):2341–8.

160. Arenz S, von Kries R. Protective effect of breastfeeding against obesity in childhood. Can a meta-analysis of observational studies help to validate the hypothesis? Adv Exp Med Biol 2005;569:40–8.

161. Owen CG, Martin RM, Whincup PH, et al. Effect of infant feeding on the risk of obesity across the life course: a quantitative review of published evidence. Pediatrics 2005;115(5):1367–77.

162. Gillman MW, Rifas-Shiman SL, Camargo CA Jr, et al. Risk of overweight among adolescents who were breastfed as infants. JAMA 2001;285(19):2461–7.

163. Li R, Jewell S, Grummer-Strawn L. Maternal obesity and breast-feeding practices. Am J Clin Nutr 2003;77(4):931–6.

164. Hediger ML, Overpeck MD, Kuczmarski RJ, et al. Association between infant breastfeeding and overweight in young children. JAMA 2001;285(19):2453–60.

165. Clifford TJ. Breast feeding and obesity. BMJ 2003;327(7420):879–80.

166. August GP, Caprio S, Fennoy I, et al. Prevention and treatment of pediatric obesity: an endocrine society clinical practice guideline based on expert opinion. J Clin Endocrinol Metab 2008;93(12):4576–99.

167. Patel MS, Srinivasan M, Laychock SG. Metabolic programming: role of nutrition in the immediate postnatal life. J Inherit Metab Dis 2009;32(2):218–28.

168. Palou A, Pico C. Leptin intake during lactation prevents obesity and affects food intake and food preferences in later life. Appetite 2009;52(1):249–52.

169. Dhurandhar NV, Israel BA, Kolesar JM, et al. Transmissibility of adenovirus-induced adiposity in a chicken model. Int J Obes Relat Metab Disord 2001;25(7):990–6.

170. Dhurandhar NV, Kulkarni P, Ajinkya SM, et al. Effect of adenovirus infection on adiposity in chicken. Vet Microbiol 1992;31(2–3):101–7.

171. Dhurandhar NV, Whigham LD, Abbott DH, et al. Human adenovirus Ad-36 promotes weight gain in male rhesus and marmoset monkeys. J Nutr 2002;132(10):3155–60.

172. van Ginneken V, Sitnyakowsky L, Jeffery JE. Infectobesity: viral infections (especially with human adenovirus-36: Ad-36) may be a cause of obesity. Med Hypotheses 2009;72(4):383–8.

173. Atkinson RL, Dhurandhar NV, Allison DB, et al. Human adenovirus-36 is associated with increased body weight and paradoxical reduction of serum lipids. Int J Obes (Lond) 2005;29(3):281–6.

174. Atkinson RL. Viruses as an etiology of obesity. Mayo Clin Proc 2007;82(10):1192–8.

175. McLachlan JA. Estrogens in the environment II. New York: Elsevier; 1995.

176. Colborn T, vom Saal FS, Soto AM. Developmental effects of endocrine-disrupting chemicals in wildlife and humans. Environ Health Perspect 1993; 101(5):378–84.

177. Colborn T, Clement C. Chemically-induced alterations in sexual and functional development: the wildlife/human connection. Princeton (NJ): Princeton Scientific; 1992.

178. Colborn T, Dumanski D, Myers JP. Our stolen future. New York: Penguin Books, Inc; 1996.

179. Newbold RR, Padilla-Banks E, Jefferson WN, et al. Effects of endocrine disruptors on obesity. Int J Androl 2008;31(2):201–8.

180. Baillie-Hamilton PF. Chemical toxins: a hypothesis to explain the global obesity epidemic. J Altern Complement Med 2002;8(2):185–92.

181. Heindel JJ. Endocrine disruptors and the obesity epidemic. Toxicol Sci 2003;76(2):247–9.

182. Heindel JJ, Levin E. Developmental origins and environmental influences—introduction. NIEHS symposium. Birth Defects Res A Clin Mol Teratol 2005;73(7):469.

183. Newbold RR, Padilla-Banks E, Snyder RJ, et al. Developmental exposure to endocrine disruptors and the obesity epidemic. Reprod Toxicol 2007; 23(3):290–6.

184. Newbold RR, Padilla-Banks E, Jefferson WN. Adverse effects of the model environmental estrogen diethylstilbestrol are transmitted to subsequent generations. Endocrinology 2006;147(Suppl 6):S11–7.

185. Newbold RR, Padilla-Banks E, Snyder RJ, et al. Perinatal exposure to environmental estrogens and the development of obesity. Mol Nutr Food Res 2007;51(7):912–7.

186. Lang IA, Galloway TS, Scarlett A, et al. Association of urinary bisphenol A concentration with medical disorders and laboratory abnormalities in adults. JAMA 2008;300(11):1303–10.

187. vom Saal FS, Myers JP. Bisphenol A and risk of metabolic disorders. JAMA 2008;300(11): 1353–5.

188. Hugo ER, Brandebourg TD, Woo JG, et al. Bisphenol A at environmentally relevant doses inhibits adiponectin release from human adipose tissue explants and adipocytes. Environ Health Perspect 2008;116(12):1642–7.

189. Penza M, Montani C, Romani A, et al. Genistein affects adipose tissue deposition in a dose-dependent and gender-specific manner. Endocrinology 2006;147(12):5740–51.

190. Stettler N, Stallings VA, Troxel AB, et al. Weight gain in the first week of life and overweight in adulthood: a cohort study of European American subjects fed infant formula. Circulation 2005; 111(15):1897–903.

191. Grun F, Blumberg B. Environmental obesogens: organotins and endocrine disruption via nuclear receptor signaling. Endocrinology 2006;147(Suppl 6):S50–5.

192. Patel SR, Malhotra A, White DP, et al. Association between reduced sleep and weight gain in women. Am J Epidemiol 2006;164(10):947–54.

193. Patel SR, Hu FB. Short sleep duration and weight gain: a systematic review. Obesity (Silver Spring) 2008;16(3):643–53.

194. Hasler G, Buysse DJ, Klaghofer R, et al. The association between short sleep duration and obesity in young adults: a 13-year prospective study. Sleep 2004;27(4):661–6.

195. Gangwisch JE, Malaspina D, Boden-Albala B, et al. Inadequate sleep as a risk factor for obesity: analyses of the NHANES I. Sleep 2005;28(10):1289–96.

196. Sturm R. The economics of physical activity: societal trends and rationales for interventions. Am J Prev Med 2004;27(Suppl 3):126–35.

197. Hill JO, Sallis JF, Peters JC. Economic analysis of eating and physical activity: a next step for research and policy change. Am J Prev Med 2004;27(Suppl 3):111–6.

198. Wing RR, Hill JO. Successful weight loss maintenance. Annu Rev Nutr 2001;21:323–41.

199. Brownell KD. Diet, exercise and behavioural intervention: the nonpharmacological approach. Eur J Clin Invest 1998;28(Suppl 2):19–21 [discussion: 22].

200. Wadden TA, Foster GD, Letizia KA. One-year behavioral treatment of obesity: comparison of moderate and severe caloric restriction and the effects of weight maintenance therapy. J Consult Clin Psychol 1994;62(1):165–71.

201. Sacks FM, Bray GA, Carey VJ, et al. Comparison of weight-loss diets with different compositions of fat, protein, and carbohydrates. N Engl J Med 2009; 360(9):859–73.

202. Dansinger ML, Gleason JA, Griffith JL, et al. Comparison of the Atkins, Ornish, Weight Watchers, and Zone

diets for weight loss and heart disease risk reduction: a randomized trial. JAMA 2005;293(1):43–53.

203. Katan MB. Weight-loss diets for the prevention and treatment of obesity. N Engl J Med 2009;360(9): 923–5.

204. Peters JC, Wyatt HR, Donahoo WT, et al. From instinct to intellect: the challenge of maintaining healthy weight in the modern world. Obes Rev 2002;3(2):69–74.

205. Romon M, Lommez A, Tafflet M, et al. Downward trends in the prevalence of childhood overweight in the setting of 12-year school- and community-based programmes. Public Health Nutr 2008;23: 1–8.

206. Economos CD, Brownson RC, DeAngelis MA, et al. What lessons have been learned from other attempts to guide social change? Nutr Rev 2001; 59(3 Pt 2):S40–56 [discussion: S57–65].

Altered Resting and Exercise Respiratory Physiology in Obesity

Akshay Sood, MD, MPH

KEYWORDS

- Obesity • Respiratory physiology • Exercise
- Expiratory reserve volume • Oxygen consumption
- Restrictive ventilatory abnormality
- Obstructive ventilatory abnormality

Obesity (body mass index [BMI] ≥ 30 kg/m^2) is the most common metabolic disease in the world, and its prevalence has increased worldwide, particularly in the United States. Data from the two National Health and Nutrition Examination Surveys show that the prevalence of obesity has increased among adults aged 20 to 74 years in the United States from 15.0% (1976–1980) to 32.9% (2003–2004).[1] Physicians are therefore routinely challenged by the comorbidities associated with obesity. Although the associations between obesity and increased risk for cancer, cardiovascular, endocrine, and rheumatologic diseases are well described, the respiratory effects of obesity, outside of sleep-related disorders, are less well known. It is now clear that respiratory function is impaired in obesity, and the magnitude of impairment is more clearly demonstrable in severe obesity.[2] This review focuses on the effect of obesity on resting and exercise-related respiratory physiology.

ALTERED RESTING RESPIRATORY PHYSIOLOGY IN OBESITY

Obesity affects various resting respiratory physiologic parameters, such as compliance, neuromuscular strength, work of breathing, lung volumes, spirometric measures, respiratory resistance, diffusing capacity, gas exchange, and airway responsiveness to methacholine (**Table 1**).

Respiratory Compliance

Respiratory compliance is the ability of the respiratory system to stretch during a change in volume relative to an applied change in pressure. Total respiratory compliance may be reduced in severe obesity with obesity-hypoventilation syndrome to as little as one third of normal.[3] In other words, there may be up to a threefold increase in elastic resistance to respiratory distention in severely obese individuals. This largely results from reduced distensibility of extrapulmonary structures from excess truncal fat.[3] Increased pulmonary blood volume and increased closure of dependent airways also contribute to the low lung compliance seen in severely obese subjects, however.[4] These physiologic changes are more pronounced during recumbency in obese subjects as compared with normal-weight subjects because of the increased gravitational effects of the large abdomen.[5]

Respiratory Muscle Strength

Obese subjects may demonstrate inefficiency of respiratory muscles, particularly the diaphragm. Reduced respiratory muscle strength and endurance, as suggested by static maximal inspiratory pressure values 60% to 70% of normal subjects, have been described in three severely obese subjects with obesity-hypoventilation syndrome in a 1974 study by Rochester and Enson.[4] Recent

This work was supported in part by University of New Mexico Clinical Translational Science Center grant NIH NCRR M01-RR-00997. The author has no financial relation to a commercial company that has an interest in the subject matter or materials discussed in this article.

Department of Medicine, 1 University of New Mexico School of Medicine, MSC 10 5550, Albuquerque, NM 87131–0001, USA

E-mail address: asood@salud.unm.edu

Clin Chest Med 30 (2009) 445–454
doi:10.1016/j.ccm.2009.05.003

Table 1
Altered resting respiratory physiology in obesity

Physiologic Parameter	Effect of Obesity
Respiratory compliance	Decreased
Respiratory muscle strength	Decreased
Work of breathing at rest	Increased
VC	Normal or decreased[a]
FEV$_1$	Normal or decreased
Ratio (FEV$_1$/VC)	Normal, increased, or decreased
Maximal expiratory flow rates at low lung volumes	Decreased
Longitudinal loss in FEV$_1$ and VC	Increased
Expiratory reserve volume	Decreased
Functional residual capacity	Usually decreased
Residual volume	Normal
Inspiratory capacity	Normal or increased
Total lung capacity	Normal or slightly decreased
Airway resistance	Increased
Specific airway conductance	Normal
Diffusing capacity	Variable
Alveolar arterial oxygen tension gradient	Increased
Airway responsiveness to methacholine	Often increased

Abbreviations: FEV$_1$, forced expiratory volume in 1 second; VC, vital capacity.
[a] The negative association between VC and obesity is better described with abdominal obesity.[30]

studies have confirmed that obese subjects are at greater risk for inspiratory muscle fatigue at rest and with exercise.[6,7] Further, weight loss in severely obese subjects is associated with improved respiratory muscle strength and endurance.[8] A possible cause of impaired respiratory muscle function in obesity includes increased elastic load, which the respiratory muscles are required to overcome during inspiration.[8] An overstretched diaphragm would place this respiratory muscle at a mechanical disadvantage, leading to decreased inspiratory muscle strength and efficiency.[9] Additionally, decreased skeletal muscle glycogen synthase activity in obese subjects may be associated with decreased isokinetic skeletal muscle endurance,[10,11] although it is not known if this phenomenon actually occurs in respiratory muscles. Further, fatty infiltration of respiratory and nonrespiratory skeletal muscle in obese subjects has been well documented,[12–14] although its clinical significance related to muscle strength is unclear.

Work of Breathing at Rest

To overcome the reduced total respiratory compliance and respiratory muscle inefficiency, severely obese subjects may breathe rapidly and shallowly.[6,15] This pattern of breathing is similar to that seen among patients with neuromuscular and musculoskeletal disorders.[16] This pattern of breathing is associated with increased oxygen cost of breathing, however.[15,17] The oxygen cost of breathing represents the oxygen consumed by the respiratory muscles per liter of ventilation and is an index of the energy required to breathe. Rochester[15] showed that the oxygen cost of breathing is 4 fold and 10 fold higher than normal among subjects with simple eucapnic obesity and obesity-hypoventilation syndrome, respectively. In a study by Kress and colleagues[17] of 18 severely obese patients, a 16% reduction in oxygen consumption ($\dot{V}_{O_2}$) was seen after elective intubation, mechanical ventilation, and anesthesia from their resting baseline values as compared with a less than 1% reduction in eight controls. This relative respiratory inefficiency among obese subjects suggests a decreased ventilatory reserve and a predisposition to respiratory failure in the setting of even mild pulmonary or systemic insults.[17]

Lung Volumes

The most common and consistent indicator of obesity is a reduction in expiratory reserve volume (ERV) (**Figs. 1** and **2**).[18] This occurs because of displacement of the diaphragm into the thorax by

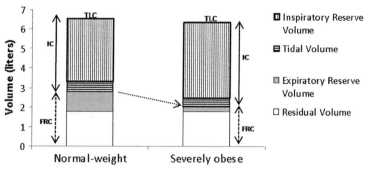

Fig. 1. Effect of obesity on lung volumes. Expiratory reserve volume (ERV) is decreased in obesity. Functional residual capacity (FRC), the sum of ERV and residual volume (RV), is usually reduced as well, often approaching RV (*arrow*). The decline in FRC in obese subjects is primarily the result of reduced ERV. Total lung capacity (TLC, the sum of FRC and inspiratory capacity [IC]) is usually preserved. Therefore, to compensate for the reduced FRC, IC, the sum of inspiratory reserve volume and tidal volume, may be increased in severe obesity.

the obese abdomen and increased chest wall mass.[19] Although this association is seen even with modest obesity,[20] ERV decreases rapidly in an exponential relation to increase in BMI (see **Fig. 2**).[21]

Conversely, obesity has fairly modest effects on the extremes of lung volumes at residual volume (RV) and total lung capacity (TLC) but a relatively larger effect in reducing functional residual capacity (FRC).[21] This reduction is often so marked that FRC approaches RV (see **Fig. 1**).[22] When the reduced FRC is equal to or lower than the closing volume, regional thoracic gas trapping may take place in obese subjects, as suggested by an elevated RV/TLC ratio.[23,24] Further, to compensate

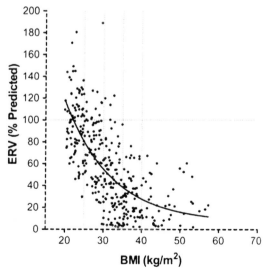

Fig. 2. ERV decreases rapidly in an exponential relation with increase in BMI. The best-fit exponential regression equation for ERV is as follows: $ERV = 587.8 \exp(-0.083 \times BMI) + 6.5$. The r^2 value for ERV was 0.49 ($P<.01$). (*From* Jones RL, Nzekwu MM. The effects of body mass index on lung volumes. Chest 2006;130:832; with permission.)

for the reduced FRC, inspiratory capacity (IC) may be increased in severe obesity (see **Fig. 1**).

As mentioned previously, TLC is usually preserved in most obese subjects, other than those with morbid obesity (weight-to-height ratio ≥ 0.9 kg/cm),[2,25] with excessive central adiposity (waist-to-hip ratio ≥ 0.95),[26] or with obesity-hypoventilation syndrome.[15] In the absence of these conditions, a restrictive defect (TLC < lower limit of normal) should not be attributed to obesity until other causes of restrictive impairment, such as interstitial lung disease, have been excluded.

Sequential studies after weight loss, usually in the context of bariatric surgery, generally show a marked improvement in ERV, intermediate improvement in RV and FRC, and a more modest improvement in TLC (**Fig. 3**).[2,8,27,28]

Spirometry

Obesity may be associated with a reduction in vital capacity (VC) and forced expiratory volume in 1 second (FEV_1) depending on the age, type of body fat distribution (with central fat distribution having a relatively greater effect),[26] and severity of obesity. Previous studies have created the impression that only morbid obesity is associated with this restriction of VC,[24,29] but a recent large French population-based study by Leone and colleagues[30] demonstrated that even mild abdominal obesity, even with a normal BMI, is associated with lower VC and FEV_1 in men and women. These findings have prompted a leading authority in this field to recommend the routine measurement of waist circumference before spirometry to allow the interpreting physician to take into account the restrictive effect of abdominal obesity on spirometric values.[31]

Possible causes of reduced VC in obese subjects may be mechanical and inflammatory.

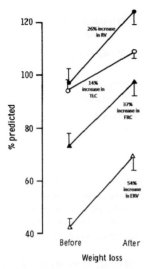

Fig. 3. Vertical banded gastroplasty in a study by Thomas and colleagues[27] was associated with a mean weight loss of 34.2 kg in 29 morbidly obese subjects. Resulting changes in static lung volumes (expressed as change in percent predicted values from baseline) are summarized. Bar lines indicate 1 SEM. The greatest improvement in ERV, intermediate improvement in RV and FRC, and least improvement in TLC were seen after surgical weight loss. (*From* Thomas PS, Cowen ER, Hulands G, et al. Respiratory function in the morbidly obese before and after weight loss. Thorax 1989;44:384; with permission.)

Mechanical causes include decreased respiratory compliance (with consequently decreased lung volumes) and increased gas trapping from premature small airway closure (particularly at the lung bases). In addition, obesity is associated with increased levels of proinflammatory adipokines (eg, leptin, interleukin-6 and tumor necrosis factor-α[32]) and decreased levels of anti-inflammatory adipokines (eg, adiponectin[32,33]). The secretion of these adipokines by adipose tissue in chronic respiratory diseases may be regulated by chronic or intermittent hypoxia.[34] These adipokines, in turn, regulate systemic inflammation, which is associated with impaired lung function.[35–37] Directly or by means of systemic inflammation, adipokines may also affect inflammation of small airways, resulting in premature closure of the inflamed and edematous small airway. Additional mechanistic studies are needed to understand better the pathophysiologic pathways by which adipokines may affect lung function.

The FEV_1/VC ratio is usually normal or increased with obesity; the latter is thought to occur because of peripheral airway closure and resulting gas trapping disproportionately, reducing the VC.[23] The implication is that although obesity may affect small airway function, it may not affect large airways. The latter impression may not be entirely true, however. A recent study by Leone and colleagues[30] suggests that abdominal obesity may be associated with a reduced FEV_1/VC ratio, suggesting an effect on large airway caliber as well. Thus, obesity may be associated with obstructive ventilatory abnormality, in addition to its well-known association with restrictive abnormality.

The effect of obesity on forced expiratory flow rates at low-lung volumes is less well described. A study by Rubinstein and colleagues[23] in 103 nonsmoking morbidly obese men showed reduced maximum expiratory flow rate at 75% of exhaled VC even after normalization for VC, implying peripheral airflow obstruction. This phenomenon is illustrated in **Fig. 4**. Possible mechanisms may include obesity-related inflammation or edema of the small airways, thus decreasing their caliber.

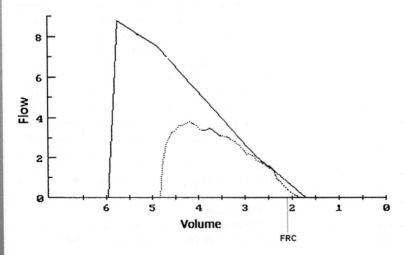

Fig. 4. Expiratory flow volume curve (*dashed line*) from a woman with a BMI of 50 kg/m^2. The solid line shows the predicted curve. The TLC (79% predicted) and FRC (68% predicted) are reduced, but maximal flows are well preserved and the FEV_1/FVC ratio is normal. Nevertheless, expiratory flows at low lung volumes are reduced relative to the predicted values derived from the VC. (*Courtesy of* Cheryl Salome, PhD, Sydney, Australia.)

Further, some but not all studies suggest that the effect of obesity on absolute lung function may be greater among men than among women, probably attributable to greater central fat distribution in men.[38–41] Yet, this absolute reduction in lung function may have a relatively greater impact on women because of their smaller initial lung volume.[19] Whether a change in lung volume of this magnitude has a relatively greater impact on dyspnea among obese women as compared with obese men is unknown and warrants further research.

Interestingly, although increased fat mass may be negatively associated with spirometric lung function, increased lean mass (ie, primarily muscle mass) may be positively associated with FEV_1, and with VC to a lesser extent, particularly among men.[19,42] This protective effect of lean mass on lung function may be associated with stronger respiratory musculature[42] or larger overall thoracic size,[19] although the mechanism remains uncertain.

Several longitudinal studies demonstrate that increasing weight gain is associated with more rapid loss of lung function (FEV_1 and VC).[43–47] Mechanical and inflammatory mechanisms related to obesity, as described previously, may contribute to this relatively rapid deterioration in airway function and may predispose obese subjects to long-term adverse effects of cigarette smoking, respiratory infections, and occupational and environmental exposures. Further, obese subjects may improve their lung function by losing weight, suggesting that these detrimental effects of obesity do not involve irreversible structural remodeling of the airways.[2,8,27,28,47,48]

In addition to these spirometric changes, severe obesity is associated with a decrease in maximum voluntary ventilation (MVV). This may be explained by respiratory muscle inefficiency, increased upper airway resistance, and inspiratory flow resistance.[2] MVV values in obese subjects usually improve after weight reduction.[49]

Airway Resistance

An increase in airway resistance (as measured by body plethysmography) is reported in obese subjects.[23,50] This may be attributable to breathing at low FRC, however, which, in turn, results in a relatively decreased airway caliber throughout the tidal breathing cycle. This conclusion is supported by normal values of specific airway conductance.[23] Some studies have suggested that the increase in airflow resistance may not be attributable entirely to the reduced lung volume

but have not described the specific cause of the additional resistance.[51,52]

Diffusing Capacity

Although diffusing capacity is usually preserved in obese subjects, decreased and increased values are reported in the literature.[2,27,53] High values of diffusing capacity may result from increased pulmonary blood volume in obesity. Conversely, diminished values may result from structural changes in the lung interstitium from lipid deposition or decreased alveolar surface area.[53]

The effect of weight loss on diffusing capacity has been examined in a few small studies; values remained largely unchanged after surgical weight loss in two separate studies of 16 and 35 morbidly obese subjects by Thomas and colleagues[27] and Zavorsky and colleagues,[54] respectively, and after medical weight loss in 35 obese men in another study by Womack and colleagues.[48]

Gas Exchange

Obese subjects have high levels of ventilation-perfusion mismatch from atelectasis of underventilated dependent lung units, which continue to be well perfused. This results in an increased alveolar-arterial oxygen tension gradient [$P(A-a)o_2$] and reduced Pao_2. This is worse in a recumbent position. Sequential studies demonstrate that weight reduction may be associated with improved Pao_2.[27,28]

Despite their greater carbon dioxide production ($\dot{V}_{CO_2}$), most obese subjects maintain a normal $Paco_2$. To maintain normal $Paco_2$ levels in the face of high $\dot{V}_{CO_2}$, obese subjects generally demonstrate higher minute ventilation (V_E). If they are eucapnic, such individuals have only simple obesity. Patients with obesity hypoventilation syndrome, conversely, are unable to augment their V_E adequately, and are therefore hypercapnic. Whether an obese individual demonstrates simple eucapnic obesity or obesity-hypoventilation syndrome depends less on the actual BMI value and more on his or her central ventilatory responses to hypoxia and hypercapnia.[55] Obesity, genetic predisposition, sleep-disordered breathing, and leptin resistance have all been proposed as possible mechanisms for this blunted ventilatory response to hypercapnia[56] (see the article by Littleton and Mokhlesi in this issue).

AIRWAY RESPONSIVENESS TO METHACHOLINE

The association between obesity and asthma has been covered elsewhere in great detail (see the article by Beuther in this issue). It is, however, worth mentioning that the mechanical effects of obesity on the lungs may alter airway smooth muscle contractility and increase airway responsiveness.[57] Breathing voluntarily at low lung volumes may increase airway responsiveness to methacholine in lean nonasthmatic subjects.[58] In obese subjects breathing at low lung volumes, the airways remain at a smaller caliber and the airway smooth muscle is at a shorter length throughout the breathing cycle. It is possible that this would change the contractile properties of the airway smooth muscle by plastic adaptation to a shorter length[59] or alterations in actin-myosin cross-bridge cycling,[60] resulting in an increase in airway smooth muscle contractility and an increase in airway responsiveness. Recent studies also raise the possibility that adipokines (high leptin and low adiponectin concentrations) may increase airway responsiveness,[56,61–64] although the mechanism remains unknown.

ALTERED EXERCISE RESPIRATORY PHYSIOLOGY IN OBESITY
Oxygen Consumption

Obesity is associated with increased rates of basal metabolism and $\dot{V}_{O_2}$ at rest (**Table 2**).[65] Because adipose tissue has a lower metabolic rate than other tissues, however, if $\dot{V}_{O_2}$ is standardized by expressing it per kilogram of actual body weight, lower than normal values are obtained in obese individuals.[65] Similarly, an active, otherwise healthy, obese subject has a reduced peak $\dot{V}_{O_2}$ if it is correlated to actual body weight but a normal or high peak $\dot{V}_{O_2}$ if it is correlated to height,[66] predicted body weight, or lean body mass.[67]

Exercise-related increase in $\dot{V}_{O_2}$ is more marked in obese subjects as compared with normal-weight subjects because additional energy is needed to move heavy body parts.[66,68] Because of the high metabolic cost of performing even modest activity, an otherwise healthy obese subject may have good cardiovascular fitness, despite the reduced work capacity.[66,68]

Interestingly, the increased oxygen cost of performing mechanical work is predictable and well worked out for a cycle ergometer.[66,68] The $\dot{V}_{O_2}$ work rate relation is displaced upward by approximately 6 mL/min/kg of extra body weight without any discernible change in the slope of the $\dot{V}_{O_2}$-work rate relation (**Fig. 5**).[66,68] This means that an appropriate peak $\dot{V}_{O_2}$ reference standard for an obese subject can be obtained by increasing the peak $\dot{V}_{O_2}$ standard obtained from the predicted body weight by 6 mL/min for each kilogram greater than the predicted weight.

It should also be noted that cardiac and ventilatory reserves in an obese subject are limited in their ability to support the increased muscle oxygen requirement during exercise because the heart and the lungs do not increase in size commensurate with the subject's added weight.[69] This imposes physiologic constraints on peak exercise performance in obese subjects, who cannot attain the same peak work rates as normal-weight subjects.[69]

Ventilatory Response to Exercise in Obesity

As discussed previously, obese subjects have increased $P(A-a)_{O_2}$ and reduced Pa_{O_2} at rest from atelectasis of peripheral lung units. This

Table 2
Altered exercise-related respiratory physiology in obesity

Physiologic Parameter	Effect of Obesity
$\dot{V}_{O_2}$ peak	Decreased (for actual weight), normal, or increased (for ideal weight)
$\dot{V}_{O_2}$-work rate relation	Displaced upward
Anaerobic threshold (percent predicted peak $\dot{V}_{O_2}$)	Normal
Peak heart rate	Normal
Peak oxygen pulse	Normal
Ventilatory reserve	Normal or decreased
Ventilatory equivalent for carbon dioxide at anaerobic threshold	Normal
Dead space-tidal volume ratio	Normal
Pa_{O_2}	Normal/may increase
Alveolar-arterial oxygen tension gradient	May decrease

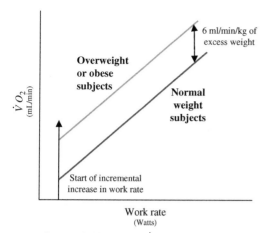

Fig. 5. Obesity displaces the $\dot{V}_{O_2}$ -work rate relation upward by approximately 6 mL/min/kg of excess body weight, but the slope itself is unchanged (*Adapted from* Wasserman K, et al. Principles of exercise testing and interpretation. 4th edition. Philadelphia: Lippincott Williams & Wilkins; 2005. p. 83; with permission.)

usually improves during exercise because of the effect of deep breathing on expansion of atelectatic lung units. It is thus the only pulmonary condition in which arterial oxygenation improves during exercise.[69] Because ventilation-perfusion relations usually normalize during exercise in the patient with uncomplicated obesity, exercise-related dead space ventilation measures (eg, ventilatory equivalent for carbon dioxide or $V_e/\dot{V}_{CO_2}$ ratio at anaerobic threshold and dead space-tidal volume ratio) and exercise-related $P(A-a)_{O_2}$ values are also normal.

Further, FRC is reduced in the resting state in obese subjects because of "chest strapping," as discussed previously. During heavy to peak exercise, however, although FRC is reduced in lean subjects, it may actually increase in obese subjects.[70] Both groups, lean subjects and obese subjects, also develop (modest and similar levels of) expiratory flow limitation at peak exercise.[70] It is important to recognize, however, that unlike lean subjects, who easily tolerate this decline in expiratory flow, obese subjects have to increase their FRC (or hyperinflate) during peak exercise to avoid significant levels of expiratory flow limitation.[70] This dynamic hyperinflation may contribute to reduced tidal volume and increased respiratory rate and may contribute to a reduced ventilatory reserve during peak exercise in obese subjects.[71]

Cardiovascular Response to Exercise in Obesity

Although work capacity is impaired in moderately obese subjects, peak oxygen pulse (a noninvasive

determinant of stroke volume) and anaerobic threshold levels (related to percent predicted peak $\dot{V}_{O_2}$) are usually normal.[66,67,69,72] This reflects the "training effect" induced consequent to the demands of performing habitual activities while "loaded" with a greater body mass.[72] Although resting heart rate is usually high in obese subjects, peak heart rate is usually normal, resulting in little heart rate reserve.[72]

Conversely, among asymptomatic severely obese subjects, abnormal indices of left ventricular diastolic filling pressures, as measured by pulse Doppler-echocardiography, more frequently develop during exercise as compared with matched lean controls.[73] This may represent a subclinical form of cardiomyopathy in severely obese subjects.[73]

SUMMARY

Obesity, particularly severe obesity, affects resting and exercise-related respiratory physiology. Obesity markedly reduces the ERV and respiratory system compliance, classically producing a restrictive ventilatory abnormality. Less often, a reduced FEV_1/VC ratio (associated with abdominal obesity) and reduced maximum expiratory flow rates at low lung volumes may produce an obstructive ventilatory abnormality as well. Arterial hypoxemia resulting from ventilation-perfusion mismatch usually improves with exercise. Increased absolute rates of oxygen consumption ($\dot{V}_{O_2}$) at rest and with exercise are seen in obese subjects. If $\dot{V}_{O_2}$ is standardized by expressing it per kilogram of actual body weight, however, lower than normal values are obtained. Decreased peak work rates are usually seen in a setting of normal or decreased ventilatory reserve and normal cardiovascular response to exercise in obese subjects. The best treatment for obesity is weight loss, which reverses many of the adverse physiologic consequences of obesity on the respiratory system.

ACKNOWLEDGMENTS

The author thanks Mark Schuyler, MD, University of New Mexico, and Cheryl Salome, PhD, Woolcock Institute of Research, University of Sydney, for their careful critique of this article.

REFERENCES

1. National Center for Health Statistics. Chartbook on trends in the health of Americans, Health, United States, 2006. Hyattsville (MD): Public Health Service; 2006.

2. Ray CS, Sue DY, Bray G, et al. Effects of obesity on respiratory function. Am Rev Respir Dis 1983; 128(3):501–6.

3. Naimark A, Cherniack RM. Compliance of the respiratory system and its components in health and obesity. J Appl Phys 1960;15:377–82.

4. Rochester DF, Enson Y. Current concepts in the pathogenesis of the obesity-hypoventilation syndrome. Mechanical and circulatory factors. Am J Med 1974;57(3):402–20.

5. Koenig SM. Pulmonary complications of obesity. Am J Med Sci 2001;321(4):249–79.

6. Chlif M, Keochkerian D, Feki Y, et al. Inspiratory muscle activity during incremental exercise in obese men. Int J Obes (Lond) 2007;31(9):1456–63.

7. Chlif M, Keochkerian D, Mourlhon C, et al. Noninvasive assessment of the tension-time index of inspiratory muscles at rest in obese male subjects. Int J Obes (Lond) 2005;29(12):1478–83.

8. Weiner P, Waizman J, Weiner M, et al. Influence of excessive weight loss after gastroplasty for morbid obesity on respiratory muscle performance. Thorax 1998;53(1):39–42.

9. Sharp JT, Druz WS, Kondragunta VR. Diaphragmatic responses to body position changes in obese patients with obstructive sleep apnea. Am Rev Respir Dis 1986;133(1):32–7.

10. Krotkiewski M, Grimby G, Holm G, et al. Increased muscle dynamic endurance associated with weight reduction on a very-low-calorie diet. Am J Clin Nutr 1990;51(3):321–30.

11. Damsbo P, Vaag A, Hother-Nielsen O, et al. Reduced glycogen synthase activity in skeletal muscle from obese patients with and without type 2 (non-insulin-dependent) diabetes mellitus. Diabetologia 1991;34(4):239–45.

12. Lennmarken C, Sandstedt S, von Schenck H, et al. Skeletal muscle function and metabolism in obese women. JPEN J Parenter Enteral Nutr 1986;10(6): 583–7.

13. Newham DJ, Harrison RA, Tomkins AM, et al. The strength, contractile properties and radiological density of skeletal muscle before and 1 year after gastroplasty. Clin Sci (Lond) 1988;74(1):79–83.

14. Fadell EJ, Richman AD, Ward WW, et al. Fatty infiltration of respiratory muscles in the Pickwickian syndrome. N Engl J Med 1962;266:861–3.

15. Rochester D. Obesity and pulmonary function. In: Alpert M, Alexander J, editors. The heart and lung in obesity. Armonk (NY): Futura Publishing Company; 1998. p. 108–32.

16. Perrin C, Unterborn JN, Ambrosio CD, et al. Pulmonary complications of chronic neuromuscular diseases and their management. Muscle Nerve 2004;29(1):5–27.

17. Kress JP, Pohlman AS, Alverdy J, et al. The impact of morbid obesity on oxygen cost of breathing (VO(2RESP)) at rest. Am J Respir Crit Care Med 1999;160(3):883–6.

18. Bedell GN, Wilson WR, Seebohm PM. Pulmonary function in obese persons. J Clin Invest 1958; 37(7):1049–60.

19. Sutherland TJ, Goulding A, Grant AM, et al. The effect of adiposity measured by dual-energy X-ray absorptiometry on lung function. Eur Respir J 2008;32(1):85–91.

20. Jenkins SC, Moxham J. The effects of mild obesity on lung function. Respir Med 1991;85(4):309–11.

21. Jones RL, Nzekwu MM. The effects of body mass index on lung volumes. Chest 2006;130(3):827–33.

22. Gibson GJ. Obesity, respiratory function and breathlessness. Thorax 2000;55(Suppl 1):S41–4.

23. Rubinstein I, Zamel N, DuBarry L, et al. Airflow limitation in morbidly obese, nonsmoking men. Ann Intern Med 1990;112(11):828–32.

24. Douglas FG, Chong PY. Influence of obesity on peripheral airways patency. J Appl Phys 1972; 33(5):559–63.

25. Biring MS, Lewis MI, Liu JT, et al. Pulmonary physiologic changes of morbid obesity. Am J Med Sci 1999;318(5):293–7.

26. Lazarus R, Sparrow D, Weiss ST. Effects of obesity and fat distribution on ventilatory function: the normative aging study. Chest 1997;111(4):891–8.

27. Thomas PS, Cowen ER, Hulands G, et al. Respiratory function in the morbidly obese before and after weight loss. Thorax 1989;44(5):382–6.

28. Refsum HE, Holter PH, Lovig T, et al. Pulmonary function and energy expenditure after marked weight loss in obese women: observations before and one year after gastric banding. Int J Obes 1990;14(2):175–83.

29. Sugerman HJ. Pulmonary function in morbid obesity. Gastroenterol Clin North Am 1987;16(2):225–37.

30. Leone N, Courbon D, Thomas F, et al. Lung function impairment and metabolic syndrome: the critical role of abdominal obesity. Am J Respir Crit Care Med 2009;179(6):509–16.

31. Enright P. Overindulgence → overweight → reduced vital capacity → reduced longevity. Am J Respir Crit Care Med 2009;179(6):432–3.

32. Cancello R, Tounian A, Poitou C, et al. Adiposity signals, genetic and body weight regulation in humans. Diabete Metab 2004;30(3):215–27.

33. Steffes MW, Gross MD, Schreiner PJ, et al. Serum adiponectin in young adults—interactions with central adiposity, circulating levels of glucose, and insulin resistance: the CARDIA study. Ann Epidemiol 2004;14(7):492–8.

34. Franssen FM, O'Donnell DE, Goossens GH, et al. Obesity and the lung: 5. Obesity and COPD. Thorax 2008;63(12):1110–7.

35. Fogarty AW, Jones S, Britton JR, et al. Systemic inflammation and decline in lung function in

a general population: a prospective study. Thorax 2007;62(6):515–20.

36. Thyagarajan B, Jacobs DR, Apostol GG, et al. Plasma fibrinogen and lung function: the CARDIA Study. Int J Epidemiol 2006;35(4):1001–8.

37. Thyagarajan B, Smith LJ, Barr RG, et al. Association of circulating adhesion molecules with lung function: the CARDIA study. Chest 2009;135(6):1481–7.

38. Carey IM, Cook DG, Strachan DP. The effects of adiposity and weight change on forced expiratory volume decline in a longitudinal study of adults. Int J Obes Relat Metab Disord 1999;23(9):979–85.

39. Chen Y, Rennie D, Cormier YF, et al. Waist circumference is associated with pulmonary function in normal-weight, overweight, and obese subjects. Am J Clin Nutr 2007;85(1):35–9.

40. Rochester DF. Respiratory muscles and ventilatory failure: 1993 perspective. Am J Med Sci 1993; 305(6):394–402.

41. Parameswaran K, Todd DC, Soth M. Altered respiratory physiology in obesity. Can Respir J 2006;13(4): 203–10.

42. Wannamethee SG, Shaper AG, Whincup PH. Body fat distribution, body composition, and respiratory function in elderly men. Am J Clin Nutr 2005;82(5): 996–1003.

43. Thyagarajan B, Jacobs DR Jr, Apostol GG, et al. Longitudinal association of body mass index with lung function: the CARDIA study. Respir Res 2008; 9:31.

44. Wise RA, Enright PL, Connett JE, et al. Effect of weight gain on pulmonary function after smoking cessation in the Lung Health Study. Am J Respir Crit Care Med 1998;157(3 Pt 1):866–72.

45. Wang ML, McCabe L, Petsonk EL, et al. Weight gain and longitudinal changes in lung function in steel workers. Chest 1997;111(6):1526–32.

46. Chen Y, Horne SL, Dosman JA. Body weight and weight gain related to pulmonary function decline in adults: a six year follow up study. Thorax 1993; 48(4):375–80.

47. Bottai M, Pistelli F, Di Pede F, et al. Longitudinal changes of body mass index, spirometry and diffusion in a general population. Eur Respir J 2002; 20(3):665–73.

48. Womack CJ, Harris DL, Katzel LI, et al. Weight loss, not aerobic exercise, improves pulmonary function in older obese men. J Gerontol A Biol Sci Med Sci 2000;55(8):M453–7.

49. Soterakis J, Glennon JA, Ishihara AM, et al. Pulmonary function studies before and after jejunoileal bypass surgery. Am J Dig Dis 1976;21(7):553–6.

50. Zerah F, Harf A, Perlemuter L, et al. Effects of obesity on respiratory resistance. Chest 1993;103(5):1470–6.

51. Watson RA, Pride NB. Postural changes in lung volumes and respiratory resistance in subjects with obesity. J Appl Phys 2005;98(2):512–7.

52. King GG, Brown NJ, Diba C, et al. The effects of body weight on airway calibre. Eur Respir J 2005; 25(5):896–901.

53. Li AM, Chan D, Wong E, et al. The effects of obesity on pulmonary function. Arch Dis Child 2003;88(4): 361–3.

54. Zavorsky GS, Kim do J, Sylvestre JL, et al. Alveolar-membrane diffusing capacity improves in the morbidly obese after bariatric surgery. Obes Surg 2008;18(3):256–63.

55. Gilbert R, Sipple JH, Auchincloss JH Jr. Respiratory control and work of breathing in obese subjects. J Appl Phys 1961;16:21–6.

56. Mokhlesi B, Tulaimat A. Recent advances in obesity hypoventilation syndrome. Chest 2007;132(4):1322–36.

57. Shore SA, Johnston RA. Obesity and asthma. Pharmacol Ther 2006;110(1):83–102.

58. Ding DJ, Martin JG, Macklem PT. Effects of lung volume on maximal methacholine-induced bronchoconstriction in normal humans. J Appl Phys 1987; 62(3):1324–30.

59. Seow CY. Myosin filament assembly in an ever-changing myofilament lattice of smooth muscle. Am J Physiol, Cell Physiol 2005;289(6):C1363–8.

60. Fredberg JJ. Airway smooth muscle in asthma: flirting with disaster. Eur Respir J 1998;12(6):1252–6.

61. Shore SA, Schwartzman IN, Mellema MS, et al. Effect of leptin on allergic airway responses in mice. J Allergy Clin Immunol 2005;115(1):103–9.

62. Shore SA, Terry RD, Flynt L, et al. Adiponectin attenuates allergen-induced airway inflammation and hyperresponsiveness in mice. J Allergy Clin Immunol 2006;118(2):389–95.

63. Sood A, Camargo CA Jr, Ford ES. Association between leptin and asthma in adults. Thorax 2006; 61(4):300–5.

64. Sood A, Cui X, Qualls C, et al. Association between asthma and serum adiponectin concentration in women. Thorax 2008;63(10):877–82.

65. Zavala DC, Printen KJ. Basal and exercise tests on morbidly obese patients before and after gastric bypass. Surgery 1984;95(2):221–9.

66. Hansen JE, Sue DY, Wasserman K. Predicted values for clinical exercise testing. Am Rev Respir Dis 1984; 129(2 Pt 2):S49–55.

67. Buskirk E, Taylor HL. Maximal oxygen intake and its relation to body composition, with special reference to chronic physical activity and obesity. J Appl Phys 1957;11(1):72–8.

68. Wasserman K, Whipp BJ. Exercise physiology in health and disease. Am Rev Respir Dis 1975; 112(2):219–49.

69. Wasserman K, Hansen JE, Sue DY, et al. Principles of exercise testing and interpretation. 4th edition. Philadelphia: Lippincott Williams & Wilkins; 2005.

70. DeLorey DS, Wyrick BL, Babb TG. Mild-to-moderate obesity: implications for respiratory mechanics at

rest and during exercise in young men. Int J Obes (Lond) 2005;29(9):1039–47.

71. Sakamoto S, Ishikawa K, Senda S, et al. The effect of obesity on ventilatory response and anaerobic threshold during exercise. J Med Syst 1993; 17(3–4):227–31.

72. Ross RM. ATS/ACCP Statement on cardiopulmonary exercise testing. Am J Respir Crit Care Med 2003; 167(2):211–77.

73. Zarich SW, Kowalchuk GJ, McGuire MP, et al. Left ventricular filling abnormalities in asymptomatic morbid obesity. Am J Cardiol 1991;68(4):377–81.

The Relationship of Obesity and Obstructive Sleep Apnea

Neomi Shah, MD, MPH[a], Francoise Roux, MD, PhD[b],*

KEYWORDS

- Sleep-disordered breathing • Obesity
- Medical weight-loss therapy • Bariatric surgery
- Dietary weight loss • Sibutramine

Obesity is a chronic disease that has become epidemic in the United States and worldwide. Approximately 127 million adults in the United States are overweight (body mass index [BMI] 25.0–29.9) and 60 million are obese (BMI >30.0).[1,2] The World Health Organization predicts that by 2015, approximately 700 million adults will be obese (at least 10% of the world's projected population).[3] Obesity is a major risk factor for various disorders, including obstructive sleep apnea (OSA), a sleep-related breathing disorder characterized by recurrent upper-airway obstruction during sleep, which results in a cycle of hypoxemia, increased respiratory effort, and frequent arousals. In addition to being a risk factor for OSA, obesity may be a consequence of OSA. This article reviews the role of obesity in the development of OSA and discusses the two-way relationship between obesity and OSA. It also reviews the evidence on the effects of treatment of both disorders on their interrelationship.

DEFINITION OF OBSTRUCTIVE SLEEP APNEA

An apnea is defined as the cessation of airflow for at least 10 seconds in the presence of thoracoabdominal ventilatory efforts. A hypopnea is a reduction in airflow of at least 30% with a decrease in oxygen saturation of 2% or more for at least 10 seconds in the presence of thoracoabdominal ventilatory efforts.[4] The apnea–hypopnea index (AHI) is the sum of apneas and hypopneas per hour of sleep. An AHI of 5 or more per hour is established as a criterion for the diagnosis of OSA according to the criteria of the American Academy of Sleep Medicine.[4] However, there are various definitions of hypopnea. A survey of American Academy of Sleep Medicine–accredited sleep centers found that no two laboratories used the same definition of hypopnea,[5] and differences include various degrees of reduction in airflow and changes in thoracoabdominal movement, associated oxygen desaturation, and arousal. Such differences have important implications for the diagnosis of OSA and the standardization of research results. Recent population studies correlating the AHI with cardiovascular disease have helped to standardize the definition of hypopnea. The Sleep Heart Health Study, which was a large, multicenter trial designed to relate cardiovascular disease with polysomnographic findings, defined hypopnea as a 30% reduction in airflow or chest wall movement from baseline movement for at least 10 seconds and accompanied by oxygen desaturation of 4% or greater.[6]

The evidence for the prevalence of OSA derives from pooled data from four large studies that used similar in-laboratory monitoring techniques, diagnostic criteria, and sampling methods. From these data, it is estimated that in Western countries 24% of men and 15% of women have OSA and 4% of men and 2% of women have OSA with symptoms of sleepiness.[7]

[a] Department of Medicine, Section of Pulmonary, Montefiore Medical Center, Albert Einstein College of Medicine, 3332 Rochambeau Avenue, Centennial Building Suite 423, Bronx, NY 10467, USA
[b] Department of Medicine, Section of Pulmonary and Critical Care Medicine, Yale Center for Sleep Medicine, Yale University School of Medicine, 333 Cedar Street, PO Box 208057, New Haven, CT 06520-8057, USA
* Corresponding author.
E-mail address: francoise.roux@yale.edu (F. Roux).

Clin Chest Med 30 (2009) 455–465
doi:10.1016/j.ccm.2009.05.012

RISK FACTORS AND HEALTH CONSEQUENCES OF OBSTRUCTIVE SLEEP APNEA

Many risk factors for OSA have been identified in addition to obesity, including increasing age, being male, abnormal craniofacial morphology, nasal obstruction, genetic factors, and endocrine abnormalities such as thyroid disorders.[8,9] However, the true difference in risk between the two sexes is not clear. In women, menopausal status is likely a factor, with postmenopausal women being at a much higher risk for OSA than premenopausal women.[10] Some studies suggest that black Americans are at greater risk than whites.[11] There are many cardiovascular[12] and other consequences of OSA (**Table 1**). Peppard and colleagues[13] found that patients who had mild OSA had a 42% greater risk for developing hypertension in 4 years compared with patients who did not have OSA and who were matched for body habitus, age, sex, smoking status, and alcohol use. Patients with more severe OSA had a much higher risk of having hypertension at a 4-year follow-up. OSA has also been strongly associated with cardiac death.[23] The relative risk of sudden death from cardiac causes during sleep was 40% higher in patients who had severe OSA (AHI $\geq$ 40/hour) than in patients who had mild to moderate OSA (AHI 5–39/hour). In a large cross-sectional study, OSA was associated with an increased prevalence of self-reported heart failure and stroke.[19] OSA has also been shown to be independently associated with coronary artery disease after adjustment for traditionally considered risk factors.[15] Mooe and colleagues[25] showed that sleep-disordered breathing in patients who had coronary artery disease was associated with a worse long-term prognosis. They found that patients who had an AHI of 10 per hour or less had a 62% relative

increase and a 10.1% absolute increase in the composite endpoints of death, stroke, and myocardial infarction. OSA has been detected in more than 50% of patients who had an acute stroke and patients after recovery from stoke, indicating that OSA had been present before the stroke.[26] In a recent, large, prospective cohort study, Yaggi and colleagues[17] found that OSA increases the risk of stroke or all-cause mortality (hazard ratio 1.97), independent of other cerebrovascular risk factors, including hypertension.

OBESITY AS A RISK FACTOR FOR OBSTRUCTIVE SLEEP APNEA

The BMI is a reliable measure of body fat and body fat mass. A normal BMI is between 18.5 and 24.9. A person who has a BMI of 25 to 29.9 is considered to be overweight, and a person who has a BMI of 30 or more is considered to be obese; there are three classes of obesity based on the BMI (**Table 2**). The prevalence of obesity in the United States has been increasing for decades (**Fig. 1**). About 60 million adults (30% of the adult population) are obese, twice the percentage from 1980.[27,28]

Obesity can affect the structure and function of the upper airway. The upper airway has three primary functions: swallowing, phonation, and breathing. In breathing, various forces promote airway collapse and airway patency. The two primary forces that tend to collapse the airway are the intraluminal negative pressure generated by the diaphragm during inspiration and the extraluminal tissue pressure, which is the pressure resulting from tissues and bony structures surrounding the airway. These forces are counterbalanced primarily by the action of the pharyngeal dilator muscles, although longitudinal traction on the airway resulting from lung inflation likely contributes as well. Upper-airway narrowing seems to be an important factor in OSA. Obesity can cause narrowing of the pharynx because of the effects of subcutaneous and periluminal fat

Table 1	
Medical consequences of obstructive sleep apnea	
Cardiovascular Consequences	**Noncardiovascular Consequences**
Hypertension[13]	Motor vehicle accidents[14]
Coronary artery disease[15]	Impaired cognitive performance[16]
Stroke[17]	Depression[18]
Heart failure[19]	Occupational accidents[20]
Arrhythmias[21]	Poor exercise tolerance[22]
Death from cardiac causes[23]	Poor marital relationship[24]

Table 2		
Classification of obesity in adults		
BMI	**Body Characteristics**	**Obesity Class**
25.0–29.9	Overweight	—
30.0–34.9	Obesity	I
35.0–39.9	Obesity	II
$\geq$ 40.0	Extreme obesity	III

Data from National Heart, Lung, and Blood Institute. Clinical guidelines on the identification, evaluation, and treatment of overweight and obesity in adults. NIH publication no. 98-4083. National Institutes of Health, 1998.

deposits; obesity can also alter compliance of the airway wall secondary to increased fat deposition, thus promoting airway collapse.[29]

Increases in weight have been associated with an increasing prevalence of OSA (**Fig. 2**). Young and colleagues[7] found a fourfold increase in the prevalence of OSA with each increase in the standard deviation of the BMI. OSA seems to be much more common in patients who have class II and III obesity. In a study of such patients, the prevalence of OSA was found to be greater than 70% and greater than 90% in patients who had a BMI of 60 of more.[30] An increase in weight has also been shown to worsen OSA. Peppard and colleagues[31] conducted a population-based, prospective cohort study from 1989 to 2000 and measured the independent association between weight change and change in the AHI (**Table 3**). They found that a 10% weight gain predicted about a 32% increase in the AHI and a sixfold increase in the risk for developing moderate to severe OSA. The Sleep Heart Health Study showed a similar relationship between BMI and OSA severity; the odds ratio for moderate to severe OSA was 1.6 for each standard deviation increment in the BMI.[32]

Central obesity (abdominal fat/visceral fat) seems to be an important risk factor for OSA. Vgontzas and colleagues[33] conducted a study to determine whether OSA correlates best with visceral, subcutaneous, or total body fat. In that study, the BMI correlated well with both subcutaneous and total body fat but not with visceral fat, and visceral fat correlated well with indices of OSA (AHI and oxygen saturation) and not with subcutaneous body fat. Other studies have found that OSA strongly correlates with intra-abdominal fat.[34] Leptin, a hormone that is made in adipose tissues and is elevated in obese people, plays a key role in energy expenditure and regulation of body weight. Serum leptin levels also appear to be elevated in patients who have OSA. Ip and colleagues[35] showed that obese people who have underlying OSA have significantly elevated serum leptin levels when compared with weight-matched controls. Animal studies have suggested that elevated leptin levels may promote hypertension[36] and platelet aggregation[37] and could thus have a role in the development of cardiovascular disease in patients who have OSA.

Weight loss has been shown to alleviate OSA, thus strengthening a causal relationship of OSA with obesity. The study by Peppard and colleagues[31] showed that a 10% weight loss was associated with a 26% decrease in the AHI. Similar effects of weight loss on the severity of OSA were detected in a study in Australia in which polysomnographic findings (including AHI) were measured before and after bariatric surgery. There was a significant decrease in the AHI with postsurgical weight loss (AHI decreased from 61.6/hour to 13.4/hour).[38] However, there is evidence that OSA does not resolve when obesity is treated appropriately by weight loss,[39] which suggests that there are other underlying mechanisms linking OSA and obesity.

OBESITY AS A CONSEQUENCE OF OBSTRUCTIVE SLEEP APNEA

OSA has many obesity-promoting effects. It reduces physical activity and exercise performance, reduces energy metabolism, and reduces motivation secondary to underlying comorbidities such as depression. Patients who have OSA have excessive daytime sleepiness, which reduces their physical activity.[40] There also seems to be an association between OSA and decreased exercise performance. Grote and colleagues[41] studied 1149 patients who had OSA and assessed their blood pressure and heart rates at rest and during

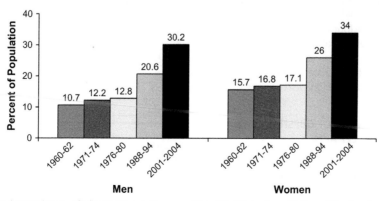

Fig. 1. Age-adjusted prevalence of obesity in adults, ages 20 to 74. (*Data from* National Center for Health Statistics, unpublished data, 2006.)

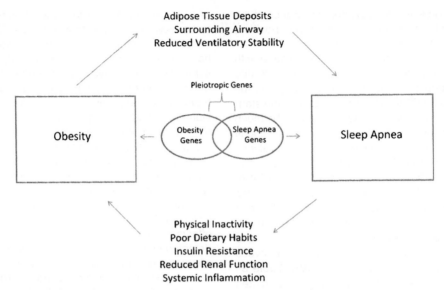

Fig. 2. Interaction between obesity and obstructive sleep apnea. (*From* Carter R, Watenpaugh DE. Obesity and obstructive sleep apnea: Or is it OSA and obesity? Pathophysiology 2008;15:72; with permission.)

graded exercise to evaluate cardiovascular reactivity during exercise and how it is affected by OSA. They found that maximal exercise capacity tended to decrease when people had OSA and concluded that OSA is associated with reduced physical work capacity and a modified hemodynamic response to exercise. Aguillard and colleagues[42] performed overnight sleep studies in 32 patients who had OSA and who also participated in a maximal exercise test, which served as an objective indicator of physical fatigue. The Fatigue Severity Scale was used as a subjective measure of fatigue. Most participants self-reported a high level of fatigue, and exercise testing revealed decreased physical work capacities. In addition to OSA resulting in reduced physical activity, there seems to be a relationship between an inadequate amount of or poor quality of sleep (commonly seen in OSA patients) and decreased energy.[43] This reduced-energy metabolism can play a role in predisposing patients who have OSA to obesity. Several studies have found an association between OSA and depression.[18] Patients who have depression often lack the motivation to exercise secondary to mood impairment, which may be yet another mechanism by which OSA causes obesity.

IMPACT OF TREATMENT OF OBESITY IN OBSTRUCTIVE SLEEP APNEA
Dietary Weight Loss

Reducing caloric intake by diet management is the most common and simplest treatment of obesity. However, dietary treatment has not been an effective long-term method in the general population,

with an overall median success rate of only 15% during up to 14 years of observation.[44] Various studies have examined the effects of weight loss in patients who have OSA. Weight loss can decrease the likelihood of upper-airway collapse by modifying its anatomy and function. A small, uncontrolled study demonstrated that a 13% weight loss decreased nasopharyngeal airway collapsibility in obese patients who had OSA after dietary treatment.[45] However, the amount of change in nasopharyngeal collapsibility varied,

Table 3
Estimated change in apnea hypopnea index by change in body weight

Percent Change in Weight (vs. No Change)	Estimated Percent Change in AHI[a] (95% Confidence Interval)[b]
−20	−48 (−58 to −35)
−10	−26 (−34 to −18)
−5	−14 (−18 to −9)
+5	15 (10 to 21)
+10	32 (20 to 45)
+20	70 (42 to 104)

[a] AHI adjusted for sex, change in cigarette packs per week, baseline body-mass index, and baseline age. All $P < .001$.
[b] In addition to change expected if weight remained stable.
Data from Peppard PE, Young T, Palta M, et al. Longitudinal study of moderate weight change and sleep-disordered breathing. JAMA 2000;284(23):3015–21.

which suggested that the critical threshold of collapsibility for OSA might be different among patients. All patients exhibited a decreased AHI on polysomnographs after weight loss. Hernandez and colleagues[46] used MRI to assess the morphologic condition of the neck in 14 patients who had a BMI of more than 40 after 3 months of weight loss and 3 months of weight maintenance. They found a significant reduction in the lateral subcutaneous neck fat after only a 10% weight loss. The average AHI was reduced from 24.3 to 2.9 per hour after weight loss in these patients. The magnitude of the decrease in the AHI after weight loss was higher in the patients who had the most severe cases of OSA. In another small study, Rubinstein and colleagues[47] showed an improvement in pharyngeal and glottic function after a 26-kg weight loss in patients who had OSA, and the improvement was accompanied by a significant reduction in the patients' AHI. These studies demonstrate that improvement in upper-airway anatomy and function achieved by weight loss can decrease apnea severity.

Sleep-disordered breathing may also be affected by weight loss. A controlled study of 15 moderately obese patients showed that even a modest mean weight loss of 10% achieved by reduced caloric intake can lead to a reduction in the AHI of 50%, from 55 to 29 per hour, in patients who have severe OSA.[48] Another small, controlled study of 15 patients found that an even smaller weight loss of about 8% after a 3-month, very-low-calorie diet reduced the nocturnal oxygen desaturation index significantly among obese (BMI 38 ± 5.9) patients who had OSA compared with normal-weight healthy controls.[49] In a large, population-based prospective cohort study of 690 people, a 10% weight loss was correlated with a 26% decrease in the AHI, showing that even minimal weight loss can be beneficial in patients who have OSA.[31] There is a preferential loss of visceral fat as opposed to subcutaneous fat after initial modest weight loss.[50] Because the visceral fat is associated with detrimental metabolic consequences, it seems that even a modest weight loss also could confer significant metabolic advantages in obese patients who have OSA. In contrast, a randomized, controlled study found that 10 weeks of dietary intervention had minimal effect on sleep-disordered breathing in most of the patients who had mild to moderate OSA, with a decrease in the AHI to less than 5 per hour in only 8 out of 34 overweight patients (BMI 27.3 ± 3).[51] Most of these studies examined the short-term effects of weight loss on sleep-disordered breathing but did not determine whether the beneficial effects of weight loss were maintained. In a recent, randomized study by Tuomilehto and colleagues[52] the effects of a low-calorie diet (600–800 kcal/day) for 12 weeks and supervised lifestyle counseling on sleep-disordered breathing were compared with the effects of a single general diet and an exercise counseling session in obese patients (BMI 28–40) who had mild OSA. The lifestyle intervention lasted for 1 year and consisted of 14 visits with a nutritionist. The control group was given general diet and exercise instructions at baseline and at 3-month and 1-year follow-ups, but without any individualized program. The intervention group had a 40% decrease in the AHI from the baseline. At the 3-month follow-up, 61% of the patients in the intervention group were considered cured of sleep apnea (AHI <5/h), compared with 32% in the control group. The changes in the AHI strongly correlated with changes in weight and waist circumference. Furthermore, this beneficial change was maintained at the 1-year follow-up, which showed the long-term efficacy of the supervised lifestyle counseling method. In contrast, a study by Sampol and colleagues[53] of 24 patients found that despite an initial cure of sleep-disordered breathing after significant weight loss resulting from a dietary intervention among obese patients who had OSA, with a decrease in the BMI from 31.5 at baseline to 25.9, sleep-disordered breathing recurred in 50% of these patients at a mean follow-up period of 94 months, regardless of whether they had regained the weight. That study suggested that the long-term success of weight loss in patients who have sleep-disordered breathing is limited and that such patients should be followed closely. Furthermore, recurrence of sleep-disordered breathing despite the maintenance of weight loss favors a multifactorial etiology of this disorder. However, most studies have had various limitations, including an absence of control groups and a lack of randomization and long-term follow-up. Some studies showed improvement in sleep-disordered breathing after weight loss but no cure of the disorder. It is unclear which patients would benefit most from weight loss and what the critical weight-loss threshold to cure sleep-disordered breathing is. It is reasonable to conclude that patients who have mild sleep-disordered breathing might be more likely to benefit.

Medical Weight-Loss Therapy

Sibutramine is a serotonin-norepinephrine reuptake inhibitor that suppresses appetite and has been shown to be effective for up to 2 years as a weight-loss agent. However, the effect overall is modest; patients taking the drug have only a 5% greater weight loss than patients taking a placebo.[54] Furthermore, sibutramine may contribute to systemic arterial hypertension and cardiac arrhythmias because of its noradrenergic activity; therefore, the drug might be not be safe to use for patients who have sleep-disordered breathing and who are already predisposed to these complications. The effects of sibutramine were investigated in an uncontrolled cohort study of 87 obese male patients who had a significant OSA-related mean respiratory disturbance index [RDI] of 46 ± 23 per hour.[55] (The RDI is a measure of sleep-disordered breathing, and the term is used interchangeably with AHI in this discussion.) After 24 weeks of the combined sibutramine-assisted dietary treatment, the weight loss in these patients was about 8% and the RDI dropped from 46 to 30 per hour. Only four patients were considered cured of their sleep-disordered breathing. There was a significant correlation between weight loss and decrease in the RDI, but most patients had persistent OSA. There were no significant changes in systolic or diastolic blood pressure, but heart rates increased slightly. Another randomized, double-blind, placebo-controlled study of 21 patients tested the effects of sibutramine on OSA severity. The study showed that 1 month of sibutramine therapy did not worsen OSA, despite the drug's effect on the central nervous system.[56]

There is insufficient evidence to justify the use of sibutramine therapy, even as an adjunct, in obese patients who have sleep-disordered breathing. (See the article in this issue by Bray regarding medical therapy of obesity.)

Bariatric Surgery

Bariatric surgery modifies the gastrointestinal tract and reduces the intake of nutrients by decreasing the capacity of the gastric pouch or inducing malabsorption. The placement of a laparoscopic adjustable gastric band is the most commonly performed procedure.

Bariatric surgery is now more commonly done because of the significant increase in the prevalence of obesity.[27,28] The National Heart, Lung, and Blood Institute guidelines recommend bariatric surgery to achieve weight loss if the patient's BMI is 40 or greater or 35 or greater in the presence of significant comorbidities such as OSA.[57] Patients should have failed to respond to nonsurgical weight-loss therapies. The prevalence of OSA in patients who have been evaluated for bariatric surgery is greater than 70%.[30] Patients being considered for bariatric surgery should be evaluated for sleep-disordered breathing to decrease the occurrence of perioperative complications; patients who have uncontrolled, severe OSA should postpone surgery until after initiation of therapy for OSA.

A prospective study[38] evaluated 49 severely obese (BMI 52.7 ± 9.5) patients using polysomnography before and after laparoscopic adjustable gastric banding. Approximately 18 months after surgery, the patients had lost a mean of 50% of their excess weight, and their AHI had decreased from a mean of 61 per hour before surgery to a mean of 13 per hour after surgery, with a corresponding improvement in sleep architecture. Perceived hypersomnia (measured using the Epworth Sleepiness Scale) also decreased after surgery. A recent cohort study[58] examined the effects of the Roux-en-Y gastric bypass procedure in 13 severely obese patients who had been diagnosed as having OSA using polysomnography at 6 months before bariatric surgery. Reevaluation of 12 of these patients 18 months after surgery revealed that the mean BMI had decreased from 55 to 34, and polysomnographic examination revealed that the mean AHI had decreased from 46 to 16 per hour, with significant improvement in oxygenation. However, despite the sustained weight loss, only 25% of the patients were considered cured of their sleep-disordered breathing 18 months after surgery. A retrospective cohort study[59] examined the effects of Roux-en-Y gastric bypass on 34 obese patients who had OSA after a longer follow-up period. Only 8 of the 34 patients returned for repeat polysomnographic examination. The mean BMI and RDI decreased by 31% and 75%, respectively, at 28 months after surgery. As a result, five of the eight patients no longer required nasal continuous positive airway pressure (CPAP) therapy. However, most of the patients in these small studies were lost to follow-up after surgery.

A much larger study[60] was performed in 289 patients who had OSA who underwent Roux-en-Y gastric bypass. At a median of 11 months postoperatively, 101 patients had a repeat evaluation and polysomnographic examination. The mean BMI decreased from 56 to 38, and the mean RDI decreased from 51 to 15 per hour, with an improvement in sleep efficiency. The greatest improvement occurred in patients who had severe OSA, in whom the mean RDI decreased from 80 to 19 per hour.

Charuzi and colleagues[61] studied 47 severely obese patients who had OSA 1 year after Roux-en-Y gastric surgery and found a marked reduction in apneas in 72% of the patients, with the mean AHI decreasing from 60 to 8 per hour

Table 4
Impact of bariatric surgery on obesity and obstructive sleep apnea severity

Authors (Reference no.)	N	Procedure	Presurgery AHI	Postsurgery AHI	Presurgery BMI	Postsurgery BMI	% Weight Loss	Follow-up
Dixon[38]	49	LAGB	61 ± 6/h	13.4 ± 13/h	52.7 ± 9.5	37.2 ± 7.2	50.1 ± 15	12–42 months
Fritscher[58]	13	Roux-en-Y	46.5/h	16/h	55.5 ± 10.1	34.1 ± 8.1	—	18 months
Guardiano[59]	8	Roux-en-Y	55 ± 31/h	14 ± 17/h	49 ± 12	34 ± 12	31	28 ± 20 months
Haines[60]	101	Roux-en-Y	51 ± 4/h	15 ± 2/h	56 ± 1	38 ± 1	—	6–42 months
Charuzi[61]	47	Roux-en-Y	60.8 ± 35.5/h	8.0 ± 11.8/h 34.5 ± 23.1/h	—	—	—	1 year 7 years
Pillar[62]	14	Roux-en-Y VBG	40 ± 28/h	11 ± 16.4/h 24 ± 23/h	45 ± 7.2	33 ± 7.5 35 ± 6	—	2–7 months 5–10 years
Lettieri[39]	24	Gastric banding	47 ± 9/h	24.5 ± 18.1/h	51.0 ± 10.4	32.1 ± 5.5	—	1 year

Abbreviations: LAGB, lapararoscopic adjustable gastric banding; VBG, vertical-banded gastroplasty.

as the mean excess body weight (over ideal body weight) decreased from 117% to 44%. Sleep apnea resolved in 40% of the patients. However, at 7 years follow-up, 22 of the patients had regained considerable weight and were diagnosed with severe OSA. The findings of Pillar and colleagues[62] raise more points of concern. Their investigation demonstrated an initial marked improvement in the BMI and AHI at 4 months after bariatric surgery. However, 7 years later, OSA had recurred without concomitant weight gain, which suggested that other mechanisms are involved in the pathophysiology of sleep-disordered breathing. Lettieri and colleagues[39] corroborated those findings, showing that significant weight loss after bariatric surgery reduced the severity of OSA, but that the disorder had resolved in only 4% of patients at 1 year after surgery. The AHI had even increased in two patients despite significant weight loss. The findings in these studies are summarized in **Table 4**.

Bariatric surgery is the most effective weight-loss therapy for morbidly obese patients; it improves sleep-disordered breathing indices in most patients and has a relatively low mortality rate. However, most patients still require CPAP therapy after surgery. Subjective resolution of hypersomnia in some studies did not correlate with the absence of sleep-disordered breathing and could promote a lack of adherence with CPAP therapy. Optimal CPAP pressure requirements can vary significantly as weight decreases after bariatric surgery. Therefore, auto-titrating CPAP devices are an attractive alternative therapeutic modality after bariatric surgery.[63] CPAP in the postoperative phase does not seem to promote gastrointestinal anatomic leaks and can reduce respiratory complications.[64] After bariatric surgery, patients should be followed closely to reassess the need for CPAP therapy in relation to weight changes, despite the lack of a strong correlation between the amount of weight loss and improvement in sleep-disordered breathing. (See the article in this issue by DeMaria regarding surgical therapy for obesity.)

IMPACT OF TREATMENT OF OBSTRUCTIVE SLEEP APNEA ON OBESITY

It is unclear whether OSA independently contributes to weight gain through sleep and metabolic disruptions. Some humoral mechanisms, such as leptin, could contribute to weight gain. A higher serum leptin level has been found in obese patients who have OSA than in matched obese controls who do not have OSA; this finding has led to the concept of leptin resistance.[65] Leptin resistance could hamper weight loss because it affects satiety. If there was a causal relationship between OSA and obesity, treatment of sleep-disordered breathing should result in weight loss. Few studies have examined the impact of CPAP therapy for OSA on obesity.

An early study[66] reported that weight loss was facilitated by CPAP therapy in obese patients who had OSA and who were adherent with CPAP therapy compared with poorly adherent CPAP users (those using CPAP less than 4 hours per night). However, CPAP adherence was based on self-reports. A more recent study examined the effects of CPAP therapy on fat partition in overweight patients who had OSA. Chin and colleagues[67] found that 6 months of CPAP therapy could reduce the amounts of intra-abdominal visceral fat even in the absence of weight loss. Metabolic indices, such as serum leptin level, were also decreased after CPAP therapy. This decrease in serum leptin levels could theoretically facilitate weight loss through decreased caloric intake. Another report[68] corroborated those findings, with decreased serum leptin level after 2 months of CPAP use in absence of weight change. Sanner and colleagues[69] found a relationship between the decrease in the serum leptin level and the degree of improvement in the AHI, independent of the change in the BMI, in 86 obese patients who had OSA and who were treated using CPAP.

In contrast, other investigations showed no change in visceral fat, weight, and serum leptin level, despite adherence to CPAP therapy, in obese patients who had OSA.[70] However, these studies were small and lacked adequate controls and information on the degree of correction of OSA, dietary habits, or sleep duration.

SUMMARY

OSA is a common condition that is closely related to obesity. The prevalence of OSA and obesity is increasing in the United States and other countries. OSA has significant consequences, including myocardial infarction, stroke, depression, and death. Obesity is not only a risk factor for the development of OSA, it also may be a consequence of OSA. This two-way relationship between obesity and OSA emphasizes the importance of treating both disorders. The achievement of weight loss using dietary modification is effective and the safest therapeutic approach for OSA, but its efficacy is limited in the long term. Bariatric surgery results in dramatic weight loss with significant improvement in sleep-disordered breathing indices in most patients. However, bariatric surgery has some inherent risks in the population of patients who have OSA and may not alleviate the need for CPAP therapy. Indeed, there is not always a good correlation between weight loss and improvement in sleep-disordered breathing. This suggests that the mechanisms underlying OSA are multifactorial and complex. CPAP is a well-established, noninvasive therapy for OSA, but it does not cure the disease. Further therapeutic trials are needed to determine whether CPAP therapy can have a sustained impact on obesity or its metabolic consequences.

REFERENCES

1. Bliwise DL, Feldman DE, Bliwise NG, et al. Risk factors for sleep disordered breathing in heterogeneous geriatric populations. J Am Geriatr Soc 1987;35(2):132–41.
2. American Obesity Association. Available at: http://obesity1.tempdomainname.com/subs/fastfacts/obesity_US.shtml.
3. World Health Organization. Available at: http://www.who.int/en/.
4. American Academy of Sleep Medicine Task Force. Sleep-related breathing disorders in adults: recommendations for syndrome definition and measurement techniques in clinical research. Sleep 1999; 22(5):667–89.
5. Moser NJ, Phillips BA, Berry DT, et al. What is hypopnea, anyway? Chest 1994;105(2):426–8.
6. Gottlieb DJ, Whitney CW, Bonekat WH, et al. Relation of sleepiness to respiratory disturbance index: the sleep heart health study. Am J Respir Crit Care Med 1999;159(2):502–7.
7. Young T, Palta M, Dempsey J, et al. The occurrence of sleep-disordered breathing among middle-aged adults. N Engl J Med 1993;328:1230–5.
8. Ancoli-Israel S, Kripke DF, Klauber MR, et al. Sleep-disordered breathing in community-dwelling elderly. Sleep 1991;14(6):486–95.
9. Redline S, Strohl KP. Recognition and consequences of obstructive sleep apnea hypopnea syndrome. Otolaryngol Clin North Am 1999;32(2): 303–31.
10. Krystal AD, Edinger J, Wohlgemuth W, et al. Sleep in peri-menopausal and post-menopausal women. Sleep Med Rev 1998;2(4):243–53.
11. Ancoli-Israel S, Klauber MR, Stepnowsky C, et al. Sleep-disordered breathing in African-American elderly. Am J Respir Crit Care Med 1995;152(6 Pt 1): 1946–9.
12. Peters RW. Obstructive sleep apnea and cardiovascular disease. Chest 2005;127(1):1–3.
13. Peppard P, Young T, Palta M, et al. Prospective study of the association between sleep-disordered breathing and hypertension. N Engl J Med 2000; 342:1378–84.
14. Mulgrew AT, Nasvadi G, Butt A, et al. Risk and severity of motor vehicle crashes in patients with obstructive sleep apnoea/hypopnoea. Thorax 2008;63(6):536–41.
15. Peker Y, Kraiczi H, Hedner J, et al. An independent association between obstructive sleep apnoea and coronary artery disease. Eur Respir J 1999;14(1): 179–84.
16. O'Donoghue FJ, Briellmann RS, Rochford PD, et al. Cerebral structural changes in severe obstructive sleep apnea. Am J Respir Crit Care Med 2005; 171(10):1185–90.
17. Yaggi H, Concato J, Kernan W, et al. Obstructive sleep apnea as a risk factor for stroke and death. N Engl J Med 2005;353:2034–41.
18. Baran AS, Richert AC. Obstructive sleep apnea and depression. CNS Spectr 2003;8(2):128–34.
19. Shahar E, Whitney C, Redline S, et al. Sleep-disordered breathing and cardiovascular disease: cross-sectional results of the Sleep Heart Health Study. Am J Respir Crit Care Med 2001;163:19–25.
20. Lindberg E, Carter N, Gislason T, et al. Role of snoring and daytime sleepiness in occupational accidents. Am J Respir Crit Care Med 2001; 164(11):2031–5.
21. Gami AS, Pressman G, Caples SM, et al. Association of atrial fibrillation and obstructive sleep apnea. Circulation 2004;110(4):364–7.
22. Lin CC, Lin CK, Wu KM, et al. Effect of treatment by nasal CPAP on cardiopulmonary exercise test in obstructive sleep apnea syndrome. Lung 2004; 182(4):199–212.
23. Gami AS, Howard DE, Olson EJ, et al. Day-night pattern of sudden death in obstructive sleep apnea. N Engl J Med 2005;352(12):1206–14.
24. Cartwright RD, Knight S. Silent partners: the wives of sleep apneic patients. Sleep 1987;10(3):244–8.
25. Mooe T, Franklin KA, Holmstrom K, et al. Sleep-disordered breathing and coronary artery disease: long-term prognosis. Am J Respir Crit Care Med 2001;164(10 Pt 1):1910–3.
26. Mohsenin V. Is sleep apnea a risk factor for stroke? A critical analysis. Minerva Med 2004;95(4):291–305.
27. Centers for Disease Control and Prevention. State-specific prevalence of obesity among adults— United States 2005. MMWR Morb Mortal Wkly Rep 2006;55:985–8.
28. Mokdad AH, Ford ES, Bowman BA, et al. Prevalence of obesity, diabetes, and obesity-related health risk factors, 2001. JAMA 2003;289(1):76–9.
29. Strobel RJ, Rosen RC. Obesity and weight loss in obstructive sleep apnea: a critical review. Sleep 1996;19(2):104–15.
30. Lopez PP, Stefan B, Schulman CI, et al. Prevalence of sleep apnea in morbidly obese patients who

presented for weight loss surgery evaluation: more evidence for routine screening for obstructive sleep apnea before weight loss surgery. Am Surg 2008; 74(9):834–8.

31. Peppard PE, Young T, Palta M, et al. Longitudinal study of moderate weight change and sleep-disordered breathing. JAMA 2000;284(23):3015–21.

32. Young T, Shahar E, Nieto FJ, et al. Predictors of sleep-disordered breathing in community-dwelling adults: the sleep heart health study. Arch Intern Med 2002;162(8):893–900.

33. Vgontzas AN, Papanicolaou DA, Bixler EO, et al. Sleep apnea and daytime sleepiness and fatigue: relation to visceral obesity, insulin resistance, and hypercytokinemia. J Clin Endocrinol Metab 2000; 85(3):1151–8.

34. Schafer H, Pauleit D, Sudhop T, et al. Body fat distribution, serum leptin, and cardiovascular risk factors in men with obstructive sleep apnea. Chest 2002; 122(3):829–39.

35. Ip MS, Lam KS, Ho C, et al. Serum leptin and vascular risk factors in obstructive sleep apnea. Chest 2000;118(3):580–6.

36. Rosmond R, Chagnon YC, Holm G, et al. Hypertension in obesity and the leptin receptor gene locus. J Clin Endocrinol Metab 2000;85(9):3126–31.

37. Konstantinides S, Schafer K, Loskutoff DJ. The prothrombotic effects of leptin possible implications for the risk of cardiovascular disease in obesity. Ann N Y Acad Sci 2001;947:134–41 [discussion 141–2].

38. Dixon JB, Schachter LM, O'Brien PE. Polysomnography before and after weight loss in obese patients with severe sleep apnea. Int J Obes (Lond) 2005; 29(9):1048–54.

39. Lettieri CJ, Eliasson AH, Greenburg DL. Persistence of obstructive sleep apnea after surgical weight loss. J Clin Sleep Med 2008;4(4):333–8.

40. Basta M, Lin HM, Pejovic S, et al. Lack of regular exercise, depression, and degree of apnea are predictors of excessive daytime sleepiness in patients with sleep apnea: sex differences. J Clin Sleep Med 2008;4(1):19–25.

41. Grote L, Hedner J, Peter JH. The heart rate response to exercise is blunted in patients with sleep-related breathing disorder. Cardiology 2004;102(2):93–9.

42. Aguillard RN, Riedel BW, Lichstein KL, et al. Daytime functioning in obstructive sleep apnea patients: exercise tolerance, subjective fatigue, and sleepiness. Appl Psychophysiol Biofeedback 1998;23(4): 207–17.

43. Van Cauter E, Holmback U, Knutson K, et al. Impact of sleep and sleep loss on neuroendocrine and metabolic function. Horm Res 2007;67(Suppl 1):2–9.

44. Ayyad C, Andersen T. Long-term efficacy of dietary treatment of obesity: a systematic review of studies published between 1931 and 1999. Obes Rev 2000;1(2):113–9.

45. Suratt PM, McTier RF, Findley LJ, et al. Changes in breathing and the pharynx after weight loss in obstructive sleep apnea. Chest 1987;92(4):631–7.

46. Hernandez TL, Ballard RD, Weil KM, et al. Effects of maintained weight loss on sleep dynamics and neck morphology in severely obese adults. Obesity (Silver Spring) 2009;17(1):84–91.

47. Rubinstein I, Colapinto N, Rotstein LE, et al. Improvement in upper airway function after weight loss in patients with obstructive sleep apnea. Am Rev Respir Dis 1988;138(5):1192–5.

48. Smith PL, Gold AR, Meyers DA, et al. Weight loss in mildly to moderately obese patients with obstructive sleep apnea. Ann Intern Med 1985;103(6 Pt 1): 850–5.

49. Kansanen M, Vanninen E, Tuunainen A, et al. The effect of a very low-calorie diet-induced weight loss on the severity of obstructive sleep apnoea and autonomic nervous function in obese patients with obstructive sleep apnoea syndrome. Clin Physiol 1998;18(4):377–85.

50. Chaston TB, Dixon JB. Factors associated with percent change in visceral versus subcutaneous abdominal fat during weight loss: findings from a systematic review. Int J Obes (Lond) 2008;32(4): 619–28.

51. Lam B, Sam K, Mok WY, et al. Randomised study of three non-surgical treatments in mild to moderate obstructive sleep apnoea. Thorax 2007;62(4):354–9.

52. Tuomilehto HP, Seppa JM, Partinen MM, et al. Lifestyle intervention with weight reduction: first-line treatment in mild obstructive sleep apnea. Am J Resp Crit Care Med 2009;179:320–7.

53. Sampol G, Munoz X, Sagales MT, et al. Long-term efficacy of dietary weight loss in sleep apnoea/hypopnoea syndrome. Eur Respir J 1998;12(5): 1156–9.

54. Li Z, Maglione M, Tu W, et al. Meta-analysis: pharmacologic treatment of obesity. Ann Intern Med 2005;142(7):532–46.

55. Yee BJ, Phillips CL, Banerjee D, et al. The effect of sibutramine-assisted weight loss in men with obstructive sleep apnoea. Int J Obes (Lond) 2007; 31(1):161–8.

56. Martinez D, Basile BR. Sibutramine does not worsen sleep apnea syndrome: a randomized double-blind placebo-controlled study. Sleep Med 2005;6(5): 467–70.

57. Kiernan M, Winkleby MA. Identifying patients for weight-loss treatment: an empirical evaluation of the NHLBI obesity education initiative expert panel treatment recommendations. Arch Intern Med 2000;160(14):2169–76.

58. Fritscher LG, Canani S, Mottin CC, et al. Bariatric surgery in the treatment of obstructive sleep apnea in morbidly obese patients. Respiration 2007;74(6): 647–52.

59. Guardiano SA, Scott JA, Ware JC, et al. The long-term results of gastric bypass on indexes of sleep apnea. Chest 2003;124(4):1615–9.
60. Haines KL, Nelson LG, Gonzalez R, et al. Objective evidence that bariatric surgery improves obesity-related obstructive sleep apnea. Surgery 2007; 141(3):354–8.
61. Charuzi I, Lavie P, Peiser J, et al. Bariatric surgery in morbidly obese sleep-apnea patients: short- and long-term follow-up. Am J Clin Nutr 1992;55(Suppl 2): 594S–6S.
62. Pillar G, Peled R, Lavie P. Recurrence of sleep apnea without concomitant weight increase 7.5 years after weight reduction surgery. Chest 1994; 106(6):1702–4.
63. Lankford DA, Proctor CD, Richard R. Continuous positive airway pressure (CPAP) changes in bariatric surgery patients undergoing rapid weight loss. Obes Surg 2005;15(3):336–41.
64. Huerta S, DeShields S, Shpiner R, et al. Safety and efficacy of postoperative continuous positive airway pressure to prevent pulmonary complications after Roux-en-Y gastric bypass. J Gastrointest Surg 2002;6(3):354–8.
65. Kapsimalis F, Varouchakis G, Manousaki A, et al. Association of sleep apnea severity and obesity with insulin resistance, C-reactive protein, and leptin levels in male patients with obstructive sleep apnea. Lung 2008;186(4):209–17.
66. Loube DI, Loube AA, Erman MK. Continuous positive airway pressure treatment results in weight less in obese and overweight patients with obstructive sleep apnea. J Am Diet Assoc 1997;97(8):896–7.
67. Chin K, Shimizu K, Nakamura T, et al. Changes in intra-abdominal visceral fat and serum leptin levels in patients with obstructive sleep apnea syndrome following nasal continuous positive airway pressure therapy. Circulation 1999;100(7):706–12.
68. Harsch IA, Konturek PC, Koebnick C, et al. Leptin and ghrelin levels in patients with obstructive sleep apnoea: effect of CPAP treatment. Eur Respir J 2003;22(2):251–7.
69. Sanner BM, Kollhosser P, Buechner N, et al. Influence of treatment on leptin levels in patients with obstructive sleep apnoea. Eur Respir J 2004;23(4):601–4.
70. Vgontzas AN, Zoumakis E, Bixler EO, et al. Selective effects of CPAP on sleep apnoea–associated manifestations. Eur J Clin Invest 2008;38(8):585–95.

The Pickwickian Syndrome—Obesity Hypoventilation Syndrome

Stephen W. Littleton, MD[a], Babak Mokhlesi, MD, MSc[b],*

KEYWORDS

- Obesity-hypoventilation syndrome
- Obstructive sleep apnea
- Hypercapnic respiratory failure
- Hypercapnia • CPAP • Bilevel PAP • Morbid obesity

HISTORY

The association between obesity and hypersomnolence has long been recognized. Of historical interest, obesity-hypoventilation syndrome (OHS) was described well before obstructive sleep apnea (OSA) was recognized as a true clinical entity in 1969.[1,2] The first published report of the association between obesity and hypersomnolence may have been as early as 1889,[3] but it was not until 1955 that Auchincloss and colleagues[4] described a case of obesity and hypersomnolence paired with alveolar hypoventilation. One year later, Burwell and colleagues[5] described a similar patient who finally sought treatment after his symptoms caused him to fall asleep during a hand of poker, despite having been dealt a full house of aces over kings. Although other clinicians had made the comparison some 50 years earlier,[3] Burwell and colleagues[5] popularized the term *Pickwickian syndrome* in their case report by noting the similarities between their patient and the boy "Joe" (**Fig. 1**), Mr. Wardle's servant in Charles Dickens' *The Posthumous Papers of the Pickwick Club*. Dickens[6] describes the first meeting of Mr. Wardle and the boy:

> "Damn that boy," said the old gentleman, "he's gone to sleep again."

> "Very extraordinary boy, that," said Mr. Pickwick, "does he always sleep in this way?"
> "Sleep!" said the old gentleman, "he's always asleep. Goes on errands fast asleep, and snores as he waits at the table."
> "How very odd!" said Mr. Pickwick.
> "Ah! Odd indeed," returned the old gentleman; "I'm proud of that boy—wouldn't part with him on any account—damme, he's a natural curiosity!"

Although OHS is rare among children,[7] it is now, unfortunately, far from a natural curiosity among adults.

DEFINITION

The salient features of OHS consist of obesity (defined as a body mass index [BMI] $\geq$30 kg/m^2), sleep-disordered breathing, and chronic daytime alveolar hypoventilation (defined as PaCO_2 $\geq$45 mm Hg and PaO_2 <70 mm Hg).[8] In approximately 90% of patients with OHS, the sleep-disordered breathing is in the form of OSA. The other 10% of patients are considered to have "sleep hypoventilation," which is defined as a 10-mm Hg increase in sleeping PaCO_2 versus wakefulness, or oxygen desaturation during sleep unexplained by obstructive apneas or hypopneas.

[a] Sleep Medicine Fellowship Program, Section of Pulmonary and Critical Care Medicine, University of Chicago, 5841 South Maryland Avenue, MC 4000, Room W438, Chicago, IL 60637, USA
[b] Department of Medicine, Section of Pulmonary and Critical Care Medicine, University of Chicago, 5841 South Maryland Avenue, MC 0999, Room L11B, Chicago, IL 60637, USA
* Corresponding author. Department of Medicine, Section of Pulmonary and Critical Care Medicine, University of Chicago, 5841 South Maryland Avenue, MC 0999, Room L11B, Chicago, IL 60637.
E-mail address: bmokhles@medicine.bsd.uchicago.edu (B. Mokhlesi).

Clin Chest Med 30 (2009) 467–478
doi:10.1016/j.ccm.2009.05.004
0272-5231/09/$ – see front matter © 2009 Elsevier Inc. All rights reserved.

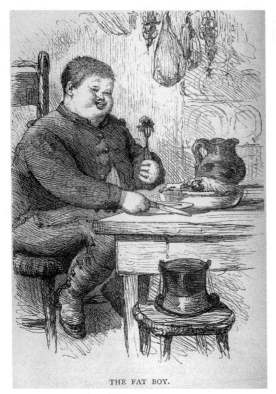

Fig. 1. Joe the "Fat Boy." Illustration by S. Etyinge, Jr. (*From* Dickens C. The posthumous papers of the Pickwick Club. Boston: Ticknor and Fields: Boston; 1867.)

OHS should be considered a diagnosis of exclusion until other causes of hypoventilation are evaluated, such as pulmonary disease (severe obstructive or restrictive), chest wall deformities, severe hypothyroidism, or neuromuscular disease. Other central hypoventilation syndromes, such as congenital central hypoventilation syndrome or Arnold-Chiari type II malformations, should also be considered.[8]

EPIDEMIOLOGY

To date, no population-based prevalence studies of OHS have been performed. The overall prevalence of OHS in patients with OSA is better studied. Multiple prospective and retrospective studies across various geographic regions with a variety of racial and ethnic populations have shown it to be between 10% and 20%.[9–18] This range is consistent among all studies performed, regardless of study design or sample size (with the two largest having 1227[18] and 1141[10] patients). The prevalence of OHS among the general adult population in the United States can, however, be estimated. If approximately 3% of the general US population has severe obesity

(BMI ≥ 40 kg/m^2),[19] half of the patients with severe obesity have OSA,[20] and 10% to 20% of the severely obese patients with OSA have OHS, a conservative estimated prevalence of OHS in the general adult population is anywhere between 0.15% and 0.3% (1.5–3 individuals among 1000 adults). If the US population is assumed to be 305 million,[21] there may be as many as half a million individuals afflicted with OHS.

Table 1 provides a summary of demographic and physiologic variables compiled from large series of patients with OHS reported in the literature. These patients are typically diagnosed in their sixth decade of life, and there is a slightly higher prevalence in men. Patients with OHS tend to be severely obese (defined as BMI ≥ 40 kg/m^2), have an apnea-hypopnea index (AHI) in the severe range, and are usually hypersomnolent.

The variable that is most strongly linked to OHS in patients with OSA is BMI. Eight of nine studies showed a significant correlation between BMI and OHS in patients with OSA.[9,11–16,18,22] Undisputedly, OHS is more prevalent in the severely obese (**Fig. 2**). The same studies also examined the relation between the AHI and the prevalence of OHS in patients with OSA. Of nine studies, five did not show a significant correlation and four did (including all three of the studies performed in Japan). The prevalence of OHS in patients with an AHI greater than 60 is approximately 25% (**Fig. 3**). The most recent study by Kawata and colleagues[18] showed, in a multivariate analysis, AHI to be strongly linked to OHS in 1227 patients with OSA (AHI of 59 in those with OHS versus AHI of 39 in those without; $P < .0001$). Although other causes of hypercapnia were not excluded in this study, the FEV$_1$ (% of predicted) was similar in the two groups.

Table 2 shows predictors of hypercapnia in patients with OSA using a logistic regression model.[17] Although BMI was associated with hypercapnia in univariate analysis, it did not remain a significant independent predictor of hypercapnia in logistic regression, possibly because of its strong correlation with the AHI and lowest oxygen saturation during sleep. **Table 3**, conversely, combines physiologic and polysomnographic features that are readily available to clinicians to assess the risk of patients with OSA for OHS.[17]

MORBIDITY AND MORTALITY

Most patients with OHS are severely obese and have severe OSA.[8] Severe obesity[23] and severe OSA (defined as AHI >30 events per hour),[24] independent of hypercapnia, are known to negatively affect quality of life, morbidity, and mortality.

Table 1
Clinical features of patients with obesity hypoventilation syndrome

Variables	Mean (Range)
Age (years)	52 (42–61)
Men (%)	60 (49–90)
BMI (kg/m^2)	44 (35–56)
pH	7.38 (7.34–7.40)
$Paco_2$ (mm Hg)	53 (47–61)
Pao_2 (mm Hg)	56 (46–74)
Serum bicarbonate level (mEq/L)	32 (31–33)
Apnea-hypopnea index	66 (20–100)
Spo_2 nadir during sleep (%)	65 (59–76)
% total sleep time Spo_2 <90%	50 (46–56)
FVC (% of predicted)	68 (57–102)
FEV_1 (% of predicted)	64 (53–92)
FEV_1/FVC	77 (74–88)
Epworth Sleepiness Scale	14 (12–16)

Data presented as mean (range) of 16 studies and include a total of 757 patients with OHS.
Abbreviations: FEV_1, forced expiratory volume in 1 second; FVC, forced vital capacity.
Data from Refs. [9–14,16,17,26–28,50–52]

OHS seems to present an additional burden for these patients above and beyond that of severe obesity and severe OSA.

Quality of Life

Hida[25] matched patients with OHS to patients with eucapnic OSA by age, BMI, and lung function, and assessed quality of life with the Short Form-36 questionnaire. There was no significant difference between the two groups, with the exception of social functioning, with those who had OHS being worse (*P*<.01). These researchers hypothesized that this was because the patients with OHS were sleepier (Epworth Sleepiness Scale: 14.6 ± 4.9 versus 12.5 ± 4.6; *P*<.05). Quality of life improved after 6 months of treatment with continuous positive airway pressure (CPAP) in both groups, but the researchers did not examine whether the patients with OHS had significantly greater improvement. Patients with OHS have a lower quality of life than those with other hypercapnic respiratory diseases, despite having a significantly lower $Paco_2$.[26] A confounding factor is that the patients with OHS were, predictably, more obese than those with other causes of hypercapnia.

Morbidity

It is also unclear whether patients with OHS experience higher morbidity than patients who are similarly obese and have OSA because no studies

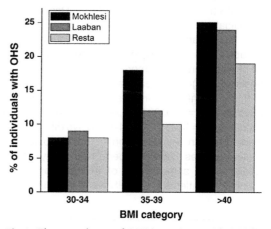

Fig. 2. The prevalence of OHS in patients with OSA by BMI categories in the United States (Moklesi) France (Labaan), and Italy (Resta). (*Data from* Laaban JP, Chailleux E. Daytime hypercapnia in adult patients with obstructive sleep apnea syndrome in France, before initiating nocturnal nasal continuous positive airway pressure therapy. Chest 2005;127:710–5; and Mokhlesi B, Tulaimat A, Faibussowitsch I, et al. Obesity hypoventilation syndrome: prevalence and predictors in patients with obstructive sleep apnea. Sleep Breath 2007;11:117–24.) The data from Italy were provided by Professor Onofrio Resta from the University of Bari, Italy.

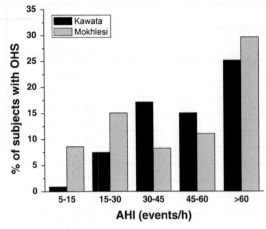

Fig. 3. Prevalence of OHS in patients with OSA distributed by various AHI categories (*Data from* Kawata N, Tatsumi K, Terada J, et al. Daytime hypercapnia in obstructive sleep apnea syndrome. Chest 2007;132:1832–8; and Mokhlesi B, Tulaimat A, Faibussowitsch I, et al. Obesity hypoventilation syndrome: prevalence and predictors in patients with obstructive sleep apnea. Sleep Breath 2007;11:117–24; previously unpublished.)

have been performed to date. Berg and colleagues[27] performed a study in which 26 patients with OHS were matched with patients of similar BMI, age, gender, and postal code (to control for socioeconomic factors). Despite the investigators' best efforts, the group with OHS was significantly more obese, although both groups were severely obese. The group with OHS was found to be more likely to carry a diagnosis of congestive heart failure (odds ratio [OR] = 9, 95% confidence interval [CI]: 2.3–35), angina pectoris (OR = 9, 95% CI: 1.4–57.10), and cor pulmonale (OR = 9, 95% CI: 1.4–57.1). No differences were found in the likelihood of having osteoarthritis, diabetes mellitus, hypertension, or hypothyroidism. The same group of investigators also found that patients with OHS were more likely to

be hospitalized and more likely to be admitted to the intensive care unit. Rates of hospital admission decreased and were equivalent to those of the control group 2 years after treatment was instituted. In another prospective study, 47 patients with OHS had higher rates of admission to the intensive care unit (40% versus 6%) and greater need for invasive mechanical ventilation (6% versus 0%) when compared with 103 patients with a similar degree of obesity but without hypoventilation.[28]

Mortality

The effect of OHS on survival, independent of obesity and OSA, is also unclear. No long-term follow-up studies have been done directly comparing survival of patients with OHS versus those with OSA, although data can be extrapolated across several studies. Budweiser and colleagues[29] conducted a retrospective analysis of 126 patients with OHS and found the 1-, 2-, and 5-year survival rates to be 97%, 92%, and 70%, respectively. Patients in this study were adherent with noninvasive positive pressure ventilation (NPPV) therapy (>6 hours per night). Likewise, in a study by Campos-Rodriguez and colleagues,[30] the 5-year survival rate in CPAP-adherent patients with OSA was 96%. No definitive conclusion can be drawn from direct comparison of the two studies because the BMI in the OHS group was higher than that in the OSA group (44.6 versus 36.7 kg/m^2).

Clearly, patients with untreated OHS have a significant risk for death. A prospective study by Nowbar and colleagues[28] followed a group of 47 severely obese patients with OHS after hospital discharge. The 18-month mortality rate for patients with untreated OHS was higher than that for the control cohort of 103 patients with obesity alone (23% versus 9%) despite the fact that the groups had similar BMI, age, and several comorbid conditions (with the exception being that

Table 2
Predictors of hypercapnia in patients with obstructive sleep apnea using a logistic regression model

Variable[a]	Odds Ratio (95% Confidence Interval)	P
BMI >40	1.8 (0.9–3.5)	0.1
AHI >50	2.2 (1.1–4.4)	0.02
Oxygen desaturation nadir <60% during polysomnography	4 (2–8)	<0.001
Moderate to severe restriction on pulmonary function testing	10 (5–24)	<0.001

[a] No significant interactions among variables.

Table 3
Independent predictors of hypercapnia in patients with obstructive sleep apnea who do not have evidence of obstructive airways disease defined as forced expiratory volume in 1 second/forced vital capacity ratio <70%

Variables		Patients	Hypercapnics[a]	
Body Mass Index >40 or Restriction on PFT	Apnea-hypopnea Index >50 or Oxygen Saturation <60%	N	n (%)	Odds Ratio
No	No	65	2 (3%)	1
Yes	No	75	9 (12%)	6
No	Yes	58	7 (12%)	6
Yes	Yes	131	47 (36%)	23
	Total	329	65 (20%)	—

Unpublished results obtained by reanalysis of data from Ref.[17]
Abbreviation: PFT, pulmonary function testing.
[a] Prevalence of hypercapnia in this prospectively obtained sample was 20%.

OSA was more prevalent in the OHS group). When adjusted for age, gender, BMI, and renal function, the hazard ratio of death in the OHS group was 4.0 in the 18-month period. Only 13% of the 47 patients were treated for OHS after their hospitalization. A retrospective study of 126 patients with OHS who were highly adherent to NPPV therapy reported an 18-month mortality rate of 3%.[8,29] Together, these two studies suggest that PAP adherence may lower the short-term mortality rates of patients with OHS.

PATHOPHYSIOLOGY

The pathogenesis of alveolar hypoventilation in morbidly obese patients is complex and likely multifactorial. There have been a variety of physiologic differences between patients with OHS and those with obesity or OSA described to date: an increased load on the respiratory system, an impaired central response to hypoxemia and hypercapnia, the presence of sleep-disordered breathing, and impaired neurohormonal responses (leptin resistance).

Increased Load on The Respiratory System

Upper airway resistance
Using impulse oscillometry, Lin and colleagues[31] found that patients with OHS have increased upper airway resistance while supine and upright when compared with an equally obese group of patients with OSA. The OSA group was found to have increased airway resistance when supine as well, albeit less than the OHS group, and the resistance decreased to that of the nonobese normal patients when upright. This finding in patients who have OSA is in agreement with previously reported data.[32] It remains unclear if increased

upper airway resistance plays a role in the development of daytime hypercapnia in this subset of patients.

Respiratory muscles
The maximal inspiratory and expiratory pressures of patients with OHS are reduced when compared with those of morbidly obese subjects.[33] This method of measuring respiratory muscle strength depends on patient cooperation, however, and is considered less reliable than diaphragmatic twitch pressures.[34] Such a study has not yet been performed. In a study by Sampson and Grassino,[33] patients with OHS were able to generate equivalent transdiaphragmatic pressures (Pdi) as eucapnic obese patients during hypercapnia-induced hyperventilation, suggesting that respiratory muscle weakness may not play a role in the development of OHS. In addition, the OHS group showed no evidence of acute diaphragmatic fatigue (or neuromuscular uncoupling) throughout the hypercapnic trial when measured by the ratio of peak electrical activity of the diaphragm to peak Pdi, which should theoretically eliminate the variable of inadequate patient cooperation. Hypercapnia is also known to have deleterious effects on diaphragmatic function; thus, it is difficult to determine whether respiratory muscle fatigue is a cause of or effect of OHS.[35]

Respiratory system mechanics
In OHS, there is an increase in the work of breathing to move the excess weight on the thoracic wall and abdomen.[36] It is unclear what contribution, if any, these altered mechanics have in the pathogenesis of OHS, however. Some other interesting differences in patients who have OHS have been described. The lung

compliance of patients who have OHS is less than that of an equally obese control group (0.122 versus 0.157 L/cm H_2O). This can be explained by the lower functional residual capacity of the group with OHS (1.71 versus 2.20 L). There is an even greater difference in chest wall compliance between the two groups (0.079 L/cm H_2O in group with OHS versus 0.196 L/cm H_2O in obese controls). The lung resistance of the two groups was equivalent but three times higher than that of a nonobese control group.[36] If the respiratory muscles are truly able to compensate for these altered mechanics, it seems unlikely that this is a significant contributor to the pathogenesis of OHS.

Central Respiratory Drive

Hypercapnic ventilatory response

Patients with OHS and eucapnic patients with morbid obesity have similar respiratory drives when measured by mouth occlusion over the first 100 milliseconds of inspiration ($P_{0.1}$ technique).[33,37] This suggests that obesity leads to an increased respiratory drive to compensate for the increased load on the respiratory muscles. Patients with OHS have a decreased hyperventilatory response to a hypercapnic challenge when compared with hypercapnic patients with chronic obstructive pulmonary disease, eucapnic obese patients, or normal subjects, however. In an elegant study by Sampson and Grassino,[33] the slope of the Pdi response to hypercapnia in patients who had OHS was equivalent to that of eucapnic subjects, suggesting that the subjects who had OHS were able to elicit the same increase in diaphragmatic work. The rate of increase of diaphragmatic activation was less than that of the eucapnic subjects, however, suggesting an inadequate central response. Most of the published literature suggests that this blunted neural response is corrected with treatment of OHS with positive airway pressure (PAP) therapy,[37–39] although there are reports of noncorrectors, even after tracheostomy.[40]

Hypoxic ventilatory response

Patients with OHS were found to have a decreased ventilatory response to hypoxemia in an observational study in 1975.[41] In 1994, Lin[39] showed that a group of hypercapnic patients with OSA had a decreased hypoxic ventilatory response when compared with patients with OSA and that the decreased response was corrected after as little as 2 weeks of therapy with PAP. However, this study was limited by the fact that the hypercapnic patients had significantly worse sleep-disordered breathing and significantly higher BMI. Then, in

2004, Han and colleagues[37] matched a small group of subjects with OHS to equally obese subjects with a similar degree of sleep-disordered breathing. Their findings confirmed those of Lin.[39] They found a decreased hypoxic ventilatory response in the subjects with OHS when compared with the controls. The hypoxic response of the subjects who had OHS improved significantly after 2 weeks of treatment with PAP and reached that of normal nonobese subjects within 6 weeks.

It is clear from the current body of literature that defects in central respiratory drive are responsible for alveolar hypoventilation in OHS and that effective treatment of sleep-disordered breathing leads to a reversal in these defects in the majority of patients. This reversal suggests that the central defects are present in OHS but are not the primary cause of the syndrome.

Leptin resistance

Leptin is a satiety hormone produced by adipocytes.[42] Mice that are deficient in leptin become morbidly obese and develop a blunted hypercapnic response, similar to patients with OHS.[43] Of note, blunting of the hypercapnic response occurs before significant weight gain. Treatment of these mice with leptin improves their ventilation.[44]

In humans, serum leptin levels correlate with increasing levels of adiposity.[45] It is postulated that as weight increases, so too does carbon dioxide production. Therefore, leptin leads to an increase in minute ventilation to maintain homeostasis and eucapnia. The contribution of OSA to leptin production, independent of obesity, is unclear. One Chinese study found higher leptin levels in patients who had OSA when matched for BMI and that the levels normalized after 6 months of treatment with CPAP therapy.[46] A Spanish study found higher levels of leptin in nonobese patients with OSA than in nonobese controls without OSA, suggesting that OSA can, independent of obesity, lead to an increase in leptin levels. Obese patients with OSA, however, were found to have similar levels to equally obese patients without OSA. In addition, the serum leptin levels of obese patients who had OSA were 2.5 times higher than those of nonobese patients who had OSA. Taken together, these data suggest that excess adiposity is a more significant contributor to elevated serum leptin levels than OSA. Leptin levels decreased in nonobese and obese patients who had OSA after treatment with CPAP but only reached statistical significance in the nonobese group.[47]

Whether OHS, independent of OSA and obesity, is associated with elevated serum leptin levels remains unclear. One study showed higher serum leptin levels in hypercapnic patients with OSA than in an equally obese eucapnic control group with OSA. Logistic regression analysis showed that serum leptin was the only predictor of hypercapnia.[48] A recent study confirmed that serum leptin levels directly correlate with the degree of hypercapnic ventilatory response (HCVR) in eucapnic patients with OSA and control subjects. These investigators showed equivalent leptin levels between eucapnic and hypercapnic patients with OSA.[49] This finding is consistent with the concept of leptin resistance as a potential contributor to lower HCVR, leading to the development of hypercapnia in patients with OHS.

Sleep-disordered breathing

Sleep-disordered breathing is considered necessary for the diagnosis of OHS and can take two forms. The first and by far the most common type is OSA, and the second type is central hypoventilation. OSA is well established in the pathophysiology of OHS by the resolution of hypercapnia in most (but not all) patients by treatment with tracheostomy or PAP therapy.[37,50–55]

Conceptually, understanding how hypoventilation during sleep leads to hypoventilation during wakefulness is not intuitive. An elegant model proposed by Norman and colleagues[56] ties the two together. In most patients with OSA, the hyperventilation that follows apneic episodes eliminates the carbon dioxide accumulated during the apnea.[57] If this inter-event hyperventilation is insufficiently adequate to do so, however, these investigators postulate that the accumulated carbon dioxide could lead to a metabolic compensation that causes a small increase in serum bicarbonate level. If the time to eliminate the accumulated serum bicarbonate is greater than the interval before the next sleep period, a small net increase in serum bicarbonate would result. This increased serum bicarbonate would lead to a blunting of the ventilatory response to hypercapnia during wakefulness.

DIAGNOSIS

The definitive test to establish hypoventilation is an arterial blood gas, although an elevated serum bicarbonate level has been suggested as an effective screening tool.[17] **Fig. 4** shows the prevalence of OHS in obese patients with OSA (BMI ≥ 30 kg/m^2 and AHI ≥ 5) using serum bicarbonate level combined with other readily available measures, such as severity of obesity, impairment of respiratory mechanics, and severity of OSA. Hypoxemia during wakefulness is not common in

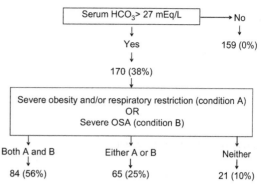

Fig. 4. Prevalence of OHS based on serum bicarbonate level in a sample of 329 adult patients with obesity (BMI ≥ 30 kg/m^2) and OSA (AHI ≥ 5). OHS was absent in 159 patients with a serum bicarbonate level lower than 27 mEq/L. In contrast, among those with a serum bicarbonate level greater than 27mEq/L, OHS was present in 38% of patients. OHS was present in 56% of the subgroup of patients with condition A (severe obesity or evidence of restrictive chest physiology based on forced vital capacity <70% of predicted) and condition B (severe OSA defined as AHI ≥ 30). (*From* Mokhlesi B, Tulaimat A, Faibussowitsch I, et al. Obesity hypoventilation syndrome: prevalence and predictors in patients with obstructive sleep apnea. Sleep Breath 2007;11:121; with permission.)

patients with simple OSA. Therefore, abnormal oxygen saturation (Spo$_2$) detected by finger pulse oximetry during wakefulness should also lead clinicians to exclude OHS in patients with OSA by obtaining a room air arterial blood gases. Once OHS is suspected, pulmonary function tests should then be performed to exclude significant obstructive or restrictive ventilatory patterns. Patients with OHS often have a minimal or mild restrictive pattern on pulmonary function testing. Chest radiography should also be performed to exclude interstitial lung disease and chest wall deformities, such as severe kyphoscoliosis. Severe hypothyroidism should also be ruled out. If not already performed, full-night polysomnography, followed by PAP titration, should be performed.

TREATMENT

Treatment of OHS has traditionally followed three modalities: reversal of sleep-disordered breathing, weight reduction, and pharmacotherapy.

Treatment of Sleep-disordered Breathing

PAP therapy (in the form of CPAP therapy) was first described as an effective treatment for OHS in 1982.[53] Although subsequent studies confirmed its efficacy, failure of CPAP in some cases has led to uncertainty as to whether CPAP should be attempted initially or if bilevel PAP therapy (more commonly known as NPPV) is a better modality.[40,51,53,58] In a recent prospective study of outpatients with severe OHS, based on the severity of obesity and OSA and the degree of hypercapnia, 57% of patients were titrated successfully with CPAP alone, and the mean pressure required was 13.9 cm H_2O.[59] The remainder had greater than 20% of total sleep time with an SpO_2 of less than 90%, although they also had a residual AHI of 25. The CPAP failure group was more obese, although both groups were extremely obese. Because this was a single-night titration study, the question of whether residual hypoxemia would resolve with long-term treatment was left unanswered.

A recent prospective randomized study performed by Piper and colleagues[60] compared the long-term efficacy of bilevel PAP versus CPAP. In this study, 45 consecutive patients with OHS underwent a full night of CPAP titration. Nine patients (20%) were excluded because of persistent hypoxemia, arbitrarily defined as 10 continuous minutes of SpO_2 less than 80% without frank apneas, during the CPAP titration. The remaining 36 patients, who had a successful CPAP titration night, were subsequently randomized to CPAP or bilevel PAP. Those randomized to bilevel PAP underwent an additional titration night to establish the effective inspiratory and expiratory pressures. Supplemental oxygen administration was necessary in 3 patients in the CPAP group and in 4 patients in the bilevel PAP group. After 3 months, there was no significant difference between the two groups in adherence to PAP therapy or in improvement in daytime sleepiness, hypoxemia, or hypercapnia. This study confirms that most patients with OHS (80%) can be successfully titrated with CPAP. Their findings also suggest that as long as OSA and nocturnal hypoxemia are effectively treated with CPAP, it makes no significant long-term difference if patients are given bilevel PAP or CPAP therapy. Therefore, bilevel PAP is not superior to CPAP a priori; rather, treatment should be individualized to each patient. Bilevel PAP should be instituted if the patient is intolerant of the higher CPAP pressures (>5 cm H_2O) that may be required to resolve apneas and hypopneas or if hypoxemia is persistent despite adequate resolution of obstructive respiratory events during the titration study.[61] During bilevel PAP titration, the inspiratory positive airway pressure (IPAP) should be at least 8 to 10 cm H_2O greater than the expiratory positive airway pressure (EPAP) to increase ventilation effectively.[50,52,62,63] In the few patients with OHS who do not have OSA, EPAP can be set at 5 cm

H_2O and IPAP can be titrated to improve ventilation.[62,63] Bilevel PAP should also be considered if the $PaCO_2$ does not normalize after 3 months of therapy with CPAP.

Average volume-assured pressure support ventilation is a hybrid mode of PAP therapy that delivers a more consistent tidal volume with the comfort of pressure support ventilation. This alternative mode of PAP therapy has proved successful in treating patients with OHS in a randomized controlled study.[64]

Adherence to PAP therapy is directly correlated with improvement in daytime arterial blood gas values. In a retrospective study of 75 outpatients with stable OHS, $PaCO_2$ decreased by 1.8 mm Hg and PaO_2 increased by 3 mm Hg per hour of daily CPAP or bilevel PAP use. Patients who used PAP therapy for more than 4.5 hours per day had a considerably greater improvement in blood gases than less adherent patients ($\Delta PaCO_2$: -7.7 versus -2.4 mm Hg, $P<.001$; ΔPaO_2: 9.2 versus 1.8 mm Hg). In addition, the need for daytime oxygen therapy decreased from 30% of patients to 6%.[51] Improvement in blood gas values may be seen as early as 1 month after the institution of PAP therapy.[37,51,65]

Tracheostomy was the first described therapy for OHS.[66] Although there have been no long-term studies to date, it is still considered a final option for a patient intolerant of PAP therapy. Although some degree of sleep-disordered breathing may persist after tracheostomy, the improvement in the AHI leads to the resolution of hypercapnia in most patients with OHS.[67] Therefore, patient reassessment after tracheostomy for residual hypercapnia is necessary because a subgroup may require nocturnal mechanical ventilation.[40]

Nocturnal oxygen therapy is necessary in approximately a third of patients with OHS, despite resolution of hypopneas and apneas with PAP therapy.[50,51,54,60,68] Patients requiring nighttime or daytime oxygen therapy should be reassessed a few months after PAP therapy is instituted, if they are adherent, because a significant proportion of patients have significant improvement in their gas exchange, obviating the need for supplemental oxygen therapy.[51] Supplemental oxygen without PAP therapy is inadequate and does not improve hypoventilation.

Weight Reduction

The weight loss experienced after bariatric surgery can lead to a significant reduction in the AHI and to significant improvement in respiratory system mechanics. These factors can lead to long-term improvements in arterial blood gases in patients with OHS. In a small series of 12 patients 5 years after bariatric surgery, Pao_2 increased from 54 to 68 mm Hg, $Paco_2$ decreased from 53 to 47 mm Hg, and the improvements in gas exchange were accompanied by significant improvements in measures of respiratory system mechanics.[69] It should be noted that patients undergoing bariatric surgery may experience weight gain in the years after surgery, however, and should still be monitored.[70] Every attempt should be made to treat OHS effectively before surgical intervention to decrease perioperative morbidity and mortality. Moreover, the use of PAP therapy in the immediate postoperative period can avoid respiratory failure without increasing the risk for intestinal leakage (see the article on obesity and bariatric surgery by DeMaria in this issue for more information on this treatment option).[71]

Pharmacotherapy

A variety of respiratory stimulants have been used in an attempt to increase respiratory drive.

Medroxyprogesterone

This agent acts as a respiratory stimulant at the hypothalamus through an estrogen-dependent progesterone receptor.[72] Overall, the studies examining medroxyprogesterone for the treatment of OHS have had mixed results. One study enrolled 10 male outpatients with OHS and administered 60 mg of sublingual medroxyprogesterone in 3 divided doses for 1 month. At baseline, all were able to correct their hypoxemia and hypercapnia with 1 to 2 minutes of voluntary hyperventilation. Medroxyprogesterone corrected daytime hypoxemia and hypercapnia and increased hypoxic respiratory drive but did not have a significant effect on hypercapnic respiratory drive.[73] Withdrawal of the agent for 1 month was followed by a return to baseline hypoxemia and hypercapnia. In another study, 8 patients admitted to the hospital were treated with intramuscular progesterone after initial therapy, which consisted of a combination of weight loss, digoxin, diuretics, intermittent PAP, or tracheostomy.[74] Their mean baseline $Paco_2$ on admission was 61.9 mm Hg, which improved to 51.0 mm Hg after medical therapy. Medroxyprogesterone therapy for a minimum of 18 days led to further improvement in $Paco_2$ to 37.9 mm Hg. Likewise, there was an improvement in Pao_2 from 54.4 mm Hg at baseline to 64.2 mm Hg after medical therapy and to 78.3 mm Hg after medroxyprogesterone therapy. In contrast, another study of 3 patients who did not respond to tracheostomy demonstrated no change in $Paco_2$, hypercapnic ventilatory response, or minute ventilation after sublingual medroxyprogesterone.[40] Progesterone therapy may have unfavorable side effects, such as impotence[73] or venous thromboembolism.[75,76]

Acetazolamide

This carbonic anhydrase inhibitor induces a metabolic acidosis; this, in turn, increases minute ventilation by 15%,[77] which could theoretically be beneficial in OHS. It also reduces the AHI in patients with moderate to severe OSA.[78,79] The only published report showed a return to eucapnia in the only patient treated with acetazolamide after tracheostomy failed to do so.[40]

Overall, pharmacotherapy for the treatment of OHS has been poorly studied and should not replace PAP therapy. Its use as adjunct therapy for OHS that is refractory to PAP therapy requires further investigation.

SUMMARY

OHS is present in 10% to 20% of patients with OSA. Despite the significant morbidity and mortality associated with this syndrome, it is often unrecognized and treatment is frequently delayed. Clinicians must maintain a high index of suspicion because early recognition and treatment may reduce the high burden of morbidity and mortality associated with this syndrome.[11,28] The most effective treatment remains PAP therapy. Therefore, early clinical follow-up with objective measurement of adherence to PAP therapy is essential. Further research is needed to answer many questions that remain, such as the following:

- Why do only some severely obese patients (with or without OSA) develop OHS?
- What is the impact of correction of daytime hypercapnia on daytime hypersomnolence and neurocognitive functioning?
- What is the true effect of untreated OHS on mortality?
- Is the morbidity associated with OHS, such as cor pulmonale, fully reversible with effective treatment?
- What is the best treatment for those who fail to respond to PAP therapy?

REFERENCES

1. Lugaresi E, Coccagna G, Tassinari CA, et al. Particularités cliniques et polygraphiques du syndrome d'impatience des membres inférieurs. Rev Neurol 1965;115:545 [in French].
2. Gastaut H, Tassinari CA, Duron B. Polygraphic study of the episodic diurnal and nocturnal (hypnic and

respiratory) manifestations of the Pickwick syndrome. Brain Res 1966;1(2):167–86.

3. Lavie P. Who was the first to use the term Pickwickian in connection with sleepy patients? History of sleep apnoea syndrome. Sleep Med Rev 2008;12(1):5–17.

4. Auchincloss JH Jr, Cook E, Renzetti AD. Clinical and physiological aspects of a case of obesity, polycythemia and alveolar hypoventilation. J Clin Invest 1955;34:1537–45.

5. Burwell CS, Robin ED, Whaley RD, et al. Extreme obesity associated with alveolar hypoventilation: a Pickwickian syndrome. Am J Med 1956;21:811–8.

6. Dickens C. The posthumous papers of the Pickwick Club. New York: The Macmillan Company; 1904.

7. Tauman R, Gozal D. Obesity and obstructive sleep apnea in children. Paediatr Respir Rev 2006;7(4): 247–59.

8. Mokhlesi B, Kryger MH, Grunstein RR. Assessment and management of patients with obesity hypoventilation syndrome. Proc Am Thorac Soc 2008;5(2): 218–25.

9. Verin E, Tardif C, Pasquis P. Prevalence of daytime hypercapnia or hypoxia in patients with OSAS and normal lung function. Respir Med 2001;95(8):693–6.

10. Laaban JP, Chailleux E. Daytime hypercapnia in adult patients with obstructive sleep apnea syndrome in France, before initiating nocturnal nasal continuous positive airway pressure therapy. Chest 2005;127(3):710–5.

11. Kessler R, Chaouat A, Schinkewitch P, et al. The obesity-hypoventilation syndrome revisited: a prospective study of 34 consecutive cases. Chest 2001;120(2):369–76.

12. Resta O, Foschino Barbaro MP, Bonfitto P, et al. Hypercapnia in obstructive sleep apnoea syndrome. Neth J Med 2000;56(6):215–22.

13. Golpe R, Jimenez A, Carpizo R. Diurnal hypercapnia in patients with obstructive sleep apnea syndrome. Chest 2002;122(3):1100–1 [author reply: 1101].

14. Akashiba T, Akahoshi T, Kawahara S, et al. Clinical characteristics of obesity-hypoventilation syndrome in Japan: a multi-center study. Intern Med 2006; 45(20):1121–5.

15. Akashiba T, Kawahara S, Kosaka N, et al. Determinants of chronic hypercapnia in Japanese men with obstructive sleep apnea syndrome. Chest 2002;121(2):415–21.

16. Leech JA, Onal E, Baer P, et al. Determinants of hypercapnia in occlusive sleep apnea syndrome. Chest 1987;92(5):807–13.

17. Mokhlesi B, Tulaimat A, Faibussowitsch I, et al. Obesity hypoventilation syndrome: prevalence and predictors in patients with obstructive sleep apnea. Sleep Breath 2007;11(2):117–24.

18. Kawata N, Tatsumi K, Terada J, et al. Daytime hypercapnia in obstructive sleep apnea syndrome. Chest 2007;132(6):1832–8.

19. Sturm R. Increases in morbid obesity in the USA: 2000–2005. Public Health 2007;121(7):492–6.

20. Lee W, Nagubadi S, Kryger MH, et al. Epidemiology of obstructive sleep apnea: a population-based perspective. Exp Rev Resp Med 2008; 2(3):349–64.

21. Available at: www.census.gov. Accessed January 24, 2009.

22. Laaban JP, Orvoen-Frija E, Cassuto D, et al. Mechanisms of diurnal hypercapnia in sleep apnea syndromes associated with morbid obesity. Presse Med 1996;25(1):12–6.

23. Flegal KM, Graubard BI, Williamson DF, et al. Excess deaths associated with underweight, overweight, and obesity. JAMA 2005;293(15):1861–7.

24. Young T, Finn L, Peppard PE, et al. Sleep disordered breathing and mortality: eighteen-year follow-up of the Wisconsin sleep cohort. Sleep 2008;31(8): 1071–8.

25. Hida W. Quality of life in obesity hypoventilation syndrome. Sleep Breath 2003;7(1):1–2.

26. Budweiser S, Hitzl AP, Jorres RA, et al. Health-related quality of life and long-term prognosis in chronic hypercapnic respiratory failure: a prospective survival analysis. Respir Res 2007;8:92–101.

27. Berg G, Delaive K, Manfreda J, et al. The use of health-care resources in obesity-hypoventilation syndrome. Chest 2001;120(2):377–83.

28. Nowbar S, Burkart KM, Gonzales R, et al. Obesity-associated hypoventilation in hospitalized patients: prevalence, effects, and outcome. Am J Med 2004;116(1):1–7.

29. Budweiser S, Riedl SG, Jorres RA, et al. Mortality and prognostic factors in patients with obesity-hypoventilation syndrome undergoing noninvasive ventilation. J Intern Med 2007;261(4):375–83.

30. Campos-Rodriguez F, Pena-Grinan N, Reyes-Nunez N, et al. Mortality in obstructive sleep apnea-hypopnea patients treated with positive airway pressure. Chest 2005;128(2):624–33.

31. Lin CC, Wu KM, Chou CS, et al. Oral airway resistance during wakefulness in eucapnic and hypercapnic sleep apnea syndrome. Respir Physiol Neurobiol 2004;139(2):215–24.

32. Kawano K, Usui N, Kanazawa H, et al. Changes in nasal and oral respiratory resistance before and after uvulopalatopharyngoplasty. Acta Otolaryngol Suppl 1996;523:236–8.

33. Sampson MG, Grassino K. Neuromechanical properties in obese patients during carbon dioxide rebreathing. Am J Med 1983;75(1):81–90.

34. Cattapan SE, Laghi F, Tobin MJ. Can diaphragmatic contractility be assessed by airway twitch pressure in mechanically ventilated patients? Thorax 2003; 58(1):58–62.

35. Laffey J, Kavanagh B. Permissive hypercapnia. In: Tobin MJ, editor. Principles and practice of

mechanical ventilation. New York: McGraw Hill; 2006. p. 373–92.

36. Sharp JT, Henry JP, Sweany SK, et al. The total work of breathing in normal and obese men. J Clin Invest 1964;43:728–39.

37. Han F, Chen E, Wei H, et al. Treatment effects on carbon dioxide retention in patients with obstructive sleep apnea-hypopnea syndrome. Chest 2001; 119(6):1814–9.

38. Berthon-Jones M, Sullivan CE. Time course of change in ventilatory response to CO_2 with long-term CPAP therapy for obstructive sleep apnea. Am Rev Respir Dis 1987;135(1):144–7.

39. Lin CC. Effect of nasal CPAP on ventilatory drive in normocapnic and hypercapnic patients with obstructive sleep apnoea syndrome. Eur Respir J 1994; 7(11):2005–10.

40. Rapoport DM, Garay SM, Epstein H, et al. Hypercapnia in the obstructive sleep apnea syndrome. A reevaluation of the "Pickwickian syndrome." Chest 1986;89(5):627–35.

41. Zwillich CW, Sutton FD, Pierson DJ, et al. Decreased hypoxic ventilatory drive in the obesity-hypoventilation syndrome. Am J Med 1975;59(3):343–8.

42. Kalra SP. Central leptin insufficiency syndrome: an interactive etiology for obesity, metabolic and neural diseases and for designing new therapeutic interventions. Peptides 2008;29(1):127–38.

43. Tankersley C, Kleeberger S, Russ B, et al. Modified control of breathing in genetically obese (ob/ob) mice. J Appl Physiol 1996;81(2):716–23.

44. Tankersley CG, O'Donnell C, Daood MJ, et al. Leptin attenuates respiratory complications associated with the obese phenotype. J Appl Physiol 1998; 85(6):2261–9.

45. Considine RV, Sinha MK, Heiman ML, et al. Serum immunoreactive-leptin concentrations in normal-weight and obese humans. N Engl J Med 1996; 334(5):292–5.

46. Ip MS, Lam KS, Ho C, et al. Serum leptin and vascular risk factors in obstructive sleep apnea. Chest 2000;118(3):580–6.

47. Barcelo A, Barbe F, Llompart E, et al. Neuropeptide Y and leptin in patients with obstructive sleep apnea syndrome: role of obesity. Am J Respir Crit Care Med 2005;171(2):183–7.

48. Shimura R, Tatsumi K, Nakamura A, et al. Fat accumulation, leptin, and hypercapnia in obstructive sleep apnea-hypopnea syndrome. Chest 2005; 127(2):543–9.

49. Makinodan K, Yoshikawa M, Fukuoka A, et al. Effect of serum leptin levels on hypercapnic ventilatory response in obstructive sleep apnea. Respiration 2008;75(3):257–64.

50. Perez de Llano LA, Golpe R, Ortiz Piquer M, et al. Short-term and long-term effects of nasal intermittent positive pressure ventilation in patients with obesity-hypoventilation syndrome. Chest 2005; 128(2):587–94.

51. Mokhlesi B, Tulaimat A, Evans AT, et al. Impact of adherence with positive airway pressure therapy on hypercapnia in obstructive sleep apnea. J Clin Sleep Med 2006;2(1):57–62.

52. Berger KI, Ayappa I, Chatr-Amontri B, et al. Obesity hypoventilation syndrome as a spectrum of respiratory disturbances during sleep. Chest 2001;120(4): 1231–8.

53. Rapoport DM, Sorkin B, Garay SM, et al. Reversal of the "Pickwickian syndrome" by long-term use of nocturnal nasal-airway pressure. N Engl J Med 1982;307(15):931–3.

54. Masa JF, Celli BR, Riesco JA, et al. The obesity hypoventilation syndrome can be treated with noninvasive mechanical ventilation. Chest 2001; 119(4):1102–7.

55. Leech JA, Onal E, Lopata M. Nasal CPAP continues to improve sleep-disordered breathing and daytime oxygenation over long-term follow-up of occlusive sleep apnea syndrome. Chest 1992;102(6):1651–5.

56. Norman RG, Goldring RM, Clain JM, et al. Transition from acute to chronic hypercapnia in patients with periodic breathing: predictions from a computer model. J Appl Physiol 2006;100(5):1733–41.

57. Ayappa I, Berger KI, Norman RG, et al. Hypercapnia and ventilatory periodicity in obstructive sleep apnea syndrome. Am J Respir Crit Care Med 2002;166(8):1112–5.

58. Schafer H, Ewig S, Hasper E, et al. Failure of CPAP therapy in obstructive sleep apnoea syndrome: predictive factors and treatment with bilevel-positive airway pressure. Respir Med 1998;92(2):208–15.

59. Banerjee D, Yee BJ, Piper AJ, et al. Obesity hypoventilation syndrome: hypoxemia during continuous positive airway pressure. Chest 2007;131(6): 1678–84.

60. Piper AJ, Wang D, Yee BJ, et al. Randomised trial of CPAP vs bilevel support in the treatment of obesity hypoventilation syndrome without severe nocturnal desaturation. Thorax 2008;63(5):395–401.

61. Kushida CA, Chediak A, Berry RB, et al. Clinical guidelines for the manual titration of positive airway pressure in patients with obstructive sleep apnea. J Clin Sleep Med 2008;4(2):157–71.

62. Redolfi S, Corda L, La Piana G, et al. Long-term noninvasive ventilation increases chemosensitivity and leptin in obesity-hypoventilation syndrome. Respir Med 2007;101(6):1191–5.

63. de Lucas-Ramos P, de Miguel-Diez J, Santacruz-Siminiani A, et al. Benefits at 1 year of nocturnal intermittent positive pressure ventilation in patients with obesity-hypoventilation syndrome. Respir Med 2004;98(10):961–7.

64. Storre JH, Seuthe B, Fiechter R, et al. Average volume-assured pressure support in obesity

hypoventilation: a randomized crossover trial. Chest 2006;130(3):815–21.

65. Piper AJ, Sullivan CE. Effects of short-term NIPPV in the treatment of patients with severe obstructive sleep apnea and hypercapnia. Chest 1994;105(2):434–40.

66. Hensley MJ, Read DJ. Intermittent obstruction of the upper airway during sleep causing profound hypoxaemia. A neglected mechanism exacerbating chronic respiratory failure. Aust N Z J Med 1976; 6(5):481–6.

67. Kim SH, Eisele DW, Smith PL, et al. Evaluation of patients with sleep apnea after tracheotomy. Arch Otolaryngol Head Neck Surg 1998;124(9):996–1000.

68. Heinemann F, Budweiser S, Dobroschke J, et al. Non-invasive positive pressure ventilation improves lung volumes in the obesity hypoventilation syndrome. Respir Med 2007;101(6):1229–35.

69. Sugerman HJ, Fairman RP, Sood RK, et al. Long-term effects of gastric surgery for treating respiratory insufficiency of obesity. Am J Clin Nutr 1992; 55(2 Suppl):597S–601S.

70. Pillar G, Peled R, Lavie P. Recurrence of sleep apnea without concomitant weight increase 7.5 years after weight reduction surgery. Chest 1994; 106(6):1702–4.

71. Mokhlesi B, Tulaimat A. Recent advances in obesity hypoventilation syndrome. Chest 2007;132(4):1322–36.

72. Bayliss DA, Millhorn DE. Central neural mechanisms of progesterone action: application to the respiratory system. J Appl Physiol 1992;73(2):393–404.

73. Sutton FD Jr, Zwillich CW, Creagh CE, et al. Progesterone for outpatient treatment of Pickwickian syndrome. Ann Intern Med 1975;83(4):476–9.

74. Lyons HA, Huang CT. Therapeutic use of progesterone in alveolar hypoventilation associated with obesity. Am J Med 1968;44(6):881–8.

75. Poulter NR, Chang CL, Farley TM, et al. Risk of cardiovascular diseases associated with oral progestagen preparations with therapeutic indications [letter]. Lancet 1999;354(9190):1610.

76. Douketis JD, Julian JA, Kearon C, et al. Does the type of hormone replacement therapy influence the risk of deep vein thrombosis? A prospective case-control study. J Thromb Haemost 2005;3(5): 943–8.

77. Swenson ER. Carbonic anhydrase inhibitors and ventilation: a complex interplay of stimulation and suppression. Eur Respir J 1998;12(6):1242–7.

78. Tojima H, Kunitomo F, Kimura H, et al. Effects of acetazolamide in patients with the sleep apnoea syndrome. Thorax 1988;43(2):113–9.

79. Whyte KF, Gould GA, Airlie MA, et al. Role of protriptyline and acetazolamide in the sleep apnea/hypopnea syndrome. Sleep 1988;11(5):463–72.

Obesity and Asthma

David A. Beuther, MD

KEYWORDS
- Asthma • Obesity • Overweight
- Pulmonary function testing • Adipokines • Inflammation

EPIDEMIOLOGIC OBSERVATIONS

Cross-sectional and case-controlled epidemiologic studies have shown a modest correlation between obesity and adult asthma prevalence, with relative risk or odds ratios ranging from 1.0 to 3.0.[1–3] These studies typically controlled for commonly known confounding variables, such as socioeconomic status, activity level, diet, and age. While this effect has been seen in children and adults and in both men and women, some investigators have reported a stronger effect in women.[4] The typical measure of obesity in these studies is body mass index (BMI), calculated as weight in kilograms divided by the square of height in meters (kg/m^2). Increasing BMI is associated with increasing prevalence of asthma, with one important exception. Because asthma risk is increased in underweight populations, the relationship between BMI and asthma is frequently J-shaped,[5,6] with increased risk seen in low BMI (<18.5 kg/m^2) in addition to overweight (25 kg/m^2–29.9 kg/m^2) and obese (≥ 30 kg/m^2). This can result in an overestimation of asthma risk in "normal weight" populations when "normal" BMI is defined as less than 25 kg/m^2, instead of a more precise definition of normal, such as 18.5 kg/m^2 to 25 kg/m^2. The lumping together of low and normal BMI can lead to an underestimation of relative asthma risk in overweight and obese BMI populations.

While these studies have been convincing in that they repeatedly demonstrate this relationship in different populations and show a dose-response effect, they have a limited ability to prove causation or enlighten us as to the direction of the relationship if it is causal. Both obesity and asthma prevalence have been increasing in the United States,[7,8] raising concern that this could be merely an epiphenomenon. Asthma can cause obesity through adverse effects of medications, social stigma, and decreased exercise tolerance,[9] and both asthma and obesity share common environmental risk factors, such as low socioeconomic status, poor diet, and the built environment.

The question that is not answered by prevalence studies is this: does excess weight increase the risk of developing asthma? Prospective epidemiologic studies have clearly shown that while the relationship is modest, the answer is yes—obesity is a risk factor for incident asthma. One of the largest prospective studies of obesity and incident asthma looked at nearly 86,000 women participating in the Nurses' Health Study, and found that over a 4-year follow-up, the odds of developing asthma were 2.7 times higher in obese (BMI ≥ 30 kg/m^2) compared with normal-weight women.[10] These investigators also reported a dose-response effect of increased odds of asthma with increasing BMI ($P<.0001$), and among those with a greater than 25-kg weight gain, the odds of asthma were 4.7 (95% confidence interval or CI 3.1–7.0).

There are several other prospective studies consistently reporting risk ratios for asthma in the range of 1.0 to 3.5, but among these studies there is heterogeneity in effect size and in the influence of sex status. Many have shown that a similar positive BMI incident-asthma relationship exists in both men and women,[11,12] but some have suggested this relationship is stronger in women,[4,13,14] while a minority of studies have shown a stronger relationship in men.[6] A recent meta-analysis of seven prospective epidemiologic studies attempted to clarify the magnitude and nature of this relationship, reporting that the pooled odds of developing asthma at 1 year for overweight and obese (BMI ≥ 25 kg/m^2) versus normal-weight individuals were 1.51 (95% CI

National Jewish Health and Department of Pulmonary and Critical Care Medicine, University of Colorado at Denver Health Sciences Programs, 1400 Jackson Street, J220, Denver, CO 80206, USA
E-mail address: beutherd@njhealth.org

Clin Chest Med 30 (2009) 479–488
doi:10.1016/j.ccm.2009.05.002
0272-5231/09/$ – see front matter © 2009 Elsevier Inc. All rights reserved.

1.27–1.80), that there was a dose-response effect of increasing asthma incidence with increasing BMI ($P<.0001$), and that while absolute odds of asthma were slightly higher in women than men, there was no significant effect of sex on this relationship ($P = .232$) (**Table 1**).[15] In addition to reporting a nearly doubling of the odds of developing asthma in obese (BMI ≥ 30 kg/m^2) compared with normal-weight individuals, they estimated that based upon the prevalence of overweight and obesity, approximately 250,000 new cases of asthma each year might be attributable to excess weight in the United States.

In both prevalence and incidence studies, the large number of study subjects frequently necessitates using self-reported and not measured weight and height. This raises concern for possible misclassification bias. To address this, some investigators have been able to incorporate measured weight and height, and in doing so found a reassuringly similar obesity-asthma relationship.[11,14] In addition, Hu and colleagues[16] performed a validation study using the Nurses' Health Study cohort, showing a strong correlation between measured and reported height and weight. This suggests that misclassification because of self-reported weight and height has not been a significant problem in these studies.

The diagnosis of asthma may be more complicated in the obese. One important limitation of a large epidemiologic study is its inability to rigorously characterize asthma using physiologic criteria. Frequently, asthma is defined as self-reported symptoms or medication use, or a self-reported physician's diagnosis of asthma. Obesity is associated with pulmonary restriction[17,18] and an increased oxygen cost of breathing,[19] raising concern as to whether some of these subjects have dyspnea because of obesity in the absence of airflow obstruction or airway hyper-responsiveness (AHR),[20] and that misdiagnosis of asthma might bias the results of epidemiologic investigations.

Reassuringly, several investigators have included rigorous physiologic criteria in their definition of asthma, and have reported similar results. For example, in a well-designed Swedish case-controlled study, where asthma was confirmed by spirometry and bronchial provocation, the odds of asthma were 2.7 times higher in obese (BMI ≥ 30 kg/m^2) versus normal-weight (BMI 20 kg/m^2–24.9 kg/m^2) individuals.[21] In addition, Aaron and colleagues[22] were able to show that overdiagnosis of asthma is similar in obese and nonobese adults. This Canadian study recruited a random telephone sample of individuals with a reported physician's diagnosis of asthma, and systematically performed spirometry and bronchial provocation. In those where an asthma diagnosis was not confirmed, asthma medications were weaned off and subjects were followed for 6 months. Asthma was ultimately excluded in 31.8% of obese and 28.7% of nonobese individuals initially given a diagnosis of asthma, a difference that was not significant ($P = .46$). Thus, asthma is over-diagnosed in developed countries, but not differentially between obese and normal-weight populations, validating the findings of epidemiologic studies that relied on self-reported physician's diagnosis of asthma.

Asthma and obesity are both chronic diseases likely contributed to by complex interactions

Table 1
Odds ratios and 95% CIs of 1-year incident asthma by BMI and sex

Comparison	Total		Men		Women	
	OR (95% CI)	P-value	OR (95% CI)	P-value	OR (95% CI)	P-value
Overweight versus normal BMI	1.38 (1.17–1.62)	<0.001	1.44 (1.01–2.04)	0.042	1.42 (1.18–1.72)	<0.001
Obese versus normal BMI	1.92 (1.43–2.59)	<0.001	1.63 (0.92–2.89)	0.094	2.30 (1.88–2.82)	<0.001
Overweight and obese versus normal BMI	1.51 (1.27–1.80)	<0.001	1.46 (1.05–2.02)	0.025	1.68 (1.45–1.94)	<0.001
Obese versus overweight	1.49 (1.20–1.85)	<0.001	1.17 (0.66–2.07)	0.590	1.58 (1.25–1.99)	<0.001

Abbreviation: OR, odds ratio.

Data from Beuther DA, Sutherland ER. Overweight, obesity and incident asthma: a meta-analysis of prospective epidemiologic studies. Am J Respir Crit Care Med 2007;175(7):663.

among multiple genetic and environmental factors. Common environmental factors, such as low socioeconomic status, smoking, age, diet, and the physical environment may predispose individuals to both asthma and obesity. There are also common genetic mechanisms that could underlie an association between the two conditions. Hallstrand and colleagues[23] reported that in same-sex monozygotic and dizygotic twins, obesity was associated with asthma, and that 8% of the genetic component of obesity was shared with asthma. One example is the β_2-receptor. The Gln$\rightarrow$Glu 27 polymorphism of the β_2-receptor has been associated with asthma[24] as well as obesity.[25] Tumor necrosis factor alpha (TNF-α) gene haplotypes have also been associated with both asthma[26] and obesity.[27] A sophisticated understanding of gene-by-environment interactions and their role in this relationship is still not well established. A more thorough understanding of these possible common determinants of disease will help to better understand the nature of the relationship between obesity and asthma.

Clinically, obesity may indirectly worsen asthma through common comorbid conditions, such as esophageal reflux and obstructive sleep apnea. While some may argue these conditions are not confounders but collinear mechanisms along the pathway through which obesity causes asthma, they are difficult to assess quantitatively and control for in large studies. Obstructive sleep apnea is to a great degree determined by obesity,[28] but it also worsens nocturnal asthma, an effect which is reversed through treatment with continuous positive airway pressure.[29] Interestingly, continuous positive airway pressure is not beneficial in nonapneic nocturnal asthma, where it may actually worsen asthma.[30] Similarly, esophageal reflux worsens with obesity and is associated with asthma, but while many investigators feel that reflux worsens asthma, the direction of this association is still of some debate.[31] Thus, whether these shared disease states are confounders or part of the mechanistic pathway, they are important considerations in both epidemiologic and pathophysiologic investigations into the obesity-asthma relationship, and most clinical studies do not adequately address them.

Finally, the demonstration of a consistent, temporally relevant, dose-response relationship between obesity and asthma would be made more compelling if it were reversible. In other words, does the excess asthma associated with obesity improve with weight loss? Both medical and surgical weight-loss studies suggest that it might, but these studies are frequently small and underpowered, and are frequently not designed with a primary outcome or rigorous characterization of asthma.

Eneli and colleagues[32] recently attempted a systematic review of this literature and found only 15 relevant studies. While the study quality and heterogeneity prevented a systematic review, they noted that there was improvement in at least one asthma outcome in every study, and there were frequent reports of dramatic improvements in asthma with weight loss. Dixon and colleagues[33] assessed asthma before and at least 1 year after laparoscopic adjustable gastric band surgery, and found that of the 10 severe asthmatics, none had severe asthma at 1 year, and there was a 57% decline in the number of patients needing daily medications for asthma. In another surgical study with 24 asthmatics, asthma medication use declined in 10 patients and was completely discontinued in 4 patients.[34] Esophageal reflux also improves dramatically following weight-loss surgery, which might explain some of the apparent dramatic improvement in asthma. In one study, there was a complete remission of asthma in 48% of patients following surgery, but about half of the asthmatics who reported reflux preoperatively had complete resolution of their reflux symptoms following surgery.[35]

Medical weight-loss results in a smaller degree of weight loss and a more modest improvement in asthma outcomes. In one of the few randomized controlled trials in asthmatics, Stenius-Aarniala and colleagues[36] reported that a dietary weight-loss intervention improved symptoms of dyspnea and health status, but there was only a small, clinically insignificant reduction in rescue medication use. Even though the frequent lack of rigorous characterization of asthma in these studies suggests it may have been over-diagnosed, the consistent improvement in asthma outcomes following surgery shows reversibility of effect, further supporting the hypothesis that obesity causes asthma.

PHYSIOLOGIC CONSEQUENCES OF OBESITY RELEVANT TO ASTHMA

The most consistently demonstrated effect of obesity on the lung is a restrictive process. Typically, obesity causes a modest reduction in total lung capacity, and a larger reduction in functional residual capacity.[17,37,38] Lung volumes are inversely proportional to the degree of adiposity, usually measured as BMI. Furthermore, weight loss is associated with significant increases total lung capacity, functional residual capacity, and expiratory reserve volume.[39]

While the BMI measure is simple and inexpensive to obtain and generally accepted in the literature, it is probably not the ideal measure of obesity for studying its effect on pulmonary disease. Body fat distribution is perhaps more relevant, not only to the metabolic effects of obesity, but also to the mechanical effects. For example, in an analysis of over 2,000 adults undergoing lung-function testing, markers of abdominal adiposity, including abdominal height, waist circumference, and waist-hip ratio, were more predictive of alterations in lung function than absolute weight or BMI.[40] Others have shown that upper or central adiposity as measured by waist-hip ratio is a better measure of obesity's effect on lung function.[41]

Obesity does not cause airflow obstruction. Being a restrictive process, the ratio of 1-second forced expiratory volume (FEV_1) to forced vital capacity (FVC) is normal to increased, rather than decreased.[20,42] Restriction leads to a reduction in airway diameter,[43] which leads to tidal breathing at or near closing volume,[44] and results in alterations in smooth muscle function, as rapidly cycling actin-myosin cross-bridges transform into slow cycling latch bridges (**Fig. 1**).[45] Thus, obesity does not cause airflow obstruction, but through its restrictive effect on the lung may lead to airway hyper-responsiveness.

The effect of obesity on AHR has been inconsistently demonstrated in clinical studies. Wang and colleagues[46] took normal (nonasthmatic) subjects and applied an external mass load to the chest to simulate obesity-associated restriction. This resulted in a reduction in lung volume and a significant increase in the maximal response to methacholine compared with the unloaded state. In the European Community Respiratory Health Survey, BMI was positively associated with increasing AHR (P = .002),[47] and in a small case-controlled study in men, the odds of having a BMI over 30 given new-onset AHR was 10 (95% CI 2.6–38).[5] However, other studies have demonstrated that while BMI is associated with asthma symptoms, it is not associated with AHR in adults[48] or children.[49] A medical weight-loss study in 58 obese women, 24 of whom had asthma, demonstrated increases in FEV_1 and FVC but not improvements in AHR.[50] Therefore, there is a plausible mechanism to explain how obesity could lead to restriction and AHR, but it is not consistently seen in clinical studies.

The three hallmark clinical findings in asthma are bronchodilator responsive airflow obstruction, airway hyper-responsiveness, and airway inflammation. Obesity does not directly cause airflow obstruction, but its ability to cause or worsen AHR is at least plausible and has been reported in some human studies. Because it is questionable whether restriction and AHR alone are adequate to constitute a diagnosis of asthma, or even a unique phenotype of asthma, it would be reassuring to also see an effect of obesity on the third major feature of asthma, airway inflammation.

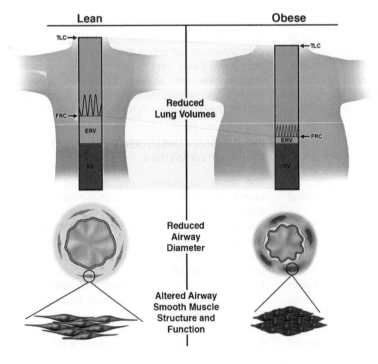

Fig. 1. Obesity leads to alterations of lung volumes (*top*), particularly expiratory reserve volume (ERV) and functional residual capacity (FRC), leading to a rapid, shallow breathing pattern that occurs close to closing volume. Obesity also causes reduced peripheral airway diameter (*middle*), which can lead to increased airway hyper-responsiveness because of alterations of smooth muscle structure and function (*bottom*). RV, residual volume; TLC, total lung capacity. (*From* Beuther DA, Weiss ST, Sutherland ER. Obesity and asthma. Am J Respir Crit Care Med. 2006;174(2):113; with permission.)

INFLAMMATORY AND IMMUNOLOGIC CONSEQUENCES OF OBESITY RELEVANT TO ASTHMA

Obesity as a disease is no longer thought of as a simple imbalance of energy intake and expenditure. In addition to its energy storage function, adipose tissue behaves like an active endocrine organ, with enhanced inflammatory activity in obesity.[51] Furthermore, adipocytes have the ability to recruit circulating monocytes, and adipose tissue macrophages interact with adipocytes to augment this inflammatory signal.[52,53] Body fat distribution is important, as the phenotype of central or visceral adiposity is associated most strongly with local and systemic inflammation, and it is the inflammation generated by the adipocytes and macrophages in adipose tissue that is thought to play a central role in insulin resistance and the metabolic syndrome.[54]

Obese individuals with this phenotype typically demonstrate elevated circulating systemic inflammatory mediators, including the adipokines (proteins produced by the adipocyte) leptin and ghrelin, TNF-α, interleukin-6 (IL-6), interleukin-18 (IL-18), transforming growth factor-β1, and C-reactive protein. With weight loss, these systemic inflammatory markers decrease. For example, Esposito and colleagues[55] reported that medical weight loss in obese women resulted in significant decreases in previously elevated IL-6, IL-18, C-reactive protein, and insulin resistance, and a significant increase in the anti-inflammatory adipokine, adiponectin. While these markers are linearly related to BMI, with increasing inflammation associated with increasing BMI, they are more closely correlated to fat distribution, particularly central or visceral adiposity.[56] While central adiposity does have a greater mechanical effect on the lung, it may be the metabolic consequences of central fat distribution that are more relevant to the pathophysiology of asthma. A recent, prospective, population-based study demonstrated that insulin resistance was a stronger predictor of developing incident wheezing (OR 1.87; 95% CI 1.38–2.54) or asthma-like symptoms (OR 1.61; CI 1.23–2.10) than was obesity or BMI.[57] Thus, body fat distribution is an important determinant of the metabolic and inflammatory effects of obesity as they pertain to asthma, and BMI may be a less meaningful measure of adiposity in this context.

In coronary artery disease, local inflammation in the atherosclerotic plaque may be central to the pathogenesis and progression of the disease,[58] and systemic inflammation is thought to contribute significantly to this process.[59] A similar hypothesis might be relevant in obese asthma, with systemic inflammation causing or enhancing airway inflammation. Leptin, a proinflammatory satiety factor produced mainly by the adipocyte, is elevated in obesity, and has been proposed to be capable of causing airway inflammation. Leptin and leptin receptor have been found in the bronchial mucosa in patients with asthma and chronic-obstructive pulmonary disease.[60] Mouse models of obesity and asthma have illuminated the possible role of leptin and other inflammatory mediators in the association between obesity and asthma.

In a murine allergic sensitization model, Shore and colleagues[61] infused ovalbumin sensitized BALB/cJ mice with either saline or leptin before ovalbumin challenge. Ovalbumin exposure increased serum leptin, even in the saline-infused mice, but the leptin-infused mice exhibited significantly increased airway reactivity and serum total immunoglobulin E level. Similarly, in a nonallergic ozone-challenge model of asthma, exogenous leptin administered to leptin-deficient mice before ozone exposure resulted in enhanced airway reactivity and inflammation.[62] Hyperleptinemia is associated with obesity in both an overfeeding mouse model[63] and in Cpe^{fat} mice,[64] and in both models ozone exposure results in increased serum leptin levels. But it is not only leptin that is responsible for obese asthma in mice. Both leptin-deficient (ob/ob) and leptin receptor-deficient (db/db) mice, given free access to food, become morbidly obese, and when exposed to ozone, show similar responses.[62,65] Adiponectin is an anti-inflammatory, insulin-sensitizing hormone that in many ways acts contrary to leptin, decreasing with increasing obesity. In a mouse model of asthma, adiponectin can suppress allergen-induced airway inflammation and reactivity,[66] suggesting that low levels of adiponectin in obesity may be permissive to the proinflammatory effects of leptin and other adipokines.

However, human studies have not consistently supported an inflammatory hypothesis to the obesity-asthma relationship. In a pediatric study involving asthmatic and nonasthmatic children, those with asthma had significantly higher serum leptin levels, and when the asthmatic children were treated with 4 weeks of inhaled corticosteroids, their serum leptin level decreased to that of the nonasthmatic controls.[67] Leptin has been associated with asthma in more than one pediatric study,[68] but none of these studies establishes that leptin causes asthma; leptin may simply be a marker for airway inflammation in poorly controlled asthma.

Recent adult studies have failed to find a consistent relationship between obesity-associated inflammation and airway inflammation or asthma. In a cross-sectional analysis of 2890 adults participating in the Coronary Artery Risk Development in Young Adults study, women with current asthma were more likely to be obese and have a lower serum adiponectin concentration compared with those women without asthma, but the obesity-asthma relationship was not affected by adjusting for serum adiponectin level.[69] Sood and colleagues[70] measured serum adiponectin in eight sensitized allergic asthmatics and six nonasthmatic controls undergoing inhalational allergen challenge, and found that while adiponectin concentrations were lower in asthmatic versus control subjects, inhalational allergen challenge did not affect adiponectin concentrations, suggesting that low adiponectin is not the result of acute asthma. Whether low adiponectin might be a result of chronic asthma or adiponectin might have a protective role in asthma is unknown. In a population-based cohort of 1000 adults, there was a significant association between obesity and asthma, but no association between obesity and airway inflammation, as measured by exhaled nitric oxide (eNO).[71] The investigators concluded that the relationship between obesity and asthma could not be mediated by airway inflammation. In a population of 136 severe adult asthmatics, 32% of whom were on oral corticosteroids, BMI was inversely correlated to sputum eosinophils and eNO, and positively correlated to comorbid factors, such as esophageal reflux, obstructive sleep apnea, and recurrent infection, suggesting that factors other than airway inflammation are responsible for the obesity-asthma relationship.[72] Finally, Sutherland and colleagues[73] studied four groups of adults: with and without obesity, each group with and without asthma. They found that systemic inflammation was increased in obesity and type-two cytokines were increased in asthma, but there were no significant interactions between these phenomena. The conclusion drawn from all four of these adult studies is that while the obesity-asthma relationship exists in some populations, the mechanism does not appear to be one of systemic inflammation causing typical asthmatic airway inflammation, and that elevated eNO and eosinophilic airway inflammation are not common characteristics of the obese asthmatic.

OBESE ASTHMA: SEVERITY VERSUS CONTROL

Asthma is a heterogeneous disease, requiring a guideline-based but customized treatment approach based upon a careful phenotyping of the patient. Obese asthma is no exception. Perhaps one way to reconcile the studies in mice and human beings is to propose that asthma in obesity represents a unique phenotype of asthma, with somewhat different pathophysiology than asthma in lean individuals. A handful of clinical studies have tried to determine whether asthma is more severe in the obese, and whether standard approaches to asthma treatment may need to be modified in the obese population.

Lessard and colleagues[74] propose that obese asthma may represent a new phenotype of asthma. They studied 88 consecutive asthmatics, half of whom were obese, and found that the obese subjects had poorer asthma control despite a similar symptom assessment. As expected, they reported obesity was associated with reductions in lung volumes, including residual volume. Induced sputum eosinophils were less common in the obese group—despite them being under poorer control—perhaps suggesting a different or more neutrophilic airway inflammation. In the National Asthma Survey, obese asthmatics appeared to be more severe, with greater prevalence of continuous symptoms, asthma-associated work absenteeism, rescue medication use, and controller medication use.[75] Obese asthmatics were also more commonly categorized as severe by the Global Initiative for Asthma severity classification.

It is important to distinguish between asthma severity and control. The issue with obese asthma may be more one of poorer control, greater risk, and greater impairment, rather than increased baseline disease severity. For example, obese asthmatics in the Emergency Department have more persistent symptoms, a longer Emergency Department stay, and greater risk for hospitalization than their nonobese counterparts.[76] In a cross-sectional survey study of 1113 adults with asthma, obese versus nonobese asthmatics reported reduced asthma-specific quality of life, less asthma control, and an increase in hospitalizations for asthma.[77] In these two studies, asthma was not well-characterized by a baseline physiologic assessment, and as a result it is unclear whether the increased morbidity in obese versus nonobese asthma is a result of more severe asthma, or whether it may be related to other comorbid physical or psychological conditions that may be more prevalent in the obese patient.

The National Heart, Lung, and Blood Institute has funded multiple studies in large, well-characterized asthma cohorts, including the Childhood Asthma Management Program (CAMP), the Asthma Clinical Research Network (ACRN), and the Severe Asthma Research Program (SARP). Unlike the previous studies, where asthma was not well characterized, in these cohorts there is little evidence that obesity is associated with a severe disease phenotype. In children participating in CAMP, BMI was not associated with airway reactivity, worsening asthma symptoms, or atopy. However, unlike some adult studies, the ratio of FEV_1 to FVC decreased with increasing BMI, leaving open the possibility that BMI may be related to disease severity in children.[78] In adults participating in ACRN studies, elevated BMI did not modify markers of asthma impairment to a clinically significant extent, although BMI was associated with altered response to therapy, lung function, and composite measures of disease activity.[79] Furthermore, there was no difference in obesity prevalence between moderate and severe asthmatics in SARP.[80] Given that the diagnosis of asthma is made more difficult in the obese, and that obesity-associated symptoms and comorbidities may complicate a clinical assessment, it is interesting to note that in the most highly characterized groups of pediatric and adult asthmatics, there appears to be little association between obesity and disease severity. Obesity might destabilize asthma, worsening asthma control, or it may modify response to asthma therapy through unique biologic mechanisms.

OBESITY: DIFFERENTIAL RESPONSE TO ASTHMA CONTROLLER THERAPY

Inhaled corticosteroids are the foundation of controller therapy for a vast majority of asthmatics. However, their effect may be attenuated in the presence of obesity. Peters-Golden and colleagues[81] performed a post-hoc analysis of four large clinical trials comparing an inhaled corticosteroid and a leukotriene modifier in adults with asthma. They reported that the placebo-adjusted clinical response to inhaled corticosteroids decreased with increasing BMI. This effect was not seen in the leukotriene modifier-treated group. Similarly, Boulet and Franssen[82] reported in another post-hoc analysis that obese asthmatics treated with inhaled corticosteroids were less likely to achieve asthma control compared with lean asthmatics similarly treated. These findings support anecdotal reports of blunted effectiveness of inhaled corticosteroids in obese asthmatics, and the question has been raised as to whether there may be impaired inhaled drug delivery or diminished biologic response to glucocorticoids in obese asthmatics.

A more recent article by Sutherland and colleagues[83] suggests that in vitro response to glucocorticoids is impaired in overweight and obese asthmatics. This group obtained peripheral blood and bronchoalveolar lavage mononuclear cells from a well-characterized group of adults with moderate to severe asthma, and stimulated them with dexamethasone. Patients were dichotomized into normal-weight (BMI <25 kg/m^2) and overweight or obese (BMI $\geq$25 kg/m^2) groups, with comparable mean baseline FEV_1 (72% vs 70% predicted, respectively, P = .1). They measured expression of mitogen-activated protein kinase phosphatase-1 (MKP-1) in response to dexamethasone, a marker of glucocorticoid sensitivity, and found that dexamethasone-induced MKP-1 induction was diminished in overweight and obese asthmatics in both peripheral blood and bronchoalveolar lavage cells. The degree of impairment in MKP-1 induction increased with increasing BMI. This trend was not observed in control subjects without asthma, suggesting that overweight and obese asthmatics demonstrate an impaired biologic response to glucocorticoids. One could speculate that some overweight asthmatics may be given increasing amounts of inhaled and oral glucocorticoids with diminishing clinical effectiveness, leading to further weight gain and glucocorticoid resistance. Alternative treatment strategies may be warranted in obese patients with asthma.

SUMMARY

Epidemiologic investigations have demonstrated that while asthma can contribute to obesity, obesity can cause or worsen asthma. Asthma incidence increases with the degree of adiposity in a dose-dependent fashion, and weight-loss studies have shown that this effect is reversible—that weight loss decreases the prevalence of asthma. While obesity does not cause airflow obstruction, it is biologically plausible that it may contribute to two of the three cardinal features of asthma: airway hyper-responsiveness and airway inflammation. While clinical evidence supporting obesity's role in AHR and airway inflammation is inconsistent, rigorously designed mouse models of asthma have consistently supported this hypothesis. Obese asthma may be a unique phenotype of asthma, characterized by lack of eosinophilic inflammation, decreased lung volumes, greater symptoms for a given degree of lung function impairment, and destabilization or lack of asthma control. Therefore, the clinical evaluation of an obese patient with asthma may require a more rigorous and objective approach. Obese asthma may respond differently than non-obese asthma to controller medication, and in particular obesity may induce a state of relative glucocorticoid resistance. Future research should focus on mechanistic studies in well-characterized clinical cohorts, and novel treatment strategies may be required to improve asthma control and quality of life in obese patients with asthma.

REFERENCES

1. Ford ES. The epidemiology of obesity and asthma. J Allergy Clin Immunol 2005;115(5):897–909, quiz 910.
2. Guerra S, Sherrill DL, Bobadilla A, et al. The relation of body mass index to asthma, chronic bronchitis, and emphysema. Chest 2002;122(4):1256–63.
3. Shaheen SO, Sterne JA, Montgomery SM, et al. Birth weight, body mass index and asthma in young adults. Thorax 1999;54(5):396–402.
4. Beckett WS, Jacobs DR Jr, Yu X, et al. Asthma is associated with weight gain in females but not males, independent of physical activity. Am J Respir Crit Care Med 2001;164(11):2045–50.
5. Litonjua AA, Sparrow D, Celedon JC, et al. Association of body mass index with the development of methacholine airway hyperresponsiveness in men: the Normative Aging Study. Thorax 2002;57(7):581–5.
6. Huovinen E, Kaprio J, Koskenvuo M. Factors associated to lifestyle and risk of adult onset asthma. Respir Med 2003;97(3):273–80.
7. Wyatt SB, Winters KP, Dubbert PM. Overweight and obesity: prevalence, consequences, and causes of a growing public health problem. Am J Med Sci 2006;331(4):166–74.
8. Rhodes L, Bailey CM, Moorman JE. Asthma prevalence and control characteristics by race/ethnicity–United States, 2002. Morb Mortal Wkly Rep 2004;53(7):145–8.
9. Pianosi PT, Davis HS. Determinants of physical fitness in children with asthma. Pediatrics 2004;113(3 Pt 1):e225–9.
10. Camargo CA Jr, Weiss ST, Zhang S, et al. Prospective study of body mass index, weight change, and risk of adult-onset asthma in women. Arch Intern Med 1999;159(21):2582–8.
11. Ford ES, Mannino DM, Redd SC, et al. Body mass index and asthma incidence among USA adults. Eur Respir J 2004;24(5):740–4.
12. Gunnbjornsdottir MI, Omenaas E, Gislason T, et al. Obesity and nocturnal gastro-oesophageal reflux are related to onset of asthma and respiratory symptoms. Eur Respir J 2004;24(1):116–21.
13. Chen Y, Dales R, Tang M, et al. Obesity may increase the incidence of asthma in women but not in men: longitudinal observations from the Canadian National Population Health Surveys. Am J Epidemiol 2002;155(3):191–7.
14. Nystad W, Meyer HE, Nafstad P, et al. Body mass index in relation to adult asthma among 135,000 Norwegian men and women. Am J Epidemiol 2004;160(10):969–76.
15. Beuther DA, Sutherland ER. Overweight, obesity and incident asthma: a meta-analysis of prospective epidemiologic studies. Am J Respir Crit Care Med 2007;175(7):661–6.
16. Hu FB, Willett WC, Li T, et al. Adiposity as compared with physical activity in predicting mortality among women. N Engl J Med 2004;351(26):2694–703.
17. Biring MS, Lewis MI, Liu JT, et al. Pulmonary physiologic changes of morbid obesity. Am J Med Sci 1999;318(5):293–7.
18. Naimark A, Cherniack RM. Compliance of the respiratory system and its components in health and obesity. J Appl Physiol 1960;15:377–82.
19. Babb TG, Ranasinghe KG, Comeau LA, et al. Dyspnea on exertion in obese women: association with an increased oxygen cost of breathing. Am J Respir Crit Care Med 2008;178(2):116–23.
20. Sin DD, Jones RL, Man SF. Obesity is a risk factor for dyspnea but not for airflow obstruction. Arch Intern Med 2002;162(13):1477–81.
21. Ronmark E, Andersson C, Nystrom L, et al. Obesity increases the risk of incident asthma among adults. Eur Respir J 2005;25(2):282–8.
22. Aaron SD, Vandemheen KL, Boulet LP, et al. Overdiagnosis of asthma in obese and nonobese adults. CMAJ 2008;179(11):1121–31.
23. Hallstrand TS, Fischer ME, Wurfel MM, et al. Genetic pleiotropy between asthma and obesity in a community-based sample of twins. J Allergy Clin Immunol 2005;116(6):1235–41.
24. Hall IP, Wheatley A, Wilding P, et al. Association of Glu 27 beta 2-adrenoceptor polymorphism with lower airway reactivity in asthmatic subjects. Lancet 1995;345(8959):1213–4.
25. Ishiyama-Shigemoto S, Yamada K, Yuan X, et al. Association of polymorphisms in the beta2-adrenergic receptor gene with obesity, hypertriglyceridaemia, and diabetes mellitus. Diabetologia 1999;42(1):98–101.
26. Moffatt MF, James A, Ryan G, et al. Extended tumour necrosis factor/HLA-DR haplotypes and asthma in an Australian population sample. Thorax 1999;54(9):757–61.
27. Norman RA, Bogardus C, Ravussin E. Linkage between obesity and a marker near the tumor necrosis factor-alpha locus in Pima Indians. J Clin Invest 1995;96(1):158–62.
28. Dempsey JA, Skatrud JB, Jacques AJ, et al. Anatomic determinants of sleep-disordered breathing across the spectrum of clinical and nonclinical male subjects. Chest 2002;122(3):840–51.
29. Guilleminault C, Quera-Salva MA, Powell N, et al. Nocturnal asthma: snoring, small pharynx and nasal CPAP. Eur Respir J 1988;1(10):902–7.

30. Martin RJ, Pak J. Nasal CPAP in nonapneic nocturnal asthma. Chest 1991;100(4):1024–7.

31. Havemann BD, Henderson CA, El-Serag HB. The association between gastro-oesophageal reflux disease and asthma: a systematic review. Gut 2007;56(12):1654–64.

32. Eneli IU, Skybo T, Camargo CA Jr. Weight loss and asthma: a systematic review. Thorax 2008;63(8):671–6.

33. Dixon JB, Chapman L, O'Brien P. Marked improvement in asthma after Lap-Band surgery for morbid obesity. Obes Surg 1999;9(4):385–9.

34. Ahroni JH, Montgomery KF, Watkins BM. Laparoscopic adjustable gastric banding: weight loss, co-morbidities, medication usage and quality of life at one year. Obes Surg 2005;15(5):641–7.

35. Macgregor AM, Greenberg RA. Effect of surgically induced weight loss on asthma in the morbidly obese. Obes Surg 1993;3(1):15–21.

36. Stenius-Aarniala B, Poussa T, Kvarnstrom J, et al. Immediate and long term effects of weight reduction in obese people with asthma: randomised controlled study. BMJ 2000;320(7238):827–32.

37. Jones RL, Nzekwu MM. The effects of body mass index on lung volumes. Chest 2006;130(3):827–33.

38. Bedell GN, Wilson WR, Seebohm PM. Pulmonary function in obese persons. J Clin Invest 1958; 37(7):1049–60.

39. Thomas PS, Cowen ER, Hulands G, et al. Respiratory function in the morbidly obese before and after weight loss. Thorax 1989;44(5):382–6.

40. Ochs-Balcom HM, Grant BJ, Muti P, et al. Pulmonary function and abdominal adiposity in the general population. Chest 2006;129(4):853–62.

41. Collins LC, Hoberty PD, Walker JF, et al. The effect of body fat distribution on pulmonary function tests. Chest 1995;107(5):1298–302.

42. Lazarus R, Sparrow D, Weiss ST. Effects of obesity and fat distribution on ventilatory function: the normative aging study. Chest 1997;111(4):891–8.

43. Rubinstein I, Zamel N, DuBarry L, et al. Airflow limitation in morbidly obese, nonsmoking men. Ann Intern Med 1990;112(11):828–32.

44. Hedenstierna G, Santesson J, Norlander O. Airway closure and distribution of inspired gas in the extremely obese, breathing spontaneously and during anaesthesia with intermittent positive pressure ventilation. Acta Anaesthesiol Scand 1976; 20(4):334–42.

45. Fredberg JJ, Inouye DS, Mijailovich SM, et al. Perturbed equilibrium of myosin binding in airway smooth muscle and its implications in bronchospasm. Am J Respir Crit Care Med 1999;159(3): 959–67.

46. Wang LY, Cerny FJ, Kufel TJ, et al. Simulated obesity-related changes in lung volume increases airway responsiveness in lean, nonasthmatic subjects. Chest 2006;130(3):834–40.

47. Chinn S, Jarvis D, Burney P. Relation of bronchial responsiveness to body mass index in the ECRHS. European Community Respiratory Health Survey. Thorax 2002;57(12):1028–33.

48. Schachter LM, Salome CM, Peat JK, et al. Obesity is a risk for asthma and wheeze but not airway hyper-responsiveness. Thorax 2001;56(1):4–8.

49. Bibi H, Shoseyov D, Feigenbaum D, et al. The relationship between asthma and obesity in children: is it real or a case of over diagnosis? J Asthma 2004;41(4):403–10.

50. Aaron SD, Fergusson D, Dent R, et al. Effect of weight reduction on respiratory function and airway reactivity in obese women. Chest 2004;125(6): 2046–52.

51. Fantuzzi G. Adipose tissue, adipokines, and inflammation. J Allergy Clin Immunol 2005;115(5): 911–9.

52. Weisberg SP, McCann D, Desai M, et al. Obesity is associated with macrophage accumulation in adipose tissue. J Clin Invest 2003;112(12):1796–808.

53. Wellen KE, Hotamisligil GS. Obesity-induced inflammatory changes in adipose tissue. J Clin Invest 2003;112(12):1785–8.

54. Xu H, Barnes GT, Yang Q, et al. Chronic inflammation in fat plays a crucial role in the development of obesity-related insulin resistance. J Clin Invest 2003;112(12):1821–30.

55. Esposito K, Pontillo A, Di Palo C, et al. Effect of weight loss and lifestyle changes on vascular inflammatory markers in obese women: a randomized trial. JAMA 2003;289(14):1799–804.

56. Wajchenberg BL. Subcutaneous and visceral adipose tissue: their relation to the metabolic syndrome. Endocr Rev 2000;21(6):697–738.

57. Thuesen BH, Husemoen LL, Hersoug LG, et al. Insulin resistance as a predictor of incident asthma-like symptoms in adults. Clin Exp Allergy 2009;39(5):700–7.

58. Ross R. The pathogenesis of atherosclerosis: a perspective for the 1990s. Nature 1993;362(6423): 801–9.

59. Pai JK, Pischon T, Ma J, et al. Inflammatory markers and the risk of coronary heart disease in men and women. N Engl J Med 2004;351(25):2599–610.

60. Bruno A, Chanez P, Chiappara G, et al. Does leptin play a cytokine-like role within the airways of COPD patients? Eur Respir J 2005;26(3):398–405.

61. Shore SA, Schwartzman IN, Mellema MS, et al. Effect of leptin on allergic airway responses in mice. J Allergy Clin Immunol 2005;115(1):103–9.

62. Shore SA, Rivera-Sanchez YM, Schwartzman IN, et al. Responses to ozone are increased in obese mice. J Appl Physiol 2003;95(3):938–45.

63. Johnston RA, Theman TA, Lu FL, et al. Diet-induced obesity causes innate airway hyperresponsiveness to methacholine and enhances ozone-induced

pulmonary inflammation. J Appl Physiol 2008; 104(6):1727–35.

64. Johnston RA, Theman TA, Shore SA. Augmented responses to ozone in obese carboxypeptidase E-deficient mice. Am J Physiol Regul Integr Comp Physiol 2006;290(1):R126–33.

65. Lu FL, Johnston RA, Flynt L, et al. Increased pulmonary responses to acute ozone exposure in obese *db/db* mice. Am J Physiol Lung Cell Mol Physiol 2006;290(5):L856–65.

66. Shore SA, Terry RD, Flynt L, et al. Adiponectin attenuates allergen-induced airway inflammation and hyperresponsiveness in mice. J Allergy Clin Immunol 2006;118(2):389–95.

67. Gurkan F, Atamer Y, Ece A, et al. Serum leptin levels in asthmatic children treated with an inhaled corticosteroid. Ann Allergy Asthma Immunol 2004;93(3): 277–80.

68. Guler N, Kirerleri E, Ones U, et al. Leptin: does it have any role in childhood asthma? J Allergy Clin Immunol 2004;114(2):254–9.

69. Sood A, Cui X, Qualls C, et al. Association between asthma and serum adiponectin concentration in women. Thorax 2008;63(10):877–82.

70. Sood A, Qualls C, Seagrave J, et al. Effect of specific allergen inhalation on serum adiponectin in human asthma. Chest 2009;135(2):287–94.

71. McLachlan CR, Poulton R, Car G, et al. Adiposity, asthma, and airway inflammation. J Allergy Clin Immunol 2007;119(3):634–9.

72. van Veen IH, Ten Brinke A, Sterk PJ, et al. Airway inflammation in obese and nonobese patients with difficult-to-treat asthma. Allergy 2008;63(5):570–4.

73. Sutherland TJ, Cowan JO, Young S, et al. The association between obesity and asthma: interactions between systemic and airway inflammation. Am J Respir Crit Care Med 2008;178(5):469–75.

74. Lessard A, Turcotte H, Cormier Y, et al. Obesity and asthma: a specific phenotype? Chest 2008;134(2): 317–23.

75. Taylor B, Mannino D, Brown C, et al. Body mass index and asthma severity in the National Asthma Survey. Thorax 2008;63(1):14–20.

76. Rodrigo GJ, Plaza V. Body mass index and response to emergency department treatment in adults with severe asthma exacerbations: a prospective cohort study. Chest 2007;132(5):1513–9.

77. Mosen DM, Schatz M, Magid DJ, et al. The relationship between obesity and asthma severity and control in adults. J Allergy Clin Immunol 2008; 122(3):507–11, e506.

78. Tantisira KG, Litonjua AA, Weiss ST, et al. Association of body mass with pulmonary function in the Childhood Asthma Management Program (CAMP). Thorax 2003;58(12):1036–41.

79. Sutherland ER, for the ACRN. Obesity, Asthma Phenotype and Response to Therapy in Asthma Clinical Research Network Trials. Presented at the American Thoracic Society International Conference. San Francisco, California, May 18–23, 2007.

80. Wenzel SE, Busse WW. Severe asthma: lessons from the Severe Asthma Research Program. J Allergy Clin Immunol 2007;119(1):14–21, quiz 22–13.

81. Peters-Golden M, Swern A, Bird SS, et al. Influence of body mass index on the response to asthma controller agents. Eur Respir J 2006; 27(3):495–503.

82. Boulet LP, Franssen E. Influence of obesity on response to fluticasone with or without salmeterol in moderate asthma. Respir Med 2007;101(11): 2240–7.

83. Sutherland ER, Goleva E, Strand M, et al. Body mass and glucocorticoid response in asthma. Am J Respir Crit Care Med 2008;178(7):682–7.

Obesity and Thromboembolic Disease

Paul D. Stein, MD[a,b,]*, Jose Goldman, MD, PhD[c]

KEYWORDS
- Obesity • Pulmonary embolism • Deep venous thrombosis
- Venous thromboembolism

Pulmonary embolism (PE) is the third most frequent cardiovascular disorder after coronary heart disease and stroke,[1] but the diagnosis is often overlooked. An important clue for establishing a suspicion of PE is the presence of risk factors. PE and deep venous thrombosis (DVT) are manifestations of the same disease and are often considered together as venous thromboembolism (VTE), that is, PE or DVT. Among patients in whom the diagnosis of DVT was made, 96% had one or more risk factors and 76% had two or more.[2] Obesity has been thought to be a risk factor for venous PE and DVT for many years, but strong data in support of this were established only recently in women[3,4] and in men and women.[5]

INCIDENCE OF PULMONARY EMBOLISM

In the years during which antithrombotic prophylaxis has been used extensively, PE was shown at autopsy in 24% of patients who died in acute-care hospitals, 22% who died in chronic-care hospitals, and 5% who died as outpatients.[6] Remarkably, even in patients who had large or fatal PE at autopsy, most cases (78%) were unsuspected or undiagnosed ante mortem, and this was true of university hospitals and tertiary care centers in addition to community hospitals.[7] In a study of unselected patients at autopsy that used postmortem pulmonary arteriography in addition to gross dissection and microscopic examination, in all 34 cases of PE, PE was found in muscular pulmonary artery branches (0.1–1 mm in diameter).[8] Only 8 cases (24%) had PE in elastic arteries (>1 mm in diameter). Microscopic examination showed PE in pulmonary arterioles (0.03–0.1 mm in diameter) in 13 (38%) of those who had grossly visible PE.[8]

Throughout the United States, from 1979 through 2001, the number of patients discharged from short-stay nonfederal hospitals with PE was 2,741,000, the number with DVT was 6,475,000, and the number with VTE (defined as PE or DVT) was 8,575,000.[9] During this 23-year period, the average population-based incidence of PE in hospitalized patients was 47 per 100,000 population, the incidence of DVT was 112 per 100,000 population, and the incidence of VTE was 148 per 100,000 population.[7] Among patients 20 years of age or older, an average of 0.4% of hospitalized patients were diagnosed with PE.[10] The incidence of PE in hospitalized patients did not change over 21 years.[10] The incidence of PE in hospitalized patients was nearly the same in men and women,[11] and it was the same in whites and blacks.[12] VTE, however, is less frequent in Asian-Pacific Islanders,[13] Alaskan Natives, and Americans Indians.[14]

DEEP VENOUS THROMBOSIS

Among patients at autopsy who had full-limb dissection in years before the general use of

[a] Department of Research, St. Joseph Mercy Oakland Hospital, 44405 Woodward Avenue, Pontiac, MI 48341–5023, USA
[b] Department of Internal Medicine, College of Osteopathic Medicine, Michigan State University, DMC Campus, Detroit, MI, USA
[c] Department of Internal Medicine, Michigan State University, B305 West Fee Hall, East Lansing, MI 48824, USA
* Corresponding author. Department of Research, St. Joseph Mercy Oakland Hospital, 44405 Woodward Avenue, Pontiac, MI 48341–5023.
E-mail address: steinp@trinity-health.org (P.D. Stein).

Clin Chest Med 30 (2009) 489–493
doi:10.1016/j.ccm.2009.05.006
0272-5231/09/$ – see front matter © 2009 Elsevier Inc. All rights reserved.

antithrombotic prophylaxis, 43% had DVT.[7] The incidence of DVT in hospitalized patients increased from 0.8% in 1979 to 1.3% in 1999.[10] This may represent an increasing availability and use of venous ultrasound during much of that period.[15] Early diagnosis and treatment of DVT may have prevented a parallel increase in the incidence of PE in hospitalized patients.

The number of patients who died from PE in 1998 based on death certificates was 24,947.[16] This equates to nine deaths attributable to PE per 100,000 population.

Among all patients with PE throughout the United States, irrespective of treatment or severity of PE, the estimated case fatality rate (death attributable to PE per 100 patients with PE) in 1998 was 7.7%.[17] The case fatality rate in short-stay hospitals in metropolitan Worcester in 1985 through 1986, 12%, was somewhat higher than calculated during those years.[18] The estimated case fatality rate from PE increased exponentially with age.[17] Various clinical investigations, such as the Prospective Investigation of Pulmonary Embolism Diagnosis (PIOPED), showed lower case fatality rates,[19] but most fatalities from PE occur within the first 2.5 hours after the diagnosis is made,[20] obviously excluding such patients from clinical investigations. Also, most investigations excluded severely ill patients, such as those in shock.

HEMOSTASIS AND OBESITY

Various abnormalities of hemostasis have been described in obesity, mainly concerning fibrinolysis, and increased plasminogen activator inhibitor-1 (PAI-1)[21–23] in particular, but other abnormalities of coagulation have been reported as well.[23] Circulating microparticles have also been observed in obesity.[24] These would suggest that obesity would be a risk factor for VTE. Microparticles are fragments shed from the plasma membrane after challenge of cells by a variety of stimuli (procoagulant, proinflammatory, or apoptogenic).[25] Some of them bear active tissue factor, and all of them expose procoagulant aminophospholipids, phosphatidylserine, and phosphatidylethanolamine, which confer a procoagulant phenotype.[24] Mean levels of microparticles, expressed as nanomolar phosphatidylserine equivalents (nMPSeq), were compared in obese patients (mean body mass index [BMI] = 42.2 kg/m^2) and controls (mean BMI = 20.9 kg/m^2).[24] Obese patients showed higher levels of microparticles (10.6 versus 3.2 nMPSeq).[24] The increased levels of circulating microparticles reflect cell activation and could account for an increased risk for thrombotic complications in obesity.[24]

Evidence in recent years has shed light on the fibrinolytic and hemostatic abnormalities in obese patients. BMI correlates with plasma levels of PAI-1.[26] Specific PAI-1 mRNA expression in human adipocytes from subcutaneous and visceral origins indicates that fat cells are a source of circulating PAI-1.[27,28] PAI-1 acts as an inhibitor of tissue- and urokinase-derived plasminogen activators, thereby interfering with the conversion of plasminogen to plasmin and decreasing fibrinolytic activity.[29] This mechanism of PAI-1–mediated inhibition of fibrinolysis is illustrated by in vitro experiments in which blockade of PAI-1 action through the addition of anti–PAI-1 monoclonal antibodies resulted in an increased rate of fibrinolysis with reduction of thrombus growth.[30] Inflammatory cytokines produced by adipose cells, namely, tumor necrosis factor-α and interleukin-1, have been reported by some[31] but not all[32] to participate in the increased production of PAI-1 in obese individuals through humoral or paracrine mechanisms. The regulation of the synthesis and release of PAI-1 from adipocytes still remains to be clarified.

Additional mechanisms contributing to prothrombosis in obesity include increased platelet aggregability[33] mediated through increases of von Willebrand factor and hypercoagulability attributable to higher levels of plasma fibrinogen, factor VII, and factor VIII.[34] In the European offspring study by the European Atherosclerosis Research Study (EARS), fibrinogen, factor VIIc, and PAI-1 were positively correlated with BMI.[35] Conversely, adjusted odds of large weight gain, defined as greater than the 90th percentile in middle-aged adults, have been associated with higher fibrinogen levels, and adjusted odds ratios for large weight gain were linked with higher levels of factor VIII and von Willebrand factor.[36] Marked weight reduction through bariatric surgery for morbid obesity leads to significant decreases of fibrinogen, factor VII, and PAI-1, although factor VIII or von Willebrand factor remained unchanged.[35]

Since 1927, obesity has been suggested to be a risk factor for fatal PE.[37] Investigations that reported an increased risk for VTE attributable to obesity have been criticized because they failed to control for hospital confinement or other risk factors.[38] High proportions of patients with VTE have been found to be obese,[18,39] but the importance of the association is diminished because of the high proportion of obesity in the general population.[40] Some investigations showed an increased risk ratio for DVT or PE in women,[3,4,41,42] but data in men were less compelling. The Nurses' Health Study showed that the age-adjusted risk ratio for PE in women with a BMI of 29.0 kg/m^2 or greater was 3.2 compared with the leanest category of less than 21.0 kg/m^2.[4] The Framingham Heart Study showed that Metropolitan relative weight was significantly and independently associated with PE among women but not among men.[3] The "Study of Men Born in 1913" showed that men in the highest decile of waist circumference ($\geq$100 cm) had an adjusted relative risk for VTE of 3.92 compared with men with a waist circumference less than 100 cm, however.[43] Among 1272 outpatients (men and women), the odds ratio for DVT, comparing obese (BMI >30 kg/m^2) with nonobese patients, was 2.39.[44] Others showed a similar odds ratio for DVT of 2.26 compared with nonobese patients.[41] Conversely, the Olmsted County, Minnesota case-control study found no evidence that current BMI was an independent risk factor for VTE in men or women.[38] Others did not show obesity to be a risk factor for VTE in men.[3,42]

Analysis of the database of the National Hospital Discharge Survey[45] showed compelling evidence that obesity is a risk factor for VTE.[5] Among patients hospitalized in short-term hospitals throughout the United States, in whom obesity was coded among the discharge diagnoses but not defined, 91,000 (0.8%) of 12,015,000 had PE (**Fig. 1**).[5] Among hospitalized patients who were not diagnosed with obesity, PE was diagnosed in 2,366,000 (0.3%) of 691,000,000. DVT was diagnosed in 243,000 (2.0%) of 12,015,000 patients diagnosed with obesity and in 5,524,000 (0.8%) of 691,000,000 who were not diagnosed with obesity.

The relative risk for PE, comparing obese patients with nonobese patients, was 2.18, and for DVT, it was 2.50.[5] The relative risks for PE and DVT depended on age. Obesity had the greatest impact on patients younger than 40 years of age, in whom the relative risk for PE in obese patients was 5.19 and the relative risk for DVT was 5.20.[5] The higher relative risk for obesity in younger patients may have reflected the fact that younger patients uncommonly have multiple confounding associated risk factors, which would make the risk for obesity inapparent.

Obese female patients had a greater relative risk for DVT than obese male patients: 2.75 versus 2.02.[5] The incidence of PE and DVT in hospitalized obese female patients was higher than in obese male patients. In female patients younger than 40 years of age, the relative risk for DVT comparing obese with nonobese patients was 6.10. In male patients younger than 40 years of age, the relative risk for DVT was 3.71.

The proportion of hospitalized patients diagnosed with obesity was within a narrow range (1.4%–2.4%) over the 21-year period of observation from 1979 through 1999, indicating consistency in the diagnostic process.[5] Previous investigators used several indices of obesity, including BMI greater than 35 kg/m^2 and BMI of 30 to 35 kg/m^2,[46] BMI of 29 kg/m^2 or greater,[4] weight greater than 20% of median recommended weight for height,[18] and (for men) waist circumference of 100 cm or greater.[43] It is likely that all patients diagnosed with obesity in the National Hospital Discharge Survey database were in fact obese, irrespective of the criteria used. Some obese patients may not have had a listed discharge diagnosis of obesity, however, and they would have been included in the nonobese group. This would have tended to reduce the relative risk for obesity in VTE.

A synergistic effect of oral contraceptives with obesity has been shown.[42,47–49] The odds ratio of DVT in obese women (BMI $\geq$30 kg/m^2) who were users of oral contraceptives ranged from 5.2 to 7.8 compared with that in with obese women who did not use oral contraceptives,[41,47,48] and among women with a BMI of 35 kg/m^2 or greater, the odds ratio was 3.1 compared with similar obese nonusers of oral contraceptives.[49]

Obesity is also a risk factor for recurrent VTE.[50] Among 1107 patients followed for an average of 46 months after a first unprovoked VTE and withdrawal of anticoagulant therapy, 168 had recurrent VTE. Mean BMI was higher in those with recurrent PE than in those without recurrence (28.5 versus 26.9). Four years after discontinuation of anticoagulation therapy, the probability of recurrent PE was 9.3% among patients with a normal weight (BMI <25 kg/m^2), 16.7% among overweight patients (BMI of 25–29 kg/m^2), and 17.5% among obese patients (BMI $\geq$30 kg/m^2). The hazard ratio of recurrence was 1.3% among overweight patients and 1.6% among obese patients.[50]

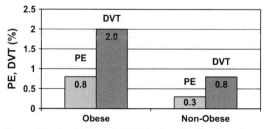

Fig. 1. Chart of PE and DVT in hospitalized patients from 1979 through 1999 shows the prevalence in obese and nonobese patients. (*From* Stein PD. Pulmonary embolism. 2nd edition. Oxford (UK): Blackwell Futura; 2007. p. 125; with permission).

Enoxaparin was shown to be effective for thromboprophylaxis in morbidly obese patients after bariatric surgery.[51] With various dosing regimens among 544 patients, PE occurred in 0.7% and none of the patients developed DVT.[51] All cases of PE occurred after the cessation of enoxaparin, 7 days to 1 month after surgery.

ACKNOWLEDGMENTS

Fadi Matta, MD, and Abdo Y. Yaekoub, MD, assisted in preparation of the manuscript.

REFERENCES

1. Giuntini C, Di Ricco G, Marini C, et al. Pulmonary embolism: epidemiology. Chest 1995;107(1 Suppl): 3S–9S.

2. Anderson FA, Spencer FA. Risk factors for venous thromboembolism. Circulation 2003;107:I9–16.

3. Goldhaber SZ, Savage DD, Garrison RJ, et al. Risk factors for pulmonary embolism. The Framingham Study. Am J Med 1983;74:1023–8.

4. Goldhaber SZ, Grodstein F, Stampfer MJ, et al. A prospective study of risk factors for pulmonary embolism in women. J Am Med Assoc 1997;277:642–5.

5. Stein PD, Beemath A, Olson RE. Obesity as a risk factor in venous thromboembolism. Am J Med 2005;118:978–80.

6. Nordstrom M, Lindblad B. Autopsy-verified venous thromboembolism within a defined urban population—the city of Malmo, Sweden. Acta Pathol Microbiol Immunol Scand 1998;106:378–84.

7. Stein PD. Pulmonary embolism. 2nd edition. Oxford (UK): Blackwell Futura; 2007. p. 3–18.

8. Smith GT, Dammin GJ, Dexter L. Postmortem arteriographic studies of the human lung in pulmonary embolization. J Am Med Assoc 1964;188:143–51.

9. Stein PD, Kayali F, Olson RE. Regional differences in rates of diagnosis and mortality of pulmonary thromboembolism. Am J Cardiol 2004;93:1194–7.

10. Stein PD, Beemath A, Olson RE. Trends in the incidence of pulmonary embolism and deep venous thrombosis in hospitalized patients. Am J Cardiol 2005;95:1525–6.

11. Stein PD, Hull RD, Patel KC, et al. Venous thromboembolic disease: comparison of the diagnostic process in men and women. Arch Intern Med 2003;163:1689–94.

12. Stein PD, Hull RD, Patel KC, et al. Venous thromboembolic disease: comparison of the diagnostic process in blacks and whites. Arch Intern Med 2003;163:1843–8.

13. Stein PD, Kayali F, Olson RE, et al. Pulmonary thromboembolism in Asian-Pacific Islanders in the United States: analysis of data from the National Hospital Discharge Survey and the United States Bureau of the Census. Am J Med 2004;116:435–42.

14. Stein PD, Kayali F, Olson RE, et al. Pulmonary thromboembolism in American Indians and Alaskan Natives. Arch Intern Med 2004;164:1804–6.

15. Stein PD, Hull RD, Ghali WA, et al. Tracking the uptake of evidence: two decades of hospital practice trends for diagnosing deep vein thrombosis and pulmonary embolism. Arch Intern Med 2003; 163:1213–9.

16. Horlander KT, Mannino DM, Leeper KV. Pulmonary embolism mortality in the United States, 1979–1998: an analysis using multiple-cause mortality data. Arch Intern Med 2003;163:1711–7.

17. Stein PD, Kayali F, Olson RE. Estimated case fatality rate from pulmonary embolism, 1979–1998. Am J Cardiol 2004;93:1197–9.

18. Anderson FA Jr, Wheeler HB, Goldberg RJ, et al. A population-based perspective of the hospital incidence and case-fatality rates of deep vein thrombosis and pulmonary embolism. Arch Intern Med 1991;151:933–8.

19. Carson JL, Kelley MA, Duff A, et al. The clinical course of pulmonary embolism. N Engl J Med 1992;326:1240–5.

20. Stein PD, Henry JW. Prevalence of acute pulmonary embolism among patients in a general hospital and at autopsy. Chest 1995;108:978–81.

21. Pannaciulli N, De Mitrio V, Marino R, et al. Effect of glucose tolerance status on PAI-1 plasma levels in overweight and obese subjects. Obes Res 2002; 10:717–25.

22. Juhan-Vague I, Alessi MC, Mavri A, et al. Plasminogen activator inhibitor-1, inflammation, obesity, insulin resistance and vascular risk. J Thromb Haemost 2003;1:1575–9.

23. De Pergola G, Pannacciulli N. Coagulation and fibrinolysis abnormalities in obesity. J Endocrinol Invest 2002;25:899–904.

24. Goichot B, Grunebaum L, Desprez D, et al. Circulating procoagulant microparticles in obesity. Diabete Metab 2006;32:82–5.

25. VanWijk MJ, VanBavel E, Sturk A, et al. Microparticles in cardiovascular diseases. Cardiovasc Res 2003;59:277–87.

26. Margaglione M, Cappuci G, d'Addedda M, et al. PAI-1 plasma levels in a general population without clinical evidence of atherosclerosis: relation to environmental and genetic determinants. Arterioscler Thromb Vasc Biol 1998;18:562–7.

27. Dusserre E, Moulin P, Vidal H. Differences in mRNA expression of the proteins secreted by the adipocytes in human subcutaneous and visceral adipose tissues. Biochim Biophys Acta 2000; 1500:88–96.

28. Alessi MC, Peiretti F, Morange P, et al. Production of plasminogen activator inhibitor 1 by human adipose

tissue: possible link between visceral fat accumulation and vascular disease. Diabetes 1997;46:860–7.

29. Kohler HP, Grant PJ. Plasminogen activator inhibitor type 1 and coronary artery disease. N Engl J Med 2000;342:1792–801.

30. Levi M, Biemond BJ, van Zonneveld, et al. Inhibition of plasminogen activator inhibitor-1 activity results in promotion of endogenous thrombolysis and inhibition of thrombus extension in models of experimental thrombosis. Circulation 1992;85:305–12.

31. Zoccali C, Mallamaci F, Tripepi G. Adipose tissue as a source of inflammatory cytokines in health and disease: focus on end stage renal disease. Kidney Int 2003;84(Suppl):S65–8.

32. Lindeman JH, Pijl H, Toet K, et al. Human visceral adipose tissue and the plasminogen activator inhibitor type 1. Int J Obes (Lond) 2007;31:1671–9.

33. Basili S, Pacini G, Guagnano MT, et al. Insulin resistance as a determinant of platelet activation in obese women. J Am Coll Cardiol 2006;48:2531–8.

34. Mertens I, Van Gaal LF. Obesity, haemostasis and the fibrinolytic system. Obes Rev 2002;3:85–101.

35. Bara L, Nicaud V, Tiret L, et al. Expression of a paternal history of premature myocardial infarction on fibrinogen, factor VIIC and PAI-1 in European offspring—the EARS study. European Atherosclerosis Research Study Group. Thromb Haemost 1994;71:434–40.

36. Duncan BB, Schmidt MI, Chambless LE, et al. Fibrinogen, other putative markers of inflammation, and weight gain in middle-aged adults—the ARIC Study. Obes Res 2000;8:279–86.

37. Snell AM. The relation of obesity to fatal postoperative pulmonary embolism. Arch Surg 1927;15:237–44.

38. Heit JA, Silverstein MD, Mohr DN, et al. The epidemiology of venous thromboembolism in the community. Thromb Haemost 2001;86:452–63.

39. Anderson FA Jr, Wheeler HB, Goldberg RJ, et al. The prevalence of risk factors for venous thromboembolism among hospital patients. Arch Intern Med 1992;152:1660–4.

40. Hedley AA, Ogden CL, Johnson CL, et al. Prevalence of overweight and obesity among US children, adolescents, and adults, 1999–2002. J Am Med Assoc 2004;291:2847–50.

41. Abdollahi M, Cushman M, Rosendaal FR. Obesity: risk of venous thrombosis and the interaction with coagulation factor levels and oral contraceptive use. Thromb Haemost 2003;89:493–8.

42. Coon WW, Coller FA. Some epidemiologic considerations of thromboembolism. Surg Gynecol Obstet 1959;109:487–501.

43. Hansson PO, Eriksson H, Welin L, et al. Smoking and abdominal obesity: risk factors for venous thromboembolism among middle-aged men: "the Study of Men Born in 1913." Arch Intern Med 1999;159:1886–90.

44. Samama MM. An epidemiologic study of risk factors for deep vein thrombosis in medical outpatients: the Sirius study. Arch Intern Med 2000;160:3415–20.

45. US Department of Health and Human Services, Public Health Service, National Center for Health Statistics National Hospital Discharge Survey 1979–1999 multi-year public-use data file documentation. Available at: http://www.cdc.gov/nchs/about/major/hdasd/nhds.htm. Accessed March 21, 2009.

46. Farmer RD, Lawrenson RA, Todd JC, et al. A comparison of the risks of venous thromboembolic disease in association with different combined oral contraceptives. Br J Clin Pharmacol 2000;49:580–90.

47. Pomp ER, le Cessie S, Rosendaal FR, et al. Risk of venous thrombosis: obesity and its joint effect with oral contraceptive use and prothrombotic mutations. Br J Haematol 2007;139:289–96.

48. Lidegaard O, Edstrom B, Kreiner S. Oral contraceptives and venous thromboembolism: a five-year national case-control study. Contraception 2002;65:187–96.

49. Nightingale AL, Lawrenson RA, Simpson EL, et al. The effects of age, body mass index, smoking and general health on the risk of venous thromboembolism in users of combined oral contraceptives. Eur J Contracept Reprod Health Care 2000;5:265–74.

50. Eichinger S, Hron G, Bialonczyk C, et al. Overweight, obesity, and the risk of recurrent venous thromboembolism. Arch Intern Med 2008;168:1678–83.

51. Hamad GG, Choban PS. Enoxaparin for thromboprophylaxis in morbidly obese patients undergoing bariatric surgery: findings of the Prophylaxis Against VTE Outcomes in Bariatric Surgery Patients Receiving Enoxaparin (PROBE) study. Obes Surg 2005;15:1368–74.

Obesity and Acute Lung Injury

Jennifer W. McCallister, MD, Eric J. Adkins, MD,
James M. O'Brien, Jr, MD, MSc*

KEYWORDS
- Acute lung injury • Acute respiratory distress syndrome
- Obesity • Mechanical ventilation • Critical care
- Disparities of care • Adiponectin

Acute lung injury (ALI) is a clinical syndrome defined by the acute onset of hypoxemic respiratory failure and bilateral pulmonary infiltrates not primarily attributable to left atrial hypertension.[1,2] When hypoxemia is more severe, the condition is termed acute respiratory distress syndrome (ARDS). ALI/ARDS is a common cause of respiratory failure with a crude incidence of 78.9 per 100,000 person-years and an age-adjusted incidence of 86.2 per 100,000 person-years.[3] In-hospital mortality remains unacceptably high between 38% and 60%.[2,3] It is estimated that there are almost 191,000 cases of ALI annually, accounting for 3.6 million hospital days and almost 75,000 deaths.[3]

Because of physiologic and biochemical changes associated with obesity, it is possible that excess weight affects the incidence and/or outcome of ALI. Alterations in thoraco-abdominal compliance and gas exchange might predispose obese patients to respiratory failure and ALI and could affect the response to therapeutic measures. The inflammation of obesity might also incline obese patients to lung injury when they suffer a secondary insult (eg, sepsis). However, provider bias and disparities in provided care could be as influential in the outcome of obese patients with ALI and require consideration in the assessment of any such association.[4,5]

PULMONARY PHYSIOLOGY IN OBESITY AND IMPLICATIONS FOR PATIENTS WITH ACUTE LUNG INJURY

The most significant change in pulmonary mechanics seen in obesity is a decrease in pulmonary compliance,[6] which has been attributed to one of several factors: fatty infiltration of the chest wall, increased pulmonary blood volume, and extrinsic compression of the thoracic cage by weight from excess soft tissue.[6-9] As a result, obese subjects exhibit an increased work of breathing[6,10] and may note a subjective increase in dyspnea.[11] In addition, respiratory resistance has been shown to be increased in obese subjects (**Table 1**) (see the article by Sood elsewhere in this issue)[9,12]

Pelosi and colleagues[12] compared the respiratory mechanics of sedated, paralyzed, morbidly obese (body mass index [BMI] ≥40) patients to normal weight subjects and found significant alterations in the obese group. Obesity resulted in a decrease in both lung and chest wall compliance and was associated with a marked increase in both airway and total lung resistance. In a separate study of 24 consecutive sedated, paralyzed patients, BMI was directly related to respiratory compliance and resistance.[10] The authors found that respiratory compliance decreased with increasing BMI, primarily as a result of the pulmonary component, while the chest wall compliance was weakly dependent on BMI. Similarly, total respiratory resistance increased with increasing BMI, largely because of an increase in lung resistance. Chest wall resistance was relatively unaffected. Zerah and associates[9] found a similar relationship between total respiratory resistance and BMI in awake, obese patients. In this series, both respiratory resistance and airway resistance correlated with BMI but chest wall resistance did not change significantly with the degree of obesity.

Division of Pulmonary, Allergy, Critical Care and Sleep Medicine, Center for Critical Care, The Ohio State University Medical Center, 201 Davis HLRI, 473 West 12th Avenue, Columbus, OH 43210, USA
* Corresponding author.
E-mail address: James.OBrien@osumc.edu (J.M. O'Brien).

Clin Chest Med 30 (2009) 495–508
doi:10.1016/j.ccm.2009.05.008

Table 1
Changes in respiratory mechanics and pulmonary function tests in obesity

Respiratory mechanics		
Total respiratory compliance	—	Decreased
	Pulmonary (lung) compliance	Decreased
	Chest wall compliance	Decreased
Total respiratory resistance	—	Increased
	Airway resistance	Increased
	Additional pulmonary (lung) resistance	Increased
	Chest wall resistance	Increased or unchanged
Pulmonary function tests		
	FVC	Decreased or unchanged
	FEV1	Decreased or unchanged
	FEV1/FVC	Decreased or unchanged
	VC	Decreased or unchanged
	FRC	Decreased
	ERV	Decreased
	TLC	Decreased or unchanged
	$D_L CO$	Increased or unchanged

Abbreviations: $D_L CO$, diffusion capacity for carbon monoxide; ERV, expiratory reserve volume; FEV1, forced expiratory volume in 1 second; FRC, functional residual capacity; FVC, forced vital capacity; TLC, total lung capacity; VC, vital capacity.

Decreased respiratory muscle function in obese patients may compound the previously mentioned changes in respiratory physiology. It has been shown that the maximum voluntary ventilation (MVV) is decreased in obesity[13–16] and is related to increasing BMI.[14] It has been suggested that this occurs as a result of upward displacement of the diaphragm within the thoracic cavity rather than as a result of true respiratory muscle weakness.[17]

The most predictable abnormalities in pulmonary function tests in obese subjects occur in the static lung volumes, with reductions in expiratory reserve volume (ERV) and functional residual capacity (FRC) most commonly described.[13,15,16,18–20] As outlined previously, these alterations are most likely attributable to the decreased respiratory compliance that occurs in response to excess soft tissue and weight. A reduction in vital capacity (VC) has been reported over a wide range of BMI by some authors[13,20–22] but others have reported a decrease in VC only with extreme obesity.[15] Total lung capacity (TLC) is often preserved in obese subjects,[13] but may be reduced with increasing BMI.[15]

Many authors have reported that the forced expiratory volume in 1 second (FEV1) and forced vital capacity (FVC) are preserved in obese subjects.[20,23,24] Others have suggested that obesity may cause airflow limitation, with reductions in both FEV1 and FVC.[13,25] In this case, the FEV1 and FVC are often symmetrically decreased, resulting in a preserved[11] or increased FEV1/FVC ratio[13] consistent with a restrictive pattern. Evidence for mild obstructive abnormalities exists, however. Rubinstein and colleagues[25] found increased airway resistance and reduced FEV1 in obese, nonsmoking men when compared with nonobese controls. Pankow and associates[26] described expiratory flow limitation (EFL) and associated intrinsic positive end-expiratory pressure (PEEPi) in obese subjects at tidal respiration that was not present in normal weight controls, which worsened in the supine position. In contrast, Ferretti and colleagues[27] showed that EFL was uncommon in obese subjects in the seated position, but noted that it was frequently identified in the same subjects in the supine position.

The diffusing capacity of carbon monoxide (DLco) is generally preserved in obesity,[13,16,17,20] supporting the concept that the pulmonary parenchyma is healthy in these individuals, and that alterations in pulmonary function are most likely related to the aforementioned changes in pulmonary mechanics. Interestingly, a few authors have identified an increase in DLco that seems to correspond to BMI.[15,19,28] Saydain and colleagues[28] hypothesized that this increase in DLco results from an increase in capillary blood volume that occurs with the increased total blood volume and cardiac output observed in obese patients.[29,30] Despite this, arterial hypoxemia and an elevated alveolar to arterial oxygen (A-a) gradient are often observed in obese subjects.[10,12,13,16,17,20] It has been hypothesized that ventilation/perfusion (V/Q) mismatching is a least partially responsible for this, with obese subjects preferentially ventilating the upper lung zones while preserving perfusion to the lung bases.[31,32] It appears that this V/Q mismatching is worsened in the supine position.[32] Others have suggested that the tendency of obese individuals to develop atelectasis is greater than in normal weight subjects[33–35] and may be explained by the previously described reduction in FRC.[10,12]

The alterations in pulmonary physiology and function have significant implications in the care of obese patients with ALI and ARDS. Alveolar overdistention and barotrauma, which may occur as a result of elevated airway pressures, may be compounded by the reduced lung volumes and increased airway resistance described above.[36] Initial tidal volume settings during mechanical ventilation should be based on ideal body weight, with a goal of limiting transpulmonary pressures to 30 to 35 cm H_2O. The development of PEEPi[26,27] and V/Q mismatching[32] seems to be worsened by the supine position, so patient positioning should be adjusted whenever possible. Accordingly, Burns and associates[37] found that the reverse Trendelenburg position at 45 degrees improved pulmonary mechanics and facilitated weaning in a small series of patients with obesity or ascites and respiratory failure. The addition of positive end-expiratory pressure should help prevent atelectasis and associated abnormalities in gas exchange[38] by improving pulmonary mechanics in obese patients.

PATHOPHYSIOLOGY OF ACUTE LUNG INJURY AND THE POSSIBLE ROLE OF OBESITY

A full description of the pathophysiology of ALI/ARDS is beyond the scope of the current review and the reader is directed to recent reviews for further details.[2,39] In brief, in ALI/ARDS imbalances occur between pro- and anti-inflammatory cytokines, oxidants and antioxidants, and coagulation factors. Alterations in neutrophil activation, recruitment, and clearance and release of proteases also are important. The net result of these changes is alveolar filling with proteinaceous fluid, alveolar and interstitial edema, surfactant inactivation, and injury of the pulmonary microvascular bed.

Endothelial injury in the pulmonary microvasculature is a major contributor to the increased permeability pulmonary edema of ALI/ARDS.[40] Two mediators thought to play a role in this endothelial dysfunction are endothelin-1 and von Willebrand factor (VWF). Endothelin-1 (ET-1) is released by endothelial cells in response to stress and injury, resulting in vasoconstriction and inflammation.[41] ET-1 is elevated in the plasma of patients with ALI/ARDS compared with healthy controls.[42]

VWF is also released in response to endothelial activation and higher levels of VWF have been associated with increased mortality in ALI/ARDS patients.[43]

Plasma levels of ET-1 and VWF are both increased in noncritically ill obese patients. ET-1 is released by subcutaneous adipose tissue and greater levels are secreted in obesity.[44] VWF is also increased in obesity[45] and appears to be linked to insulin resistance and endothelial dysfunction.[46] Despite this, it is unknown if ET-1 and VWF are increased in obese ALI/ARDS patients or if alterations in these proinflammatory mediators predispose obese patients to the syndrome.

In addition to endothelial injury, ALI/ARDS is characterized by damage to the alveolar epithelium. Characteristic lesions in the alveolar epithelium lead to loss of epithelial integrity and result in pulmonary edema and impaired clearance of lung water. Injury to type II cells leads to impaired surfactant production and lung repair.[47] A comparison of the underlying mechanisms of damage to the alveolar epithelium and the degree to which it occurs in obese versus nonobese ALI/ARDS patients is lacking.

Neutrophils play a critical role in the development of ALI/ARDS with increased neutrophils found in the lung and bronchoalveolar lavage fluid of ALI/ARDS patients.[47,48] There are a number of putative mechanisms thought to be involved in neutrophil recruitment and activation, which may contribute to the development of ALI/ARDS, including up-regulation of adhesion molecules, induced neutrophil deformation, release of neutrophil-derived proteases and dysregulated neutrophil clearance.[39] Alterations in neutrophil recruitment in the obese ALI/ARDS patient may exist, but evidence is inconclusive. There appears to be an increase in multiple adhesion molecule markers in the blood of obese patients, including intracellular adhesion molecule-1 (ICAM-1) and E-selectin, which correlates with the degree of obesity.[49] However, other studies find that selected neutrophil adhesion antigens, such as CD62L (L-selectin), are reduced in obese patients, suggesting the possibility of impaired neutrophil recruitment.[50] As with endothelial damage, we are unaware of studies directed at differences in recruitment or activation of neutrophils in obese and nonobese ALI/ARDS patients.

The inflammatory condition in ALI/ARDS is promoted and modulated by a complex interplay of cytokines produced by a wide variety of cell types.[51] Interleukin-1 (IL-1) and tumor necrosis factor-α (TNF-α) are early-response cytokines that promote subsequent inflammation.[39] IL-8 is thought to enhance this initial inflammation through recruitment of neutrophils.[52] These inflammatory markers are accompanied by anti-inflammatory cytokines, such as IL-10 and IL-11, and inhibitors of proinflammatory cytokines, such as soluble TNF receptors, IL-1 receptor antagonist, and auto-antibodies against IL-8.[39] In response to inflammatory stimuli, a number of cells release reactive oxygen and nitrogen species, which may be responsible for much of the cellular damage occurring in ALI/ARDS.[53]

Data linking obesity and ALI/ARDS is, perhaps, most convincing on the basis of chronic excessive inflammation and oxidative stress in obese patients compared with nonobese patients.[54] There is a significant increase in abnormal cytokine production and acute-phase reactants and an up-regulation of proinflammatory signaling pathways in otherwise-healthy obese patients.[55] Additional weight gain stimulates further induction of proinflammatory cytokines and mediators, such as TNF-α, IL-6, pre-B-cell-enhancing factor (PBEF), plasminogen activator inhibitor -1 (PAI-1), angiotensinogen, retinol-binding protein-4 (RBP-4), leptin, and IL-1β.[54] In fact, adipose cells can contribute up to 30% of circulating IL-6 in obese individuals.[56]

Obesity is associated with an increase in oxidative stress and formation of reactive oxygen species.[57] Reactive oxygen species cause cellular injury through direct damage to cellular membranes and by cellular adhesion of monocytes and release of chemotactic factors and vasoactive substances.[58] Oxidative stress has been associated with diaphragmatic dysfunction.[59] Diaphragmatic dysfunction has also been described in obesity,[60] but a direct link between oxidative stress, obesity, and diaphragm function has not been reported.

ADIPOCYTOKINES AND ACUTE LUNG INJURY/ ACUTE RESPIRATORY DISTRESS SYNDROME

In addition to classic cytokines, adipose tissue releases adipocytokines that act as mediators of subsequent proinflammatory and anti-inflammatory pathways.[54] Although there are a number of known adipocytokines, of primary importance are leptin and adiponectin.[54] Leptin is a polypeptide hormone secreted by adipocytes that is elevated in states of obesity and functions as a mediator of energy balance.[61] It is secreted mainly by adipose tissue and meant to signal adequate stores of energy and feelings of satiety. When energy levels diminish, leptin levels fall to stimulate feelings of hunger. Leptin levels are increased in patients with obesity and are thought to play a role in the development and maintenance of obesity and its morbid complications. These increased levels may be a result of leptin-resistance, which is present in more than 90% of patients with type 2 diabetes and is believed to be attributable to receptor down-regulation.[62]

In addition to its regulation of energy balance, leptin also functions as an adipocytokine to affect inflammatory cells. Leptin can induce the production of TNF-α, IL-1β, IL-1RA, IL-R2, and IL-6 as well as that of reactive oxygen species, and to increase phagocytosis in some antigen-presenting cells.[63] Leptin has a structural similarity to other cytokines, such as IL-6, which is known to serve a proinflammatory role. However, leptin's role in acute inflammatory conditions leading to ALI/ ARDS, such as sepsis, is unproven. For example, in healthy volunteers, plasma leptin is not increased above baseline after intravenous endotoxin administration at 6 or 24 hours.[64] Similarly, studies exploring an association between leptin levels and outcomes from sepsis are conflicting. One showed an association between elevated leptin levels and higher mortality,[65] another found no association,[66] and others showed higher leptin levels in sepsis survivors.[67,68]

One recent study attempted to evaluate the role of leptin and leptin resistance and its potential protective properties in mice with hyperoxia-induced acute lung injury.[69] With hyperoxia, lung leptin levels were increased in wild-type and leptin-receptor deficient mice. However, leptin resistant mice developed less lung edema and lung injury and had improved survival compared with mice with normally functioning leptin receptors. This suggests that the activation of the leptin receptor plays a role in the development of acute lung injury from hyperoxia and leptin resistance may be protective in preventing acute lung injury and associated morbidity and mortality. The relevance in alternate models of ALI/ARDS and in patients with ALI/ARDS is unknown.

Patients with diabetes mellitus, many of whom have elevated leptin levels, appear to be protected from acute lung injury. Several studies have suggested that diabetic patients are at lower risk for developing ARDS when suffering an acute insult associated with ALI/ARDS.[70,71] It is unknown if this apparent protection from ALI/ARDS in diabetic patients at risk is attributable to an effect of leptin resistance, excess weight, or alternate mechanisms.

Adiponectin is another adipocytokine that might play a role in the pathogenesis of ALI/ARDS of obese patients. It stimulates fatty acid oxidation, decreases plasma triglyceride levels, and improves insulin sensitivity.[72] Adiponectin levels are generally decreased in obese individuals.[73] Adiponectin has anti-inflammatory effects, including suppression of TNF-α, IL-6, and nuclear factor-κB and up-regulation of IL-10 and IL-1RA.[74]

Studies using animal models (most commonly transgenic rodents with dysfunctional leptin receptors) have begun to explore a possible interaction between obesity and acute inflammation. In an experimental model of acute pancreatitis, pulmonary levels of TNF-α mRNA were significantly higher in obese than lean rats. However, there were no significant differences in pulmonary mRNA levels of IL-6, IL-10, or pancreatitis-associated protein.[75] In a study exploring bronchial hyper-responsiveness seen in obese mice lacking the leptin receptor, investigators measured bronchoalveolar (BAL) levels of cytokines and adipocytokines.[76] There were minimal differences between the wild-type and transgenic mice in regards to BAL inflammatory cytokines. However, BAL leptin levels were higher in obese than lean mice and there was a trend toward lower adiponectin levels in the obese mice. It remains unknown if these differences might also affect the murine response to stimuli causing ALI/ARDS.

OBESITY AND OUTCOMES FROM ACUTE LUNG INJURY

Although a number of studies explore the association between obesity and outcome for critically ill adults (see article in this issue by Honiden and McArdle), few articles have focused specifically on patients with ALI/ARDS (**Table 2**). The first such study[77] reported a secondary analysis of patients enrolled in the National Heart, Lung and Blood Institute's (NHLBI) multicenter, randomized trials of the Acute Respiratory Distress Syndrome Network.[80–82] These studies included comparisons of lower and higher tidal volumes (6 mL/kg versus 12 mL/kg predicted body weight, respectively) and ketoconazole or lisofylline versus placebo. Of note, patients with a weight-to-height ratio (kilograms divided by centimeters) of greater than 1.0 were excluded from these studies. BMI calculated from height and weight at the time of study enrollment was used as the measure of excess weight with a variety of variable formats used in the analyses; risk-adjusting methods incorporated multivariable logistic regression with survival to 28 days being the primary outcome.

BMI data were missing for 6.1% (n = 55) of subjects enrolled in the initial studies. The investigators also excluded subjects with an underweight BMI (<18.5 kg/m^2, 4.7%, n = 40). Ultimately, 807 subjects were included in the analysis. Based on

NHLBI categories of BMI, 31.5% (n = 254) of subjects had an overweight BMI and 27.1% (n = 219) had an obese BMI. In unadjusted analyses, there were no significant differences in 28-day or 180-day mortality, achieving unassisted ventilation by day 28 or ventilator-free days between patients with overweight or obese BMIs and those with normal BMIs. After adjusting for the effects of age, severity of illness, PaO$_2$/FiO$_2$ ratio, study group assignment, peak airway pressure, primary lung injury category, and gender, there was no significant increase in the adjusted odds of 28-day mortality for subjects with overweight (adjusted odds ratio 1.10 [95% confidence interval 0.71–1.69]) or obese BMIs (adjusted odds ratio 1.11 [95% confidence interval 0.69–1.78]), compared with subjects with normal BMIs. There was also no significant association in multivariable analysis including BMI as a continuous variable, when severe obesity (BMI $\geq$40 kg/m^2) was considered or when the subject's BMI was adjusted for the fluid balance for the 24 hours preceding study enrollment. The same risk-adjusting model was refit for 180-day mortality, achieving unassisted ventilation by day 28, and ventilator-free days. In no analysis were overweight or obese BMIs associated with outcomes.

A second retrospective study by the same authors used data from Project IMPACT, a subscription database designed for ICU benchmarking (www.cerner.com/piccm/products_pi.html), to further explore any possible association between obesity and outcomes among ALI patients.[78] The investigators analyzed data from 1488 patients admitted from December 1995 to September 2001. Subjects were included if (1) admission data allowed for a BMI calculation, (2) there was an admission diagnosis consistent with ALI, and (3) the subject required mechanical ventilation within 24 hours of ICU admission. Again, BMI was used as an indicator of excess weight and was calculated from data included in the admitting record. The primary outcome was hospital mortality and multivariable logistic regression was used to account for possible confounding. Underweight patients were included in the analysis.

Of the included subjects, 26.8% (n = 399) had an overweight BMI, 21.9% (n = 326) had an obese BMI, and 8.8% (n = 131) were severely obese, by NHLBI categorization.[83] In unadjusted analyses, there was a significant association between BMI and hospital mortality (P < .001). Crude hospital mortality was highest in patients with underweight BMIs (54.6%) and lowest in the severely obese patients (29.0%). Hospital mortality was intermediate in the other BMI categories. ICU and hospital length of stay and discharge destination were not

Table 2
Studies examining the association between outcome and obesity in ALI/ARDS patients

	O'Brien et al.[77]	O'Brien et al.[78]	Morris et al.[79]
Setting	Retrospective analysis of randomized clinical trial	Retrospective cohort study of subscription database	Prospective cohort study of ICU patients in King County, WA
Definition of ALI/ARDS	AECC	Diagnostic codes	AECC
Years of study	1996–1999	1995–2001	1999–2000
Sample size	807	1488	825
Measure(s) of excess weight	BMI, fluid-adjusted BMI by NHLBI categories, continuous	BMI by NHLBI categories, continuous and quadratic transformation	BMI by NHLBI categories
Percentage of obese subjects	27.1%	30.7%	28.7%
Primary outcome	28-day mortality	Hospital mortality	Hospital mortality
Crude association with primary outcome	Not statistically significant	Highest mortality in underweight (54.6%) and lowest in severely obese (29.0%)	Highest mortality in underweight (44.0%) with lowest in severely obese (25.9%)
Risk-adjusted association with primary outcome	Not statistically significant	Statistically significant with highest adjusted odds of hospital mortality in underweight and lowest adjusted odds ratio in obese BMI groups, relative to normal BMI	Not statistically significant
Secondary outcome(s)	180-day mortality, achieving unassisted ventilation, ventilator-free days	None	Hospital length of stay, ICU length of stay, duration of mechanical ventilation
Risk-adjusted association with secondary outcome(s)	Not statistically significant	N/A	Statistically significantly longer length of stay in severely obese relative to normal BMI patients; statistically significantly longer ICU length of stay and duration of ventilation among severely obese hospital survivors relative to normal BMI survivors
Miscellaneous findings	Lower tidal volume ventilation appeared to have similar benefit for all BMI groups; 14% of subjects changed BMI category when adjusted for fluid balance; higher pre-enrollment tidal volumes in higher BMI groups	Higher BMI patients more likely to receive heparin prophylaxis and this mediated some of "benefit" of higher BMI	Day 3 tidal volumes were higher with higher BMIs; severely obese patients more likely to be discharged to a higher level of care on hospital discharge

Abbreviations: ALI/ARDS, acute lung injury/acute respiratory distress syndrome; AECC, American-European Consensus Conference; BMI, body mass index; N/A, not applicable; NHLBI, National Heart, Lung and Blood Institute.

different between the various BMI categories. The best fit of the noncategorized BMI variable with hospital mortality was found to be a quadratic transformation and this was also significantly associated with hospital mortality in unadjusted analyses ($P < .0001$). After adjustment for an assortment of possible confounders found in preliminary analyses, BMI category remained associated with hospital mortality ($P < .0001$) when the group with normal BMIs was considered the referent group. The highest adjusted odds for mortality were in the patients with underweight BMIs (adjusted odds ratio 1.94 [95% confidence interval 1.05–3.60]) and patients with an obese BMI had significantly lower adjusted odds of death (adjusted odds ratio 0.67 [95% confidence interval 0.46–0.97]). A trend toward lower mortality for the overweight and severely obese BMI groups was also suggested in risk-adjusted analyses (adjusted odds ratios, 0.72 and 0.78, respectively) but failed to reach statistical significance. A similar association was observed when the transformed BMI variable was included in the risk-adjusting model with the highest adjusted odds seen at underweight BMI levels and the lowest odds seen at a BMI of 35 to 40 kg/m^2.

The most recent study examining the association between obesity and acute lung injury used data gathered as part of a population-based, prospective cohort study among 21 hospitals in and around King County, Washington, between April 1999 and July 2000 (KCLIP).[3] All patients receiving mechanical ventilation in the participating hospitals were screened for enrollment based on the American-European Consensus Conference definition of ALI.[1] In the analysis of these data examining obesity,[79] BMI was calculated from height and weight recorded at hospital admission and NHLBI categories were used. Outcomes included ICU and hospital mortality, ICU and hospital length of stay, duration of mechanical ventilation, and discharge disposition. Multivariable logistic and linear regression models were used for risk adjusting.

As in the prior studies examining excess weight and ALI, most subjects were either overweight (28.7%, n = 237) or obese (28.7%, n = 237). Crude mortality was highest in the patients with underweight BMIs (44.0%) and decreased as BMI increased. ICU and hospital lengths of stay and duration of mechanical ventilation were similar among all BMI categories in unadjusted analyses. After adjustment for age, severity of illness, and ALI risk factor, there were no statistically significant differences in mortality between the underweight, overweight, obese, or severely obese BMI groups and the reference group (patients

with normal BMIs). ICU and hospital lengths of stay were markedly increased among the severely obese patients (BMI $\geq$ 40) compared with patients with normal BMIs. Moreover, compared with survivors with normal BMIs, the risk-adjusted duration of mechanical ventilation among surviving severely obese patients was increased by 4.1 days (95% confidence interval 0.4 to 7.7 days). Finally, severely obese patients were more likely to be discharged to rehabilitation facilities and skilled nursing facilities. These differences in lengths of stay, duration of ventilation, and discharge location among the severely obese were not observed among the patients with overweight and obese BMIs compared with those with normal BMIs.

OBESITY AS A RISK FACTOR FOR ACUTE LUNG INJURY AND MULTIORGAN FAILURE IN AT-RISK PATIENTS

Because of changes in physiology and inflammation associated with excess weight, it is conceivable that obese patients might be at greater risk for ALI/ARDS when suffering a predisposing acute event, such as sepsis or trauma. One of the earliest studies exploring an association between obesity and outcome among the critically ill reviewed data from 184 patients admitted to a trauma service over 6 months.[84] In this study, mortality was significantly higher in patients with a BMI greater than 31 kg/m^2 (42.1% versus 5.0% in patients with BMI <27) and this increased mortality remained after adjustment for severity of injury. The authors also noted that the higher BMI group had a significantly higher rate of complications per patient and this "was predominantly accounted for by an increase in pulmonary complications." The details of these pulmonary complications were not provided. However, the authors also presented the cause of death among the 17 patients who died. Seven of eight higher BMI patients had ARDS listed as the primary factor leading to death. No patients in the lower BMI group (BMI <27) had ARDS listed as the primary factor leading to death, although three of six had multiorgan system failure listed.

A more recent retrospective cohort study reexplored this association among 242 consecutive patients admitted to an intensive care unit following blunt trauma.[85] There were no differences in the development of ARDS between subjects with an obese (BMI $\geq$ 30 kg/m^2) or a nonobese BMI (8% versus 6%, $P = .55$) but obese subjects had a higher rate of multiorgan system failure (13% versus 3%). After adjustment for head injury, pulmonary contusion, injury severity, and age, the subjects with obese BMIs had significantly higher mortality (adjusted odds ratio 5.7 [95% confidence interval 1.9–19.6]). However, only one death in the study was attributed to respiratory failure. Multiorgan system failure was a more common cause of death among the obese-BMI subjects than the nonobese-BMI subjects (35.0% versus 17.2%).

A secondary analysis of a prospective cohort study of critically injured adults sought to determine if obese and severely obese patients were at increased risk of pulmonary complications, including ARDS.[86] The study cohort included 1219 adults admitted to an ICU following trauma. ARDS occurred in 21% of normal-BMI patients, 32% of obese-BMI patients, and 11% of severely obese-BMI patients. After adjustment for age, gender, and severity of injury, the patients with severe obesity had a statistically significant decrease in the risk of ARDS (adjusted odds ratio 0.36 [95% confidence interval 0.13–0.99]) compared with the normal-BMI group. A similar effect was not seen among the overweight- (adjusted odds ratio 0.97) and obese-BMI groups (adjusted odds ratio 1.0). When BMI was explored as a continuous variable, the peak of unadjusted risk for ARDS occurred between a BMI of 20 and 30. Ventilator management practices, including tidal volume, were not reported.

Although there are hypothetical reasons that obesity could create a pathologic milieu promoting the development of ALI/ARDS in patients otherwise at risk, definitive data are lacking. Most studies have focused on less specific outcomes such as length of stay and mortality for obese ICU patients. As discussed subsequently, even those studies focusing on the development of ALI/ARDS in obese patients suffer from potential bias owing to the definition of ALI/ARDS and lack of standard care practices.

LIMITATIONS OF HUMAN STUDIES EXPLORING AN ASSOCIATION BETWEEN OBESITY AND ACUTE LUNG INJURY
Measures of Excess Weight and the Heterogeneity of Obesity

Existing studies of excess weight and ALI have examined BMI as the only measure of excess weight. Although this measure is highly reliable and associated with adult body fat in ambulatory patients,[87] BMI might not be the best representation of risk (or benefit) for critically ill patients. For example, the distribution of excess weight may have particular relevance for mechanically ventilated patients kept in a supine or semi-supine position.[88] In selected epidemiologic studies,

waist circumference is a better marker of cardiovascular risk than BMI.[83] Because centripetal obesity is more likely to affect thoraco-abdominal compliance than excess weight distributed elsewhere in the body, it is possible that measures of the distribution of excess weight may be more strongly associated with outcome than BMI in mechanically ventilated patients, such as those with ALI. Further research is needed to explore alternate measures of excess weight. Such efforts would be an initial effort to consider the heterogeneity of pathogenesis and pathophysiology in the construct lumped together as "obesity."

Fluid Balance

Studies of the association between excess weight and acute lung injury have used height and weight as recorded at ICU[78] or hospital admission[79,86] or at the time of study enrollment.[77] However, many of the conditions that lead to ALI (eg, sepsis, trauma) are accompanied by fluid resuscitation and changes that may alter fluid handling (eg, "third-spacing," acute renal failure). The administration of fluid or induced diuresis before weight measurement might, therefore, affect the calculated BMI. Furthermore, the course of illness leading to ALI (eg, anorexia attributable to infection) might alter the patient's weight before intervention and may not reflect the patient's true BMI.

The previously discussed study using data from the ARDS Network considered the effects of therapeutic fluid manipulation on measured BMI in the analysis.[77] For the 24 hours before study enrollment (and weight measurement), fluid balance was determined. There was a wide range in net fluid balance (mean balance, 2591 mL gained [95% confidence interval 5527 mL lost to 10,709 mL gained]). In other words, based on net fluid balance alone, on average, subjects were 2.6 kg (5.7 pounds) heavier on the day of study enrollment compared with the prior day. The adjustment for individual fluid balances resulted in 14.4% of subjects changing BMI category. When BMI was adjusted for this fluid balance, there remained no association with outcome.

Differences in net fluid balance before BMI calculation could explain some of the variation in observed results across studies. Early appropriate resuscitation may be important for outcome in patients with ALI and its predisposing conditions.[89–91] Patients receiving earlier volume resuscitation will likely gain more fluid (and weight) before BMI calculation. They are then more likely to migrate into higher BMI categories and this could bias the results. Additionally, because obese patients are less tolerant of fluid loading than the nonobese,[92,93] similar resuscitation practices might then affect obese and nonobese patients differently. This could also confound the observed association.

Diagnosis of Acute Lung Injury/Acute Respiratory Distress Syndrome in Obesity

The current clinical definition of ALI or ARDS is based on the American-European Consensus Conference statement, which requires the presence of bilateral pulmonary infiltrates on chest radiograph.[1] Obesity often decreases the quality of chest radiographs,[94] and may limit the usefulness of this definition in many patients. Typical settings used to obtain chest radiographs may not allow adequate penetration of the x-ray beams in an obese patient, resulting in lower image contrast and increased background scatter.[95] In addition, the increased body thickness through which x-ray beams must travel in obese patients requires increased exposure time and may result in excessive motion artifact. Accordingly, the distinction between infiltrates and overlying soft tissue may be difficult, and the presence of mediastinal adipose tissue may produce abnormalities on chest radiograph that mimic other clinical conditions.[36] Finally, when a large surface area is imaged, the area of clinical interest may lie outside the field of view.[94] A computed tomography scan may provide better visualization of the pulmonary parenchyma, but factors such as the difficulty transporting obese patients and the weight and aperture limitations of available equipment may limit the usefulness of these studies in many patients.[36,95]

Disparities in Processes of Care

Observational studies rely on appropriate risk adjusting to reach unbiased conclusions about the measured results. Among patients with ALI, several care practices have high-level evidence supporting their use. If such practices are differentially applied to nonobese and obese patients, this disparity in care might bias the results. The use of lower tidal volume ventilation (eg, 6 mL/kg predicted body weight and plateau airway pressure <30) was associated with an 8.8% absolute risk-reduction in hospital mortality[80] compared with traditional tidal volumes (eg, 12 mL/kg predicted body weight). In a secondary analysis of the data from this randomized controlled trial, the tidal volumes used just before the institution of the study protocol were analyzed by BMI category.[77] Patients with obese BMIs had significantly higher tidal volumes (10.76 mL/kg predicted body weight) than patients with normal BMIs (10.05 mL/kg predicted body weight). This study also concluded

that there was no significant interaction between patient BMI and the benefit of lower tidal volumes, arguing that lower tidal volumes should be used for ALI patients of all BMIs.

The King Country study also found significantly higher tidal volumes on day 3 of mechanical ventilation among obese and severely obese patients (10.5 and 11.4 mL/kg predicted body weight, respectively) than among patients with normal BMIs (9.9 mL/kg predicted body weight).[79] Noting the possible effect of such disparities in ventilator practices, the authors did not include tidal volume in their risk-adjusting estimates because they could be in the causal pathway to worse outcomes for obese patients. Based on existing data, clinicians should be attentive to tidal volumes based on predicted body weight for *all* ALI patients. Particular attention should be paid to obese ALI patients because they seem most prone to the use of potentially injurious tidal volumes.

In a retrospective cohort study of ALI patients in an observational database, other care practices were observed to be used differently for obese and nonobese patients.[78] For example, heparin prophylaxis for thromboembolic disease was used more frequently for obese and severely obese patients (46.0% and 57.2% of patients, respectively) than for normal BMI patients (43.8%). Importantly, this increased use of what is considered best-practice for prevention of venous thromboembolism in mechanically ventilated patients[96] mediated approximately 10% of the observed protective effect of severe obesity in this study. Said another way, a significant portion of the apparent "protective" effect of severe obesity in this study was attributable to an increased use of appropriate thromboembolism prophylaxis in the severely obese patients. Whether this is a causal effect of thromboembolism prophylaxis or if this observation is merely a marker for other unmeasured disparities in provided care is unknown. However, it emphasizes the need to consider differences in clinical care in observational studies determining an association between obesity and outcome.

Increasing evidence points to excessive use of sedatives and/or analgesics to be major causes of poorer outcomes, including prolonged time requiring mechanical ventilation, increased rates of delirium, and higher mortality among mechanically ventilated patients.[97-99] Because many of these medications are extremely fat soluble, their volume of distribution is altered in obese patients.[100] Although most data on the pharmacokinetic and pharmacodynamic properties of these agents in obese patients are based on their use in elective surgery or healthy volunteers, rather than in critically ill mechanically ventilated patients, differences in response to these medications could confound any observed association between obesity and outcome for ALI patients.

Benzodiazepines are highly lipophilic drugs that are commonly used in mechanically ventilated patients. Among obese patients, there is a significant increase in volume of distribution and elimination half-life for benzodiazepines.[101] The increase in volume of distribution into excess fat appears to be directly associated with the lipid solubility of the drug. For example, after a single 5-mg intravenous bolus, midazolam has a total volume of distribution more than three times larger in obese than nonobese subjects.[102] The elimination half-life was also almost four times longer (8.4 hours versus 2.7 hours) in the obese subjects. This was because of the dramatic increase in volume of distribution, rather than changes in clearance of drug. Therefore, whereas single doses of midazolam should be based on total body weight, continuous infusions should be adjusted based on ideal body weight However, in the ICU, infusions are usually titrated to effect (eg, level of sedation) rather than dose. If bolus doses of midazolam are not based on actual body weight, there may be a delay in the desired level of sedation. This could leave a patient at risk for complications from under-sedation. Furthermore, we have anecdotally noted an increased reliance on higher infusion rates in these instances to mitigate the apparent resistance to the inadequately dosed bolus. This might then produce an overshoot in the depth of sedation and a subsequent delay in drug washout.

Obesity's effects on distribution and elimination of synthetic opioids and alternative sedatives are less consistent than those observed for benzodiazepines. Sufenatil and alfentanil have increased volumes of distribution in obese subjects and prolonged elimination half-lives when compared with nonobese patients.[103,104] However, the pharmacokinetics of fentanyl do not appear to be appreciably altered by obesity while the volume of distribution is increased.[104] Propofol is a highly lipophilic drug commonly used for mechanically ventilated adults. Although there is an increase in the volume of distribution of propofol in obese patients, it is paralleled by an increase in drug clearance. Therefore, the elimination half-life of propofol is similar in nonobese and obese patients.[105] We are unaware of a published study that compares various strategies of sedation and analgesia among obese versus nonobese patients. Known alterations in pharmacokinetics of these commonly used drugs could affect outcomes by producing prolonged sedation and increased incidence of delirium, even if identical practices are used for obese and nonobese patients.

SUMMARY

ALI/ARDS is a common cause of acute respiratory failure with a high mortality rate. Although current data are premature, obesity and ALI/ARDS appear to share alterations in inflammation, endothelial dysfunction, and oxidative stress. This raises the possibility that obese patients may be at higher risk of developing ALI/ARDS and have poorer outcomes from ALI/ARDS. However, data supporting such an association are inconclusive. Additionally, obese ALI/ARDS patients may receive different care than nonobese patients. These disparities in provided care might worsen (eg, tidal volumes influenced by total body weight) or improve (eg, greater use of appropriate thromboembolism prophylaxis) outcomes in obese ALI/ARDS and bias observed results. With the epidemic of obesity, a greater number of ALI/ARDS patients will be obese and greater understanding of the mechanisms underlying lung injury in these patients is needed to better characterize the syndrome and improve treatment.

REFERENCES

1. Bernard GR, Artigas A, Brigham KL, et al. The American-European Consensus Conference on ARDS. Definitions, mechanisms, relevant outcomes, and clinical trial coordination. Am J Respir Crit Care Med 1994;149(3 Pt 1):818–24.
2. Ware LB, Matthay MA. The acute respiratory distress syndrome. N Engl J Med 2000;342(18):1334–49.
3. Rubenfeld GD, Caldwell E, Peabody E, et al. Incidence and outcomes of acute lung injury. N Engl J Med 2005;353(16):1685–93.
4. Hebl MR, Xu J. Weighing the care: physicians' reactions to the size of a patient. Int J Obes Relat Metab Disord 2001;25(8):1246–52.
5. Adams CH, Smith NJ, Wilbur DC, et al. The relationship of obesity to the frequency of pelvic examinations: do physician and patient attitudes make a difference? Women Health 1993;20(2):45–57.
6. Naimark A, Cherniack RM. Compliance of the respiratory system and its components in health and obesity. J Appl Physiol 1960;15:377–82.
7. Barrera F, Hillyer P, Ascanio G, et al. The distribution of ventilation, diffusion, and blood flow in obese patients with normal and abnormal blood gases. Am Rev Respir Dis 1973;108(4):819–30.
8. Fadell EJ, Richman AD, Ward WW, et al. Fatty infiltration of respiratory muscles in the Pickwickian syndrome. N Engl J Med 1962;266:861–3.

9. Zerah F, Harf A, Perlemuter L, et al. Effects of obesity on respiratory resistance. Chest 1993; 103(5):1470–6.

10. Pelosi P, Croci M, Ravagnan I, et al. The effects of body mass on lung volumes, respiratory mechanics, and gas exchange during general anesthesia. Anesth Analg 1998;87(3):654–60.

11. Sin DD, Jones RL, Man SF. Obesity is a risk factor for dyspnea but not for airflow obstruction. Arch Intern Med 2002;162(13):1477–81.

12. Pelosi P, Croci M, Ravagnan I, et al. Total respiratory system, lung, and chest wall mechanics in sedated-paralyzed postoperative morbidly obese patients. Chest 1996;109(1):144–51.

13. Biring MS, Lewis MI, Liu JT, et al. Pulmonary physiologic changes of morbid obesity. Am J Med Sci 1999;318(5):293–7.

14. Ladosky W, Botelho MA, Albuquerque JP Jr. Chest mechanics in morbidly obese non-hypoventilated patients. Respir Med 2001;95(4):281–6.

15. Ray CS, Sue DY, Bray G, et al. Effects of obesity on respiratory function. Am Rev Respir Dis 1983; 128(3):501–6.

16. Sahebjami H, Gartside PS. Pulmonary function in obese subjects with a normal FEV1/FVC ratio. Chest 1996;110(6):1425–9.

17. Unterborn J. Pulmonary function testing in obesity, pregnancy, and extremes of body habitus. Clin Chest Med 2001;22(4):759–67.

18. Bedell GN, Wilson WR, Seebohm PM. Pulmonary function in obese persons. J Clin Invest 1958; 37(7):1049–60.

19. Jones RL, Nzekwu MM. The effects of body mass index on lung volumes. Chest 2006;130(3): 827–33.

20. Thomas PS, Cowen ER, Hulands G, et al. Respiratory function in the morbidly obese before and after weight loss. Thorax 1989;44(5):382–6.

21. Refsum HE, Holter PH, Lovig T, et al. Pulmonary function and energy expenditure after marked weight loss in obese women: observations before and one year after gastric banding. Int J Obes 1990;14(2):175–83.

22. Wadstrom C, Muller-Suur R, Backman L. Influence of excessive weight loss on respiratory function. A study of obese patients following gastroplasty. Eur J Surg 1991;157(5):341–6.

23. Crapo RO, Kelly TM, Elliott CG, et al. Spirometry as a preoperative screening test in morbidly obese patients. Surgery 1986;99(6):763–8.

24. Kollias J, Boileau RA, Barlett HL, et al. Pulmonary function and physical conditioning in lean and obese subjects. Arch Environ Health 1972;25(2): 146–50.

25. Rubinstein I, Zamel N, DuBarry L, et al. Airflow limitation in morbidly obese, nonsmoking men. Ann Intern Med 1990;112(11):828–32.

26. Pankow W, Podszus T, Gutheil T, et al. Expiratory flow limitation and intrinsic positive end-expiratory pressure in obesity. J Appl Physiol 1998;85(4): 1236–43.

27. Ferretti A, Giampiccolo P, Cavalli A, et al. Expiratory flow limitation and orthopnea in massively obese subjects. Chest 2001;119(5):1401–8.

28. Saydain G, Beck KC, Decker PA, et al. Clinical significance of elevated diffusing capacity. Chest 2004;125(2):446–52.

29. Licata G, Scaglione R, Barbagallo M, et al. Effect of obesity on left ventricular function studied by radionuclide angiocardiography. Int J Obes 1991;15(4): 295–302.

30. Karason K, Wallentin I, Larsson B, et al. Effects of obesity and weight loss on cardiac function and valvular performance. Obes Res 1998;6(6):422–9.

31. Holley HS, Milic-Emili J, Becklake MR, et al. Regional distribution of pulmonary ventilation and perfusion in obesity. J Clin Invest 1967;46(4): 475–81.

32. Tucker DH, Sieker HO. The effect of change in body position on lung volumes and intrapulmonary gas mixing in patients with obesity, heart failure, and emphysema. Am Rev Respir Dis 1960;82:787–91.

33. Fox GS, Whalley DG, Bevan DR. Anaesthesia for the morbidly obese. Experience with 110 patients. Br J Anaesth 1981;53(8):811–6.

34. Salem MR, Dalal FY, Zygmunt MP, et al. Does PEEP improve intraoperative arterial oxygenation in grossly obese patients? Anesthesiology 1978; 48(4):280–1.

35. Vaughan RW, Wise L. Intraoperative arterial oxygenation in obese patients. Ann Surg 1976; 184(1):35–42.

36. El Solh AA. Clinical approach to the critically ill, morbidly obese patient. Am J Respir Crit Care Med 2004;169(5):557–61.

37. Burns SM, Egloff MB, Ryan B, et al. Effect of body position on spontaneous respiratory rate and tidal volume in patients with obesity, abdominal distension and ascites. Am J Crit Care 1994; 3(2):102–6.

38. Pelosi P, Ravagnan I, Giurati G, et al. Positive end-expiratory pressure improves respiratory function in obese but not in normal subjects during anesthesia and paralysis. Anesthesiology 1999;91(5): 1221–31.

39. Ware LB. Pathophysiology of acute lung injury and the acute respiratory distress syndrome. Semin Respir Crit Care Med 2006;27(4):337–49.

40. Zimmerman GA, Albertine KH, Carveth HJ, et al. Endothelial activation in ARDS. Chest 1999; 116(1 Suppl):18S–24S.

41. Fagan KA, McMurtry IF, Rodman DM. Role of endothelin-1 in lung disease. Respir Res 2001;2(2): 90–101.

42. Druml W, Steltzer H, Waldhausl W, et al. Endothelin-1 in adult respiratory distress syndrome. Am Rev Respir Dis 1993;148(5):1169–73.

43. Ware LB, Conner ER, Matthay MA. von Willebrand factor antigen is an independent marker of poor outcome in patients with early acute lung injury. Crit Care Med 2001;29(12):2325–31.

44. van Harmelen V, Eriksson A, Astrom G, et al. Vascular peptide endothelin-1 links fat accumulation with alterations of visceral adipocyte lipolysis. Diabetes 2008;57(2):378–86.

45. Blann AD, Bushell D, Davies A, et al. von Willebrand factor, the endothelium and obesity. Int J Obes Relat Metab Disord 1993;17(12):723–5.

46. Charles MA, Morange P, Eschwege E, et al. Effect of weight change and metformin on fibrinolysis and the von Willebrand factor in obese nondiabetic subjects: the BIGPRO1 Study. Biguanides and the prevention of the risk of obesity. Diabetes Care 1998;21(11):1967–72.

47. Bachofen M, Weibel ER. Structural alterations of lung parenchyma in the adult respiratory distress syndrome. Clin Chest Med 1982;3(1):35–56.

48. Matthay MA, Eschenbacher WL, Goetzl EJ. Elevated concentrations of leukotriene D4 in pulmonary edema fluid of patients with the adult respiratory distress syndrome. J Clin Immunol 1984;4(6):479–83.

49. Pontiroli AE, Frige F, Paganelli M, et al. In morbid obesity, metabolic abnormalities and adhesion molecules correlate with visceral fat, not with subcutaneous fat effect of weight loss through surgery. Obes Surg 2009;19(6):745–50.

50. Cottam DR, Schaefer PA, Fahmy D, et al. The effect of obesity on neutrophil Fc receptors and adhesion molecules (CD16, CD11b, CD62L). Obes Surg 2002;12(2):230–5.

51. Goodman RB, Pugin J, Lee JS, et al. Cytokine-mediated inflammation in acute lung injury. Cytokine Growth Factor Rev 2003;14(6):523–35.

52. Miller EJ, Cohen AB, Matthay MA. Increased interleukin-8 concentrations in the pulmonary edema fluid of patients with acute respiratory distress syndrome from sepsis. Crit Care Med 1996;24(9):1448–54.

53. Pittet JF, Mackersie RC, Martin TR, et al. Biological markers of acute lung injury: prognostic and pathogenetic significance. Am J Respir Crit Care Med 1997;155(4):1187–205.

54. Tilg H, Moschen AR. Role of adiponectin and PBEF/visfatin as regulators of inflammation: involvement in obesity-associated diseases. Clin Sci (Lond) 2008;114(4):275–88.

55. Wellen KE, Hotamisligil GS. Inflammation, stress, and diabetes. J Clin Invest 2005;115(5):1111–9.

56. Fantuzzi G. Adipose tissue, adipokines, and inflammation. J Allergy Clin Immunol 2005;115(5):911–9.

57. Keaney JF Jr, Larson MG, Vasan RS, et al. Obesity and systemic oxidative stress: clinical correlates of oxidative stress in the Framingham Study. Arterioscler Thromb Vasc Biol 2003;23(3):434–9.

58. Avogaro A, De Kreutzenberg SV. Mechanisms of endothelial dysfunction in obesity. Clin Chim Acta 2005;360(1–2):9–26.

59. Lopez LC, Escames G, Tapias V, et al. Identification of an inducible nitric oxide synthase in diaphragm mitochondria from septic mice: its relation with mitochondrial dysfunction and prevention by melatonin. Int J Biochem Cell Biol 2006;38(2):267–78.

60. De Vito EL, Montiel GC, Semeniuk GB. [Diaphragmatic reserve strength in obese patients]. Medicina (B Aires) 1991;51(6):524–8 [in Spanish].

61. Ahima RS, Flier JS. Leptin. Annu Rev Physiol 2000; 62:413–37.

62. Friedman JM. Modern science versus the stigma of obesity. Nat Med 2004;10(6):563–9.

63. Lam QL, Lu L. Role of leptin in immunity. Cell Mol Immunol 2007;4(1):1–13.

64. Bornstein SR, Preas HL, Chrousos GP, et al. Circulating leptin levels during acute experimental endotoxemia and antiinflammatory therapy in humans. J Infect Dis 1998;178(3):887–90.

65. Arnalich F, Lopez J, Codoceo R, et al. Relationship of plasma leptin to plasma cytokines and human survival in sepsis and septic shock. J Infect Dis 1999;180(3):908–11.

66. Papathanassoglou ED, Moynihan JA, Ackerman MH, et al. Serum leptin levels are higher but are not independently associated with severity or mortality in the multiple organ dysfunction/systemic inflammatory response syndrome: a matched case control and a longitudinal study. Clin Endocrinol (Oxf) 2001; 54(2):225–33.

67. Bornstein SR, Licinio J, Tauchnitz R, et al. Plasma leptin levels are increased in survivors of acute sepsis: associated loss of diurnal rhythm, in cortisol and leptin secretion. J Clin Endocrinol Metab 1998; 83(1):280–3.

68. Torpy DJ, Bornstein SR, Chrousos GP. Leptin and interleukin-6 in sepsis. Horm Metab Res 1998; 30(12):726–9.

69. Bellmeyer A, Martino JM, Chandel NS, et al. Leptin resistance protects mice from hyperoxia-induced acute lung injury. Am J Respir Crit Care Med 2007;175(6):587–94.

70. Gong MN, Thompson BT, Williams P, et al. Clinical predictors of and mortality in acute respiratory distress syndrome: potential role of red cell transfusion. Crit Care Med 2005;33(6):1191–8.

71. Moss M, Guidot DM, Steinberg KP, et al. Diabetic patients have a decreased incidence of acute respiratory distress syndrome. Crit Care Med 2000;28(7):2187–92.

72. Beltowski J. Adiponectin and resistin—new hormones of white adipose tissue. Med Sci Monit 2003;9(2):RA55–61.

73. Arita Y, Kihara S, Ouchi N, et al. Paradoxical decrease of an adipose-specific protein, adiponectin, in obesity. Biochem Biophys Res Commun 1999;257(1):79–83.

74. Wolf AM, Wolf D, Rumpold H, et al. Adiponectin induces the anti-inflammatory cytokines IL-10 and IL-1RA in human leukocytes. Biochem Biophys Res Commun 2004;323(2):630–5.

75. Segersvard R, Tsai JA, Herrington MK, et al. Obesity alters cytokine gene expression and promotes liver injury in rats with acute pancreatitis. Obesity (Silver Spring) 2008;16(1):23–8.

76. Holguin F, Rojas M, Hart CM. The peroxisome proliferator activated receptor gamma (PPARgamma) ligand rosiglitazone modulates bronchoalveolar lavage levels of leptin, adiponectin, and inflammatory cytokines in lean and obese mice. Lung 2007;185(6):367–72.

77. O'Brien JM Jr, Welsh CH, Fish RH, et al. Excess body weight is not independently associated with outcome in mechanically ventilated patients with acute lung injury. Ann Intern Med 2004;140(5):338–45.

78. O'Brien JM Jr, Phillips GS, Ali NA, et al. Body mass index is independently associated with hospital mortality in mechanically ventilated adults with acute lung injury. Crit Care Med 2006;34(3):738–44.

79. Morris AE, Stapleton RD, Rubenfeld GD, et al. The association between body mass index and clinical outcomes in acute lung injury. Chest 2007;131(2):342–8.

80. Ventilation with lower tidal volumes as compared with traditional tidal volumes for acute lung injury and the acute respiratory distress syndrome. The Acute Respiratory Distress Syndrome Network. N Engl J Med 2000;342(18):1301–8.

81. Randomized, placebo-controlled trial of lisofylline for early treatment of acute lung injury and acute respiratory distress syndrome. Crit Care Med 2002;30(1):1–6.

82. Ketoconazole for early treatment of acute lung injury and acute respiratory distress syndrome: a randomized controlled trial. The ARDS Network. JAMA 2000;283(15):1995–2002.

83. Clinical guidelines on the identification, evaluation, and treatment of overweight and obesity in adults–The Evidence Report. National Institutes of Health. Obes Res 1998;2(6 Suppl):51S–209S.

84. Choban PS, Weireter LJ Jr, Maynes C. Obesity and increased mortality in blunt trauma. J Trauma 1991;31(9):1253–7.

85. Neville AL, Brown CV, Weng J, et al. Obesity is an independent risk factor of mortality in severely injured blunt trauma patients. Arch Surg 2004;139(9):983–7.

86. Dossett LA, Heffernan D, Lightfoot M, et al. Obesity and pulmonary complications in critically injured adults. Chest 2008;134(5):974–80.

87. Deurenberg P, Weststrate JA, Seidell JC. Body mass index as a measure of body fatness: age- and sex-specific prediction formulas. Br J Nutr 1991;65(2):105–14.

88. Perilli V, Sollazzi L, Bozza P, et al. The effects of the reverse Trendelenburg position on respiratory mechanics and blood gases in morbidly obese patients during bariatric surgery. Anesth Analg 2000;91(6):1520–5.

89. Rivers E, Nguyen B, Havstad S, et al. Early goal-directed therapy in the treatment of severe sepsis and septic shock. N Engl J Med 2001;345(19):1368–77.

90. Bilkovski RN, Rivers EP, Horst HM. Targeted resuscitation strategies after injury. Curr Opin Crit Care 2004;10(6):529–38.

91. Otero RM, Nguyen HB, Huang DT, et al. Early goal-directed therapy in severe sepsis and septic shock revisited: concepts, controversies, and contemporary findings. Chest 2006;130(5):1579–95.

92. Alpert MA, Lambert CR, Panayiotou H, et al. Relation of duration of morbid obesity to left ventricular mass, systolic function, and diastolic filling, and effect of weight loss. Am J Cardiol 1995;76(16):1194–7.

93. Alpert MA, Terry BE, Mulekar M, et al. Cardiac morphology and left ventricular function in normotensive morbidly obese patients with and without congestive heart failure, and effect of weight loss. Am J Cardiol 1997;80(6):736–40.

94. Uppot RN, Sahani DV, Hahn PF, et al. Effect of obesity on image quality: fifteen-year longitudinal study for evaluation of dictated radiology reports. Radiology 2006;240(2):435–9.

95. Uppot RN, Sahani DV, Hahn PF, et al. Impact of obesity on medical imaging and image-guided intervention. AJR Am J Roentgenol 2007;188(2):433–40.

96. Geerts WH, Bergqvist D, Pineo GF, et al. Prevention of venous thromboembolism: American College of Chest Physicians Evidence-Based Clinical Practice Guidelines (8th Edition). Chest 2008;133(6 Suppl):381S–453S.

97. Kress JP, Pohlman AS, O'Connor MF, et al. Daily interruption of sedative infusions in critically ill patients undergoing mechanical ventilation. N Engl J Med 2000;342(20):1471–7.

98. Girard TD, Kress JP, Fuchs BD, et al. Efficacy and safety of a paired sedation and ventilator weaning protocol for mechanically ventilated patients in intensive care (Awakening and Breathing Controlled trial): a randomised controlled trial. Lancet 2008;371(9607):126–34.

99. Pandharipande P, Shintani A, Peterson J, et al. Lorazepam is an independent risk factor for

transitioning to delirium in intensive care unit patients. Anesthesiology 2006;104(1):21–6.

100. Casati A, Putzu M. Anesthesia in the obese patient: pharmacokinetic considerations. J Clin Anesth 2005;17(2):134–45.

101. Cheymol G. Clinical pharmacokinetics of drugs in obesity. An update. Clin Pharmacokinet 1993;25(2): 103–14.

102. Greenblatt DJ, Abernethy DR, Locniskar A, et al. Effect of age, gender, and obesity on midazolam kinetics. Anesthesiology 1984;61(1):27–35.

103. Schwartz AE, Matteo RS, Ornstein E, et al. Pharmacokinetics of sufentanil in obese patients. Anesth Analg 1991;73(6):790–3.

104. Scholz J, Steinfath M, Schulz M. Clinical pharmacokinetics of alfentanil, fentanyl and sufentanil. An update. Clin Pharmacokinet 1996;31(4):275–92.

105. Servin F, Farinotti R, Haberer JP, et al. Propofol infusion for maintenance of anesthesia in morbidly obese patients receiving nitrous oxide. A clinical and pharmacokinetic study. Anesthesiology 1993; 78(4):657–65.

Role of Obesity in Cardiomyopathy and Pulmonary Hypertension

Charles S. Dela Cruz, MD, PhD, Richard A. Matthay, MD*

KEYWORDS
- Obesity • Cardiomyopathy • Congestive heart failure
- Right-heart dysfunction • Pulmonary hypertension

Obesity is a medical problem of epidemic and worldwide proportions. The U.S. Surgeon General has identified obesity as a major health problem, with more than one billion overweight adults (body mass index [BMI] 25–29.9 kg/m^2) and at least 300 million obese adults (BMI >30 kg/m^2).[1] The number of overweight children has doubled and number of overweight adolescents has tripled since 1980. Obese persons have a 50% to 100% greater risk for death from any cause than normal-weight persons.[2] Obese patients often present with symptoms, such as dyspnea, shortness of breath, wheezing, exercise intolerance, orthopnea, or leg swelling, that may be caused by primary pulmonary or primary cardiac disorders. In this article, the authors explore the role of obesity in the development of heart failure as a result of obesity cardiomyopathy and pulmonary hypertension.

OBESITY CARDIOMYOPATHY

Obesity cardiomyopathy is under-recognized and underdiagnosed, especially in obese patients who have not previously been diagnosed with dyslipidemia, coronary artery disease, systemic hypertension, or diabetes mellitus. The association between obesity and heart failure has only recently been established, and the 2005 guidelines of the American College of Cardiology and American Heart Association have recognized obesity as an important risk factor for heart failure.[3]

Wong and Marwick[4,5] have suggested that the definition of obesity-related cardiomyopathy should encompass myocardial disease in obese patients that cannot be explained by systemic hypertension, coronary artery disease, diabetes mellitus, or other causes. Obesity itself is thought to be an independent risk factor for heart failure and myocardial dysfunction.[6] This form of myocardial disease presents as heart failure, either in the form of systolic dysfunction or diastolic dysfunction resulting from impaired left heart filling and relaxation.[6] Patients with obesity cardiomyopathy may present with range of disorders from asymptomatic left ventricular (LV) dysfunction to dilated cardiomyopathy.

THE EVIDENCE FOR THE ASSOCIATION BETWEEN OBESITY AND HEART FAILURE

The association between obesity and heart failure was initially suggested from the results of autopsy studies. Smith and Willius in 1933[7] described four patients with an average body weight of 150 kg and no known comorbidities who had all died of heart failure. Kasper and colleagues[8] reported a higher incidence of idiopathic, dilated cardiomyopathy in obese patients (average body weight of 130 kg), compared with lean patients (average body weight of 71 kg) (76.7% versus. 35.5%, $P<.0001$). A study by Duflou and colleagues[9] reported 22 severely obese, relatively young patients (average body weight 175 kg; mean age 34 years)

Section of Pulmonary and Critical Care Medicine, Department of Internal Medicine, Yale University School of Medicine, 333 Cedar Street, PO Box 208057, New Haven, CT 06520-8057, USA
* Corresponding author.
E-mail address: richard.matthay@yale.edu (R.A. Matthay).

Clin Chest Med 30 (2009) 509–523
doi:10.1016/j.ccm.2009.06.001
0272-5231/09/$ – see front matter © 2009 Published by Elsevier Inc.

chestmed.theclinics.com

who died of sudden cardiac death, with the most common cause being dilated cardiomyopathy.

Various epidemiologic studies have also provided evidence for a link between obesity and heart failure. The Framingham Heart Study report[10] in 1984 identified obesity as a major risk factor for heart failure for both men and women, noting that excessive body weight adversely affects ventricular function. Other large long-term epidemiologic studies have shown that obesity is an important risk factor for LV dysfunction or heart failure, after adjustment for other known risk factors such as hypertension, coronary artery disease, and diabetes mellitus.[11,12] The risk for heart failure in obese persons can be increased by as much as 100%.[13] Kenchaiah and colleagues[13] reported that the population attributable risk for heart failure caused by obesity was 13.9% in women and 10.9% in men. After controlling for other risk factors, for every one increment in BMI, the incurred risk of heart failure is increased by 5% in men and 7% in women.[13]

Increased body weight, especially in the form of visceral fat, is an important risk factor for obesity-related heart dysfunction.[14] Other risk factors include increased age and the duration of obesity.[15,16] The duration of morbid obesity is one of the strongest predictors of heart failure among obese persons (**Fig. 1** and **Table 1**); the

probability of developing heart failure is 66% with 20 years of obesity and 93% with 25 years of obesity.[17]

OBESITY-RELATED STRUCTURAL AND FUNCTIONAL CHANGES OF THE HEART

Obesity has been shown to increase LV wall thickening, ventricular mass, dilatation, and remodeling.[18-22] Increased right ventricular (RV) wall thickening and volume have also been described in obese patients.[22] Initial studies of right-heart dysfunction and obesity were confounded by patients having coexisting obstructive sleep apnea (OSA) and pulmonary hypertension. However, more recent studies have shown a correlation between right-heart dysfunction and increased weight.[23,24] The role of obesity in pulmonary hypertension is briefly discussed later in this article.

In one of the earliest descriptions of the effect of obesity on the heart, Smith and Willius[7] described myopathic changes in postmortem specimens of obese patients. A later autopsy study[25] of 12 severely obese patients who had an average body weight of 173 kg confirmed the earlier findings of increased heart mass, biventricular hypertrophy, and diffuse myocyte hypertrophy. In animal models and in obese humans,

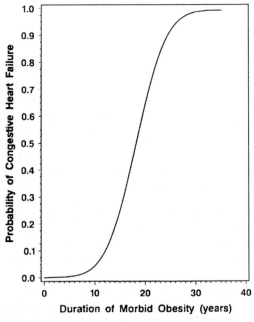

Fig.1. Probability of congestive heart failure as a function of duration of morbid obesity. (*Adapted from* Alpert M, Terry B, Mulekar M, et al. Cardiac morphology and left ventricular function in normotensive morbidly obese patients with and without congestive heart failure, and effect of weight loss. Am J Cardiol 1997;80(6):736–40; with permission.)

Table 1
Factors associated with CHF in morbidly obese patients

Factor	P-value
Duration of morbid obesity	<0.00000002
Left ventricular (LV) internal dimension in diastole	<0.00003
LV end-systolic wall stress	<0.00004
Left atrial dimension	<0.000001
Right ventricular (RV) internal dimension	<0.00004

Abbreviations: CHF, congestive heart failure; LV, left ventricular; RV, right ventricular.
  Data from Alpert M, Terry B, Mulekar M, et al. Cardiac morphology and left ventricular function in normotensive morbidly obese patients with and without congestive heart failure, and effect of weight loss. Am J Cardiol 1997;80(6):736–40.

cardiovascular changes involving myocardial fibrosis have been described.[26] In animal models of obesity, inflammatory cell recruitment as well as myocardial damage and fibrosis have been described and are associated with depressed myocardial contractility.[27]

LV diastolic dysfunction characterized by resistance to LV filling and/or difficulty in ventricular relaxation leading to an increase in LV end-diastolic blood pressures has been described in obese patients.[28] Alpert and colleagues[29] have found that normotensive, morbidly obese patients with CHF have significantly higher LV internal dimensions, LV end-systolic wall stress, and LV mass/height indices, and have significantly more impaired LV systolic function and diastolic filling compared with morbidly obese patients without CHF (see **Table 1**). A study by Wong and colleagues[30] showed that such LV diastolic dysfunction is common in obese patients without obvious other causes such as coronary artery disease, diabetes mellitus, or systemic hypertension. Other studies have provided evidence of subclinical depressed LV systolic function in morbidly obese patients.[31,32] Echocardiographic measurements of myocardial tissue velocity and strain index decrease with increasing degrees of obesity, suggesting early myocardial depression.[30] The use of such new echocardiographic techniques has allowed for the detection of such subclinical findings in obese patients.

PATHOPHYSIOLOGY OF OBESITY CARDIOMYOPATHY

Excessive adipose tissue can lead to increased blood volume and cardiac output. Cardiac output increases because of increased stroke volume, because heart rate does not change with increased body weight.[33–36] As a response to

increased cardiac output, systemic vascular resistance decreases. The increase in cardiac output can also lead to ventricular dilatation.[33,34] Increased LV mass and LV dilatation correlate with obesity, and the dilatation can diminish myofibril shortening and lead to reduced systolic myocardial contraction.[33–36] If ventricular hypertrophic changes correspond with dilatation, cardiac wall stress may normalize and enable systolic function to be preserved. However, if hypertrophy is inadequate for a given ventricular dilatation, systolic dysfunction ensues. Eventual myocardial hypertrophy and fibrosis, myocyte injury, and accumulation of collagen can potentiate diastolic impairment. Subsequent prolonged LV failure can lead to pulmonary venous hypertension and eventual pulmonary arterial hypertension.

Obese patients with OSA and/or obesity hypoventilation syndrome (OHS) can have pulmonary hypertension, and in some of these patients, concurrent LV and RV dysfunction develops.[37] **Fig. 2** shows the proposed pathophysiology of obesity cardiomyopathy.[38] Obesity cardiomyopathy is likely multifactorial. One factor is ventricular and myocardial remodeling in response to an altered hemodynamic load that results from increased body weight.[39] High metabolic activity of adipose tissue and increased lean mass can lead to an increase in the preload and afterload of the circulatory system.[38] These metabolic and hemodynamic changes, in turn, can predispose a person to ventricular remodeling and dilatation, and increased myocardial wall stress and oxygen consumption, which can lead to eventual LV dysfunction.[38]

Various obesity-related metabolic alterations (for example, insulin resistance) may also mediate the development of cardiomyopathy.[40] For example, in patients who have insulin resistance—which is commonly seen in obese patients—myocardial oxygen consumption and

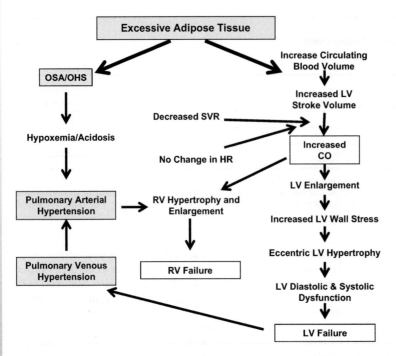

Fig. 2. Pathophysiology of obesity cardiomyopathy. CO, cardiac output; HR, heart rate; LV, left ventricular; OHS, obesity hypoventilation syndrome; OSA, obstructive sleep apnea; RV, right ventricular; SVR, systemic vascular resistance. (*Adapted from* Alpert M. Obesity cardiomyopathy: pathophysiology and evolution of the clinical syndrome. Am J Med Sci 2001;321(4):225–36; with permission.)

efficiency are impaired.[41] The presence of insulin resistance also correlates with myocardial fatty acid uptake, use and oxidation.[41] Excessive use and uptake of myocardial fatty acid can lead to lipotoxic heart disease, a condition in which increased myocardial oxygen consumption and accumulation of potentially toxic intermediates of fatty acid metabolism impair myocardial performance.[42] Excessive fatty acids may cause cardiac myocyte dysfunction owing to the accumulation of toxic long-chain nonesterified fatty acids and their byproducts, such as diacylglerols and ceramides.[43] Elevated myocardial triglyceride content may also alter myocardial structure and function.[44] In addition, insulin-like growth factor 1 (IGF-1) contributes to obesity cardiomyopathy as the level of IGF-1 is reduced with increased body mass.[44] The exact mechanism of how low levels of IGF-1 contribute to cardiomyopathy is not clear, but it has been suggested that obese hearts are resistant to IGF-1 induced cardiac contractile function, possibly mediated by decreased IGF-1 receptor levels.[45]

Obesity-related elevation of various circulating proteins has also been implicated in the pathogenesis of obesity cardiomyopathy. Adiponectin, which is derived from adipose tissues, has a protective effect on cardiac myocytes by limiting the action of insulin in causing adrenergic receptor-mediated cardiac myocyte hypertrophy.[46] In obese persons, tumor necrosis factor (TNF), which suppresses adiponectin, is overexpressed in adipose tissues, thus inhibiting the cardioprotective effects of adiponectin.[46] Obese persons are also insensitive to leptin, a hormone that attenuates contraction of cardiac myocytes.[47] Animal models with nonfunctional leptin receptors show accumulation of myocardial fat, triggering apoptosis and subsequent ventricular dysfunction, which can be reversed when leptin stores are repleted.[48] In addition, various genes for inflammatory mediators and macrophages are up-regulated in adipose tissues.[49] Persistent inflammation can lead to fibrotic changes, particularly in the heart.[50] However, the role of inflammation in myocardial dysfunction is not clear.

Other mechanisms have been postulated for the development of obesity cardiomyopathy.[4] Insulin resistance and hyperinsulinemia can affect the renin-angiotensin-aldosterone (RAA) system by increasing the levels of the renin substrate angiotensinogen. Elevated angiotensinogen increases levels of angiotensin II, a potent cardiac myocyte growth factor that can result in increased cellular proliferation, hypertrophy, fibrotic changes, and subsequent myocardial dysfunction.[51] Elevated levels of aldosterone, also common in obesity, can facilitate interstitial myocardial and perivascular fibrotic changes,[52] effects of which can be reversed by using anti-aldosterone agents. The sympathetic nervous system is activated in patients with myocardial dysfunction, leading to a potentially vicious cycle of signaling cascade that results in the progressive loss of cardiac myocytes and further myocardial dysfunction.[53] Other effects on myocardial function include impairment of the signaling transduction of the β-adrenergic receptor and down-regulation of sarcoplasmic reticular calcium ATPase, an important inotropic protein.[53]

Microvascular disease and endothelial dysfunction have also been described in the cardiac vasculature of obese individuals.[54] Episodic vasoconstriction caused by this endothelial dysfunction as well as tissue microinfarction and reperfusion injuries all contribute to myocardial dysfunction.[55]

DIAGNOSIS OF OBESITY CARDIOMYOPATHY
Clinical Manifestations

Approximately 10% of persons with a BMI ≥40 kg/m^2 or with an actual body weight more than 75% over ideal body weight develop signs and symptoms of obesity cardiomyopathy.[35,36,56,57] It is especially typical in persons with a duration of such obesity of more than 10 years (see **Fig. 1**).[17] Symptoms of obesity cardiomyopathy include progressive: dyspnea on exertion; fatigue; orthopnea; paroxysmal nocturnal dyspnea; and lower extremity edema. Affected patients often have normal LV systolic function.[8] However, some obese patients have combined left-sided diastolic and systolic dysfunction.[58] Arrhythmias, such as atrial fibrillation and atrial flutter, occur in some patients. OSA and OHS, which occur in approximately 10% of morbidly obese patients, contribute to right-sided cardiac dysfunction and, in severe cases, can lead to abdominal congestion and swelling, lower extremity edema, and symptoms of right-sided heart failure.[59] Patients with obesity cardiomyopathy may present with pulmonary crackles, elevated jugular venous distention, an S$_3$ and S$_4$, hepatojugular reflux, lower extremity edema, and ascites; such findings are most common in patients with established heart failure.[60] For patients with concurrent OSA or OHS, additional signs of Cheyne-Stokes respiration, cyanosis, retinal venous congestion, and papilledema can be observed.[60] However, because such features are nonspecific, history and physical examination alone are not reliable for the diagnosis of obesity cardiomyopathy.

Patients with obesity cardiomyopathy die either of progressive heart failure[7] or of sudden cardiac death.[9,61–63] In most cases of the sudden cardiac deaths, the patients have had established heart failure and developed terminal ventricular tachyarrhythmias.[63] Fatty and mononuclear cell infiltration and fibrotic changes involving the sinus node have

been postulated to be responsible for fatal arrhythmias.[64]

Electrocardiography

The electrocardiogram of morbidly obese patients is often characterized by low QRS voltage and a mild leftward shift in P, QRS, and T-wave axes.[65] Excessive adipose tissue makes diagnosis of LV hypertrophy difficult. Changes consistent with RV hypertrophy as well as T-wave flattening in the inferior and lateral leads may also occur; these changes may be caused by the heart being in the horizontal position in obese patients.[66]

Imaging

Cardiomegaly is commonly observed on chest radiograph in morbidly obese patients, with a 1 mm increase in cardiac diameter for each 3-lb increase in body weight.[38,67] Transthoracic echocardiography is used routinely for the measurement of systolic and diastolic function, but the use of echocardiography is limited in obese patients because of their body habitus. Only 70% of morbidly obese patients can have a complete and reliable transthoracic echocardiogram.[60] Conventional two-dimensional echocardiography can reliably measure global LV function and LV and RV volumes and dimensions.[40]

With newer Doppler imaging techniques, the function of the myocardium can be directly assessed more sensitively.[30,68] Using ultrasonographic tissue characterization with tissue Doppler, subclinical changes of LV structure and function in obese persons without overt heart disease can be detected.[30] Another study showed that increases in BMI in overweight and obese persons without overt heart disease were associated with increasing severity of RV dysfunction, independent of sleep apnea.[23] Incorporating myocardial integrated backscatter parameters with cardiac ultrasonography enables myocardial tissue density to be measured; myocardial tissue density is a marker of myocardial contractile function and abnormal density suggests fibrotic changes.[69] This technique has been useful to detect hypertrophic cardiomyopathy, characterized by an abnormally increased wall reflectivity.[70] Using such techniques to measure subclinical myocardial dysfunction, Wong and colleagues[24] found that in obese patients (BMI >30 kg/m^2), weight loss (average of 4.5 kg) due to lifestyle intervention correlated with modest improvement in myocardial reflectivity and diastolic function as measured by an increase in diastolic mitral annular velocity (Em) (**Fig. 3**). These patients had normal pre-intervention systolic ejection fractions and no

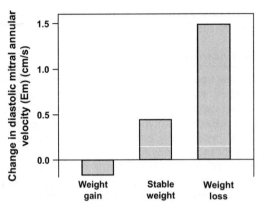

Fig. 3. Change in diastolic mitral annular velocity (Em) as a function of weight changes. Improved diastolic parameter (with an increased Em) is associated with weight loss. Lowest tertile shows minor weight change; middle tertile shows stable weight; and highest tertile shows weight loss in obese patients. (*Adapted from* Wong C, Byrne N, O'Moore-Sullivan T, et al. Effect of weight loss due to lifestyle intervention on subclinical cardiovascular dysfunction in obesity (body mass index >30 kg/m2). Am J Cardiol 2006; 98(12):1593–8; with permission.)

known history of cardiovascular disease. Weight loss was not associated with a significant change in LV systolic parameters, such as global heart strain, strain rate, or regional myocardial systolic velocity.[23,24]

Dynamic parameters such as ventricular ejection fraction with exercise enable myocardial contractile reserve to be measured.[23] For example, Alpert and colleagues[71] used echocardiography and radionuclide ventriculography to study 22 patients who weighed more than twice their ideal body weight and had no evidence of underlying heart or pulmonary disease; the study found a significant negative correlation between percent over ideal body weight and RV exercise response, as defined by the change in RV ejection fraction during peak exercise. In morbidly obese individuals without obvious RV dilatation, evaluation of RV exercise response could be an important marker for early cardiomyopathy.[71,72] A study of morbidly obese patients (mean BMI ~50 kg/m²) awaiting bariatric surgery demonstrated impaired cardiac response to fluid challenge and exercise characterized by increased LV end-diastolic volume and decreased LV ejection fraction.[20] After surgery and weight loss of a mean of ~54 kg, cardiac function improved with reduced filling pressures and increased LV work during fluid and exercise challenges, suggesting the presence of noncompliant ventricles in these patients with obesity cardiomyopathy.

Nuclear ventriculography can assess global and regional systolic function, but the images can be compromised in obese patients because of background and scattering of signals as a result of body habitus and adiposity.[73] Other imaging modalities, including CT and MRI, can evaluate ventricular structure and function. Multidetector row computed tomography (MDCT) can identify coronary artery disease and assess global and regional systolic function.[74] MDCT has superior spatial resolution for the analysis of ventricular size, mass, and systolic function, but it lacks temporal resolution for optimal detection of end-diastolic function.[74] However, MDCT is being improved with newer technologies that incorporate multisegment reconstruction and dual-source scanning.[75] The procedure requires contrast enhancement and exposure to radiation, and currently its use is not recommended for routine cardiovascular assessment.[74] MRI, which has excellent spatial and temporal resolution, remains the reference imaging standard for the assessment of LV function.[76]

Biomarkers

The measurement of biomarkers, such as brain natriuretic peptide (BNP) and N-terminal pro-BNP (NT-proBNP), to screen for elevated ventricular filling pressures is now a mainstay in the management of patients with heart failure.[77] However, serum levels of these biomarkers are often decreased in obese patients, even in those with elevated ventricular filling pressures; in fact, the levels of BNP and NT-proBNP are inversely proportional to BMI, irrespective of the presence or severity of heart failure in the obese patients (**Fig. 4**).[78–80] This relationship has been attributed to reduced synthesis or secretion of the peptides, rather than increased clearance.[78–80] In contrast, a recent review concluded that NT-proBNP levels in patients with acute dyspnea can be equally useful to rule out heart failure in obese and in lean patients, and no adjustment of NT-proBNP thresholds for BMI is recommended.[81]

MANAGEMENT OF OBESITY CARDIOMYOPATHY

Weight reduction is the only effective long-term management for obesity cardiomyopathy. Weight loss can be achieved by: (1) dieting and moderate exercise; (2) pharmacologic therapies for direct weight loss or that control diabetes mellitus, hypertension, and sleep disorders; and, (3) especially for the morbidly obese, bariatric surgical procedures. The role and effect of weight loss interventions on cardiac function have been reviewed.[5,60] Loss of as little as 5% to 10% of

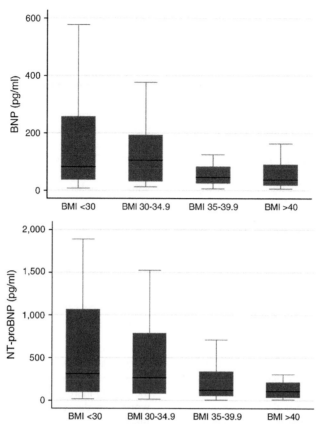

Fig. 4. Relationship of BNP and NT-proBNP with increasing BMI. There is incremental decrease in both levels of BNP and NT-proBNP with increasing BMI. BNP, brain natriuretic peptide; NT-proBNP, N-terminal pro-BNP; BMI, body mass index (kg/m²). (*Adapted from* Taylor J, Christenson R, Rao K, et al. B-type natriuretic peptide and N-terminal pro B-type natriuretic peptide are depressed in obesity despite higher left ventricular end diastolic pressures. Am Heart J 2006;152(6):1071–6; with permission.)

body weight in obese patients can improve glucose metabolism, lipid profile, and cardiovascular risk.[82,83] There have been few studies of the relationship between nonsurgical weight loss measures and myocardial changes. In one such study, 106 asymptomatic obese persons (BMI >30 kg/m²), who had cardiovascular risk factors but no structural heart disease on echocardiography or ischemic heart disease on stress testing, were enrolled in a weight loss program consisting of dietary modification, caloric limitation, and moderate exercise.[24] Diastolic myocardial velocities improved in 48 subjects, with documented weight loss of ~4.5 kg after 8 to 12 weeks.[24] However, there was no improvement in blood pressure or LV mass index. In another study of 41 young, overweight hypertensive patients, dietary weight loss resulted in improved diastolic function and LV mass index.[84] Therefore, there is evidence that weight loss through nonsurgical means can improve LV diastolic dysfunction, with or without improvement in LV mass.[84] There is also evidence that weight loss from combined

dietary changes and exercise leads to a more long-term weight loss maintenance and that involvement of physical activity helps improve LV wall thickness more than diet alone.[85,86]

Pharmacologic weight-loss therapies include drugs such as: sibutramine, a serotonin reuptake inhibitor; orlistat, a lipase; and rimonabant, a blocker of cannabinoid-1 receptor.[87] (Also see the article by Bray in this issue.)The effects of pharmacologic weight loss on the cardiovascular system are not clear, and the mechanism is not well established. There is some reduction in LV mass index after sertraline-related weight loss.[88] Rimonabant has been shown to reduce cardiovascular risk, but its effect on the myocardium is not known.[89] In one study, weight loss with sibutramine did not significantly improve LV structure and function.[90]

Bariatric surgical weight loss has been shown to have significant beneficial effects on the heart, most likely because patients who undergo the procedure are usually morbidly obese and have a postoperative weight loss often of more than 20% of their initial body weight.[91] (Also see the article by Yurcisin, Gaddor and DeMaria in this issue.) Bariatric surgery has been shown to reduce LV wall thickness and size,[18] improve systolic[18] and diastolic function,[92] improve RV function,[93] and reduce ventricular filling pressures and LV work during exercise and fluid challenge.[20] Obese patients with preexisting LV abnormalities tend to have improvement in LV function after bariatric weight loss surgery.[94] The cardiovascular benefit from weight loss likely depends on the severity of obesity, the amount of weight loss achieved, and the duration of obesity.[95]

The beneficial effects of weight loss on LV structure and function can be attributed to improved hemodynamics and decreased oxygen consumption requirements. However, the metabolic effects of weight reduction, especially in the mildly obese, may also be important.[5] Weight loss improves myocardial function by improving insulin sensitivity,[96] modulation of the RAA system,[97] and alteration of the peroxisome proliferators-activated receptors (PPARγ),[98] transcriptions factors that are important in adipocyte differentiation and cardiac energy metabolism and remodeling.[99] For example, weight loss has been shown to have a beneficial effect on plasma renin activity and plasma aldosterone levels in obese patients.[97] Weight loss-associated induction of PPARγ correlates with improved cardiovascular function as measured by improved ejection fraction.[100] Studies on weight loss resulting from liposuction alone have shown to have favorable hemodynamic benefits, such as improvement in systolic blood pressures;[101] however, liposuction did not have an effect on insulin action or risk factors for coronary artery disease.[102]

Because obesity cardiomyopathy is not well studied or well understood, obese patients with heart failure are treated with conventional regimens consisting of diuretics, angiotensin converting enzyme inhibitors, angiotensin-receptor blockers, digoxin, and β-blockers. Blocking the RAA system with angiotensin-receptor blockers has a favorable effect on ventricular chamber size and may improve glucose metabolism and prevent myocardial fibrosis.[103]

The role of β-blockers in nonischemic cardiomyopathy is unknown. Generally, β-blocker therapy improves myocardial contractility, up-regulates β-adrenergic receptors, and reverses cardiac remodeling processes.[104] β-blockers, especially β1-selective β-blockers, have potential adverse effects of inducing weight gain and peripheral vasoconstriction, and unfavorably altering lipid and carbohydrate metabolism, and should therefore be prescribed with caution in obese patients.[105] Nonselective β-blockers, such as carvedilol, may be more appropriate for obese patients with heart failure.[106]

Some of the medications that obese patients with diabetes mellitus take have potential beneficial effects on the myocardium. The thiazolidinediones often used by obese diabetic patients can help increase insulin sensitivity by increasing GLUT4 expression (an insulin-regulated glucose transporter in adipose tissues) and decrease myocardial free fatty acid and triglyceride levels.[107] Thiazolidinediones also have an important role in regulating peroxisome proliferator-activated receptor (PPARγ), increasing myocardial glucose oxidation, and improving endothelial function.[107,108] Because obesity is often associated with such comorbidities as diabetes mellitus, hypertension, and OSA, management of obesity cardiomyopathy should also address each of these comorbidities.

THE ROLE OF OBESITY IN PULMONARY HYPERTENSION

OSA is common in obese patients; it has been reported that a BMI >25 kg/m^2 has a sensitivity of 93% and a specificity of 74% for OSA.[109] Increasing increments of BMI are associated with worsening degrees of OSA in a dose dependent fashion.[110,111] It has been postulated that OSA can contribute to pulmonary hypertension and RV failure (see **Fig. 2**).[38,112] Repetitive chronic upper airway collapse and oxygen desaturation can lead to hypoxic pulmonary vasoconstriction that eventually can result in pulmonary hypertension.[113,114] Frequent episodes of increased pulmonary artery pressure during sleep have been documented in patients with OSA.[115] However, it is not known how much OSA, independent of coexisting pulmonary or heart disease, contributes to sustained daytime pulmonary hypertension (Also see article by Shah and Roux in this issue.). It is even more difficult to determine the role that obesity, itself, independent of OSA, plays in the development of pulmonary hypertension. In 2008, the American Heart Association and American College of Cardiology expert consensus scientific statement on sleep apnea and cardiovascular disease recognizes sleep apnea as a risk factor for pulmonary arterial hypertension.[116]

Defining the role of OSA in pulmonary hypertension has been difficult: pulmonary hypertension is diagnosed by various methods, including conventional echocardiography and varying right heart and pulmonary artery pressure cutoffs; accurate echocardiographic measurements are difficult to obtain in obese patients;[117] and OSA and pulmonary hypertension share common risk factors, such as aging and obesity. It has been reported that 5% of normal individuals with a BMI >30 kg/m² have pulmonary arterial systolic pressure (PASP) over 50 mm Hg.[118] The reported prevalence of pulmonary hypertension in OSA has ranged from 17% to 52%,[115,119,120] with the largest study of 220 subjects with OSA showing 17% meeting the criteria for pulmonary hypertension.[115] Most of these patients had relatively mild disease, with only two of 37 patients having a PASP >35 mm Hg.[115] A small study that excluded patients with clinically significant pulmonary or cardiac disease showed that 41% (11 out of 27) of patients with OSA had mild pulmonary hypertension, with a mean pulmonary artery pressure of 26 mm Hg.[121] There was no significant difference in BMI and apnea-hypopnea index (AHI) between OSA patients with pulmonary hypertension and those without pulmonary hypertenstion. Two other studies that also excluded patients with significant cardiopulmonary diseases found that approximately 20% of patients with OSA (mostly with AHI >30) had mild pulmonary hypertension.[122,123]

There is mounting evidence that treatment of OSA with continuous positive airway pressure (CPAP) can lower daytime pulmonary artery pressure, suggesting that it is plausible that OSA may be an independent cause of pulmonary hypertension.[124] OSA has been associated with increases in pulmonary arterial pressure during obstructive breathing events.[112] Elevated pulmonary arterial pressure has been attributed to increased pulmonary vascular resistance caused by hypoxemia and hypercapnia.[121,125,126] Relief of upper airway obstruction and hypoxemia with continuous positive airway pressure (CPAP),[124] or with tracheostomy,[125] can lead to improvement and/or resolution of pulmonary hypertension. Studies on the effects of 6-month CPAP therapy showed reduction in mean pulmonary arterial pressure in patients with OSA and pulmonary hypertension.[127,128] OSA patients without pulmonary hypertension also had demonstrable improvement in mean pulmonary arterial pressure after CPAP use.[127] The same study showed that patients with OSA and pulmonary hypertension tended to have a greater BMI those without pulmonary hypertension (BMI 41 kg/m² ± 7 versus 32 kg/m² ± 4).[127]

A more recent randomized crossover, placebo-controlled trial confirmed the beneficial effect of CPAP therapy versus sham treatment on pulmonary hypertension in a subset of patients with OSA.[129] In this study, patients with pulmonary hypertension also tended to have a greater BMI and more severe sleep apnea, and showed a greater reduction of mean pulmonary arterial pressure with CPAP therapy than patients without pulmonary hypertension.[129] Severe OSA was found to be independently associated with pulmonary hypertension and to be directly related to severity of disease and the presence of diastolic dysfunction.[129] Another study, however, showed no significant improvement in pulmonary arterial pressure after CPAP therapy, although the patients with OSA studied had such comorbidities as chronic obstructive pulmonary disease, and in many patients the pulmonary artery pressure was relatively normal before CPAP therapy.[130] It is unclear whether nocturnal hypoxemia alone can lead to daytime pulmonary arterial hypertension or whether it is necessary to have concomitant daytime hypoxemia, such as in patients with severe obesity and obesity hypoventilation syndrome. Nevertheless, the most recent pulmonary hypertension classification has included sleep-disordered breathing in the respiratory disorder category that is associated with pulmonary hypertension.[131] Larger studies are needed to evaluate the association between OSA and pulmonary hypertension and whether CPAP therapy has sustained benefits on pulmonary hypertension.

Primary pulmonary hypertension, which is more common in young persons, is now seen in those patients who are obese. A review of patients referred to a pulmonary hypertension center

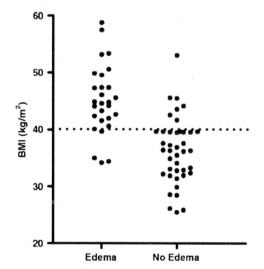

Fig. 5. Increased BMI is associated with increased evidence of right heart failure manifested by leg edema. BMI, body mass index. (*Adapted from* O'Hearn D, Gold A, Gold M, et al. Lower extremity edema and pulmonary hypertension in morbidly obese patients with obstructive sleep apnea. Sleep Breath 2009;13(1):25–4; with permission.)

showed that 48% with severe pulmonary hypertension were obese.[132] However, there is a lack of evidence to support a causal relationship between pulmonary hypertension and obesity in the absence of other comorbidities. Obese patients are known to have a higher incidence of pulmonary hypertension when they have a history of anorexigenic agent use.[133] In a small study following patients with unexplained lower leg edema and pulmonary hypertension, almost all were obese and most had OSA without daytime somnolence.[134] Another study[59] found that lower extremity edema and pulmonary hypertension were common in morbidly obese patients (BMI >40 kg/m^2) with OSA (**Fig. 5**). It can be postulated that obesity can worsen existing pulmonary hypertension by providing an additional burden of altered pulmonary mechanics on a failing right ventricle. Unfortunately, at the present time, not much is known about the precise role obesity itself has on the development of pulmonary hypertension independent of OSA or history of anorexigen use.

SUMMARY

Obesity has significant effects on the cardiovascular system and produces various structural cardiac changes and hemodynamic changes that can lead to heart failure. There is evidence to support the existence of obesity cardiomyopathy, independent of other known risk factors for heart failure, such as coronary artery disease, systemic hypertension, diabetes mellitus, and obstructive sleep apnea. Mechanisms for the development of obesity cardiomyopathy include obesity-related metabolic disturbances. The use of more sophisticated myocardial imaging techniques may help in the detection of subclinical obesity-related myocardial changes. Significant weight reduction has been shown to reverse some of the myocardial effects of obesity.

Defining the role of obesity in pulmonary hypertension is difficult. There is mounting evidence that OSA, which is frequently present in obese patients, can be an independent cause of pulmonary hypertension. The prevalence of pulmonary hypertension in OSA has been reported to range from 17% to 52%. Treatment of OSA with CPAP or tracheostomy can lower daytime pulmonary artery pressures.

This review emphasizes the potential importance of obesity in the development of both left-sided and right-sided heart failure. More research is needed to define the pathophysiology of obesity cardiomyopathy and the relationship between obesity and pulmonary hypertension.

REFERENCES

1. Puska P, Nishida C, Porter D. Obesity and overweight. In: World Health Organization: Global strategy on diet physical activity and health. Geneva: WHO; 2003. p. 1–2.
2. Allison D, Fontaine K, Manson J, et al. Annual deaths attributable to obesity in the United States. JAMA 1999;282(16):1530–8.
3. Hunt S. ACC/AHA 2005 guideline update for the diagnosis and management of chronic heart failure in the adult: a report of the American College of Cardiology/American Heart Association Task Force on Practice Guidelines (Writing committee to update the 2001 guidelines for the evaluation and management of heart failure). J Am Coll Cardiol 2005;46(6):e1–82.
4. Wong C, Marwick T. Obesity cardiomyopathy: pathogenesis and pathophysiology. Nat Clin Pract Cardiovasc Med 2007;4(8):436–43.
5. Wong C, Marwick T. Obesity cardiomyopathy: diagnosis and therapeutic implications. Nat Clin Pract Cardiovasc Med 2007;4(9):480–90.
6. Poirier P, Giles T, Bray G, et al. Obesity and cardiovascular disease: pathophysiology, evaluation, and effect of weight loss: an update of the 1997 American Heart Association Scientific Statement on Obesity and Heart Disease from the Obesity Committee of the Council on Nutrition, Physical Activity, and Metabolism. Circulation 2006;113(6):898–918.
7. Smith H, Willius F. Adiposity of the heart: a clinical and pathologic study of one hundred and thirty-six obese patients. Arch Intern Med 1933;52:911–31.
8. Kasper E, Hruban R, Baughman K. Cardiomyopathy of obesity: a clinicopathologic evaluation of 43 obese patients with heart failure. Am J Cardiol 1992;70(9):921–4.
9. Duflou J, Virmani R, Rabin I, et al. Sudden death as a result of heart disease in morbid obesity. Am Heart J 1995;130(2):306–13.
10. Hubert H, Feinleib M, McNamara P, et al. Obesity as an independent risk factor for cardiovascular disease: a 26-year follow-up of participants in the Framingham Heart Study. Circulation 1983;67(5):968–77.
11. He J, Ogden L, Bazzano L, et al. Risk factors for congestive heart failure in US men and women: NHANES I epidemiologic follow-up study. Arch Intern Med 2001;161(7):996–1002.
12. Murphy N, MacIntyre K, Stewart S, et al. Long-term cardiovascular consequences of obesity: 20-year follow-up of more than 15,000 middle-aged men and women (the Renfrew-Paisley study). Eur Heart J 2006;27(1):96–106.
13. Kenchaiah S, Evans J, Levy D, et al. Obesity and the risk of heart failure. N Engl J Med 2002; 347(5):305–13.

14. Malavazos A, Ermetici F, Coman C, et al. Influence of epicardial adipose tissue and adipocytokine levels on cardiac abnormalities in visceral obesity. Int J Cardiol 2007;121(1):132–4.

15. Alpert M, Lambert C, Panayiotou H, et al. Relation of duration of morbid obesity to left ventricular mass, systolic function, and diastolic filling, and effect of weight loss. Am J Cardiol 1995;76(16):1194–7.

16. Licata G, Scaglione R, Paterna S, et al. Left ventricular function response to exercise in normotensive obese subjects: influence of degree and duration of obesity. Int J Cardiol 1992;37(2):223–30.

17. Alpert M, Terry B, Mulekar M, et al. Cardiac morphology and left ventricular function in normotensive morbidly obese patients with and without congestive heart failure, and effect of weight loss. Am J Cardiol 1997;80(6):736–40.

18. Karason K, Wallentin I, Larsson B, et al. Effects of obesity and weight loss on left ventricular mass and relative wall thickness: survey and intervention study. BMJ 1997;315(7113):912–6.

19. Lauer M, Anderson K, Kannel W, et al. The impact of obesity on left ventricular mass and geometry. The Framingham Heart Study. JAMA 1991;266(2):231–6.

20. Alaud-din A, Meterissian S, Lisbona R, et al. Assessment of cardiac function in patients who were morbidly obese. Surgery 1990;108(4):809–18 [discussion: 818–20].

21. Nakajima T, Fujioka S, Tokunaga K, et al. Noninvasive study of left ventricular performance in obese patients: influence of duration of obesity. Circulation 1985;71(3):481–6.

22. Amad K, Brennan J, Alexander J. The cardiac pathology of chronic exogenous obesity. Circulation 1965;32(5):740–5.

23. Wong C, O'Moore-Sullivan T, Leano R, et al. Association of subclinical right ventricular dysfunction with obesity. J Am Coll Cardiol 2006;47(3):611–6.

24. Wong C, Byrne N, O'Moore-Sullivan T, et al. Effect of weight loss due to lifestyle intervention on subclinical cardiovascular dysfunction in obesity (body mass index >30 kg/m2). Am J Cardiol 2006;98(12):1593–8.

25. Warnes C, Roberts W. The heart in massive (more than 300 pounds or 136 kilograms) obesity: analysis of 12 patients studied at necropsy. Am J Cardiol 1984;54(8):1087–91.

26. Cittadini A, Mantzoros C, Hampton T, et al. Cardiovascular abnormalities in transgenic mice with reduced brown fat: an animal model of human obesity. Circulation 1999;100(21):2177–83.

27. Mizushige K, Yao L, Noma T, et al. Alteration in left ventricular diastolic filling and accumulation of myocardial collagen at insulin-resistant prediabetic stage of a type II diabetic rat model. Circulation 2000;101(8):899–907.

28. Powell B, Redfield M, Bybee K, et al. Association of obesity with left ventricular remodeling and diastolic dysfunction in patients without coronary artery disease. Am J Cardiol 2006;98(1):116–20.

29. Alpert M, Lambert C, Terry B, et al. Influence of left ventricular mass on left ventricular diastolic filling in normotensive morbid obesity. Am Heart J 1995;130(5):1068–73.

30. Wong C, O'Moore-Sullivan T, Leano R, et al. Alterations of left ventricular myocardial characteristics associated with obesity. Circulation 2004;110(19):3081–7.

31. Peterson L, Waggoner A, Schechtman K, et al. Alterations in left ventricular structure and function in young healthy obese women: assessment by echocardiography and tissue Doppler imaging. J Am Coll Cardiol 2004;43(8):1399–404.

32. Ferraro S, Perrone-Filardi P, Desiderio A, et al. Left ventricular systolic and diastolic function in severe obesity: a radionuclide study. Cardiology 1996;87(4):347–53.

33. Lavie C, Messerli F. Cardiovascular adaptation to obesity and hypertension. Chest 1986;90(2):275–9.

34. Contaldo F, Pasanisi F, Finelli C, et al. Obesity, heart failure and sudden death. Nutr Metab Cardiovasc Dis 2002;12(4):190–7.

35. Alexander J. Obesity and the heart. Heart Dis Stroke 1993;2(4):317–21.

36. Alexander J. Obesity and coronary heart disease. Am J Med Sci 2001;321(4):215–24.

37. Bradley T, Floras J. Obstructive sleep apnoea and its cardiovascular consequences. Lancet 2009;373(9657):82–93.

38. Alpert M. Obesity cardiomyopathy: pathophysiology and evolution of the clinical syndrome. Am J Med Sci 2001;321(4):225–36.

39. Schram K, Sweeney G. Implications of myocardial matrix remodeling by adipokines in obesity-related heart failure. Trends Cardiovasc Med 2008;18(6):199–205.

40. Banerjee S, Peterson L. Myocardial metabolism and cardiac performance in obesity and insulin resistance. Curr Cardiol Rep 2007;9(2):143–9.

41. Peterson L, Herrero P, Schechtman K, et al. Effect of obesity and insulin resistance on myocardial substrate metabolism and efficiency in young women. Circulation 2004;109(18):2191–6.

42. Zhou Y, Grayburn P, Karim A, et al. Lipotoxic heart disease in obese rats: implications for human obesity. Proc Natl Acad Sci U S A 2000;97(4):1784–9.

43. Listenberger L, Schaffer J. Mechanisms of lipoapoptosis: implications for human heart disease. Trends Cardiovasc Med 2002;12(3):134–8.

44. McGavock J, Victor R, Unger R, et al. Adiposity of the heart, revisited. Ann Intern Med 2006;144(7):517–24.

45. Ren J, Samson W, Sowers J. Insulin-like growth factor I as a cardiac hormone: physiological and pathophysiological implications in heart disease. J Mol Cell Cardiol 1999;31(11):2049–61.

46. Shibata R, Ouchi N, Ito M, et al. Adiponectin-mediated modulation of hypertrophic signals in the heart. Nat Med 2004;10(12):1384–9.

47. Nickola M, Wold L, Colligan P, et al. Leptin attenuates cardiac contraction in rat ventricular myocytes. Role of NO. Hypertension 2000;36(4):501–5.

48. Minhas K, Khan S, Raju S, et al. Leptin repletion restores depressed {beta}-adrenergic contractility in ob/ob mice independently of cardiac hypertrophy. J Physiol 2005;565(Pt 2):463–74.

49. Rasouli N, Kern P. Adipocytokines and the metabolic complications of obesity. J Clin Endocrinol Metab 2008;93(11 Suppl 1):S64–73.

50. Xu H, Barnes G, Yang Q, et al. Chronic inflammation in fat plays a crucial role in the development of obesity-related insulin resistance. J Clin Invest 2003;112(12):1821–30.

51. Harte A, McTernan P, Chetty R, et al. Insulin-mediated upregulation of the renin angiotensin system in human subcutaneous adipocytes is reduced by rosiglitazone. Circulation 2005;111(15):1954–61.

52. Brilla C, Matsubara L, Weber K. Anti-aldosterone treatment and the prevention of myocardial fibrosis in primary and secondary hyperaldosteronism. J Mol Cell Cardiol 1993;25(5):563–75.

53. Corry D, Tuck M. Obesity, hypertension, and sympathetic nervous system activity. Curr Hypertens Rep 1999;1(2):119–26.

54. Sundell J, Laine H, Luotolahti M, et al. Obesity affects myocardial vasoreactivity and coronary flow response to insulin. Obes Res 2002;10(7):617–24.

55. Sivitz W, Wayson S, Bayless M, et al. Obesity impairs vascular relaxation in human subjects: hyperglycemia exaggerates adrenergic vasoconstriction arterial dysfunction in obesity and diabetes. J Diabetes Complications 2007;21(3):149–57.

56. Estes EJ, Sieker H, Mcintosh H, et al. Reversible cardiopulmonary syndrome with extreme obesity. Circulation 1957;16(2):179–87.

57. MacGregor M, Block A, Ball WJ. Topics in clinical medicine: serious complications and sudden death in the Pickwickian syndrome. Johns Hopkins Med J 1970;126(5):279–95.

58. Desai A, Fang J. Heart failure with preserved ejection fraction: hypertension, diabetes, obesity/sleep apnea, and hypertrophic and infiltrative cardiomyopathy. Heart Fail Clin 2008;4(1):87–97.

59. O'Hearn D, Gold A, Gold M, et al. Lower extremity edema and pulmonary hypertension in morbidly obese patients with obstructive sleep apnea. Sleep Breath 2009;13(1):25–34.

60. Alpert M. Management of obesity cardiomyopathy. Am J Med Sci 2001;321(4):237–41.

61. Drenick E, Fisler J. Sudden cardiac arrest in morbidly obese surgical patients unexplained after autopsy. Am J Surg 1988;155(6):720–6.

62. Bharati S, Lev M. Cardiac conduction system involvement in sudden death of obese young people. Am Heart J 1995;129(2):273–81.

63. Messerli F, Nunez B, Ventura H, et al. Overweight and sudden death. Increased ventricular ectopy in cardiopathy of obesity. Arch Intern Med 1987;147(10):1725–8.

64. Nishida N, Kudo K, Esaki R, et al. Two cases of sudden death in obese psychiatric patients with microscopic cardiopulmonary abnormalities. Fukuoka Igaku Zasshi 2003;94(4):66–74.

65. Eisenstein I, Edelstein J, Sarma R, et al. The electrocardiogram in obesity. J Electrocardiol 1982;15(2):115–8.

66. Okin P, Roman M, Devereux R, et al. ECG identification of left ventricular hypertrophy. Relationship of test performance to body habitus. J Electrocardiol 1996;29(Suppl):256–61.

67. Ungerleider HE, Clark CP. A study of the transverse diameter of the heart silhouette with prediction based on teleroentgenogram. Am Heart J 1939;17:92–8.

68. Garcia M, Thomas J, Klein A. New Doppler echocardiographic applications for the study of diastolic function. J Am Coll Cardiol 1998;32(4):865–75.

69. Wickline S, Thomas LR, Miller J, et al. A relationship between ultrasonic integrated backscatter and myocardial contractile function. J Clin Invest 1985;76(6):2151–60.

70. Lucarini A, Talarico L, Di Bello V, et al. Increased myocardial ultrasonic reflectivity is associated with extreme hypertensive left ventricular hypertrophy: a tissue characterization study in humans. Am J Hypertens 1998;11(12):1442–9.

71. Alpert M, Singh A, Terry B, et al. Effect of exercise and cavity size on right ventricular function in morbid obesity. Am J Cardiol 1989;64(19):1361–5.

72. Alpert M, Singh A, Terry B, et al. Effect of exercise on left ventricular systolic function and reserve in morbid obesity. Am J Cardiol 1989;63(20):1478–82.

73. Abidov A, Hachamovitch R, Berman D. Modern nuclear cardiac imaging in diagnosis and clinical management of patients with left ventricular dysfunction. Minerva Cardioangiol 2004;52(6):505–19.

74. Orakzai S, Orakzai R, Nasir K, et al. Assessment of cardiac function using multidetector row computed tomography. J Comput Assist Tomogr 2006;30(4):555–63.

75. Sigurdsson G. CT for assessing ventricular remodeling: is it ready for prime time? Curr Heart Fail Rep 2008;5(1):16–22.

76. Epstein F. MRI of left ventricular function. J Nucl Cardiol 2007;14(5):729–44.

77. Lainscak M, von Haehling S, Anker S. Natriuretic peptides and other biomarkers in chronic heart failure: from BNP, NT-proBNP, and MR-proANP to routine biochemical markers. Int J Cardiol 2009; 132(3):303–11.

78. Wang T, Larson M, Levy D, et al. Impact of obesity on plasma natriuretic peptide levels. Circulation 2004;109(5):594–600.

79. Taylor J, Christenson R, Rao K, et al. B-type natriuretic peptide and N-terminal pro B-type natriuretic peptide are depressed in obesity despite higher left ventricular end diastolic pressures. Am Heart J 2006;152(6):1071–6.

80. Iwanaga Y, Kihara Y, Niizuma S, et al. BNP in overweight and obese patients with heart failure: an analysis based on the BNP-LV diastolic wall stress relationship. J Card Fail 2007;13(8):663–7.

81. Bayes-Genis A, DeFilippi C, Januzzi JJ. Understanding amino-terminal pro-B-type natriuretic peptide in obesity. Am J Cardiol 2008;101(3A): 89–94.

82. Mertens I, Van Gaal L. Overweight, obesity, and blood pressure: the effects of modest weight reduction. Obes Res 2000;8(3):270–8.

83. Tuomilehto J, Lindström J, Eriksson J, et al. Prevention of type 2 diabetes mellitus by changes in lifestyle among subjects with impaired glucose tolerance. N Engl J Med 2001;344(18): 1343–50.

84. MacMahon S, Wilcken D, Macdonald G. The effect of weight reduction on left ventricular mass. A randomized controlled trial in young, overweight hypertensive patients. N Engl J Med 1986;314(6): 334–9.

85. Wirth A, Kröger H. Improvement of left ventricular morphology and function in obese subjects following a diet and exercise program. Int J Obes Relat Metab Disord 1995;19(1):61–6.

86. Hinderliter A, Sherwood A, Gullette E, et al. Reduction of left ventricular hypertrophy after exercise and weight loss in overweight patients with mild hypertension. Arch Intern Med 2002;162(12): 1333–9.

87. Bray G, Ryan D. Drug treatment of the overweight patient. Gastroenterology 2007;132(6):2239–52.

88. Jordan J, Messerli F, Lavie C, et al. Reduction of weight and left ventricular mass with serotonin uptake inhibition in obese patients with systemic hypertension. Am J Cardiol 1995;75(10):743–4.

89. Aronne L, Isoldi K. Cannabinoid-1 receptor blockade in cardiometabolic risk reduction: efficacy. Am J Cardiol 2007;100(12A):18P–26P.

90. Godoy-Matos A, Carraro L, Vieira A, et al. Treatment of obese adolescents with sibutramine: a randomized, double-blind, controlled study. J Clin Endocrinol Metab 2005;90(3):1460–5.

91. O'Brien P, Brown W, Dixon J. Obesity, weight loss and bariatric surgery. Med J Aust 2005;183(6): 310–4.

92. Kanoupakis E, Michaloudis D, Fraidakis O, et al. Left ventricular function and cardiopulmonary performance following surgical treatment of morbid obesity. Obes Surg 2001;11(5):552–8.

93. Willens H, Chakko S, Byers P, et al. Effects of weight loss after gastric bypass on right and left ventricular function assessed by tissue Doppler imaging. Am J Cardiol 2005;95(12):1521–4.

94. Alpert M, Terry B, Kelly D. Effect of weight loss on cardiac chamber size, wall thickness and left ventricular function in morbid obesity. Am J Cardiol 1985;55(6):783–6.

95. Ashrafian H, le Roux C, Darzi A, et al. Effects of bariatric surgery on cardiovascular function. Circulation 2008;118(20):2091–102.

96. Vidal-Puig A, Considine R, Jimenez-Liñan M, et al. Peroxisome proliferator-activated receptor gene expression in human tissues. Effects of obesity, weight loss, and regulation by insulin and glucocorticoids. J Clin Invest 1997;99(10):2416–22.

97. Tuck M, Sowers J, Dornfeld L, et al. The effect of weight reduction on blood pressure, plasma renin activity, and plasma aldosterone levels in obese patients. N Engl J Med 1981;304(16):930–3.

98. Bastard J, Hainque B, Dusserre E, et al. Peroxisome proliferator activated receptor-gamma, leptin and tumor necrosis factor-alpha mRNA expression during very low calorie diet in subcutaneous adipose tissue in obese women. Diabetes Metab Res Rev 1999;15(2):92–8.

99. Barger P, Kelly D. PPAR signaling in the control of cardiac energy metabolism. Trends Cardiovasc Med 2000;10(6):238–45.

100. Verreth W, De Keyzer D, Pelat M, et al. Weight-loss-associated induction of peroxisome proliferator-activated receptor-alpha and peroxisome proliferator-activated receptor-gamma correlate with reduced atherosclerosis and improved cardiovascular function in obese insulin-resistant mice. Circulation 2004;110(20):3259–69.

101. Giese S, Bulan E, Commons G, et al. Improvements in cardiovascular risk profile with large-volume liposuction: a pilot study. Plast Reconstr Surg 2001;108(2):510–9 [discussion: 520–11].

102. Klein S, Fontana L, Young V, et al. Absence of an effect of liposuction on insulin action and risk factors for coronary heart disease. N Engl J Med 2004;350(25):2549–57.

103. Duprez D. Role of the renin-angiotensin-aldosterone system in vascular remodeling and

inflammation: a clinical review. J Hypertens 2006; 24(6):983–91.

104. Satwani S, Dec G, Narula J. Beta-adrenergic blockers in heart failure: review of mechanisms of action and clinical outcomes. J Cardiovasc Pharmacol Ther 2004;9(4):243–55.

105. Jacob S, Rett K, Henriksen E. Antihypertensive therapy and insulin sensitivity: do we have to redefine the role of beta-blocking agents? Am J Hypertens 1998;11(10):1258–65.

106. Al-Hesayen A, Azevedo E, Floras J, et al. Selective versus nonselective beta-adrenergic receptor blockade in chronic heart failure: differential effects on myocardial energy substrate utilization. Eur J Heart Fail 2005;7(4):618–23.

107. Raji A, Seely E, Bekins S, et al. Rosiglitazone improves insulin sensitivity and lowers blood pressure in hypertensive patients. Diabetes Care 2003; 26(1):172–8.

108. Wang T, Chen W, Lin J, et al. Effects of rosiglitazone on endothelial function, C-reactive protein, and components of the metabolic syndrome in nondiabetic patients with the metabolic syndrome. Am J Cardiol 2004;93(3):362–5.

109. Grunstein R, Wilcox I, Yang T, et al. Snoring and sleep apnoea in men: association with central obesity and hypertension. Int J Obes Relat Metab Disord 1993;17(9):533–40.

110. Lopez P, Stefan B, Schulman C, et al. Prevalence of sleep apnea in morbidly obese patients who presented for weight loss surgery evaluation: more evidence for routine screening for obstructive sleep apnea before weight loss surgery. Am Surg 2008;74(9):834–8.

111. Peppard P, Young T, Palta M, et al. Longitudinal study of moderate weight change and sleep-disordered breathing. JAMA 2000;284(23): 3015–21.

112. Golbin J, Somers V, Caples S. Obstructive sleep apnea, cardiovascular disease, and pulmonary hypertension. Proc Am Thorac Soc 2008;5(2): 200–6.

113. Voelkel N. Mechanisms of hypoxic pulmonary vasoconstriction. Am Rev Respir Dis 1986;133(6): 1186–95.

114. Presberg K, Dincer H. Pathophysiology of pulmonary hypertension due to lung disease. Curr Opin Pulm Med 2003;9(2):131–8.

115. Chaouat A, Weitzenblum E, Krieger J, et al. Pulmonary hemodynamics in the obstructive sleep apnea syndrome. Results in 220 consecutive patients. Chest 1996;109(2):380–6.

116. Somers V, White D, Amin R, et al. Sleep apnea and cardiovascular disease: an American Heart Association/American College of Cardiology Foundation Scientific Statement from the American Heart Association Council for High Blood Pressure Research Professional Education Committee, Council on Clinical Cardiology, Stroke Council, and Council on Cardiovascular Nursing. In collaboration with the National Heart, Lung, and Blood Institute National Center on Sleep Disorders Research (National Institutes of Health). Circulation 2008; 118(10):1080–111.

117. Finkelhor R, Moallem M, Bahler R. Characteristics and impact of obesity on the outpatient echocardiography laboratory. Am J Cardiol 2006;97(7): 1082–4.

118. McQuillan B, Picard M, Leavitt M, et al. Clinical correlates and reference intervals for pulmonary artery systolic pressure among echocardiographically normal subjects. Circulation 2001;104(23): 2797–802.

119. Bady E, Achkar A, Pascal S, et al. Pulmonary arterial hypertension in patients with sleep apnoea syndrome. Thorax 2000;55(11):934–9.

120. Krieger J, Sforza E, Apprill M, et al. Pulmonary hypertension, hypoxemia, and hypercapnia in obstructive sleep apnea patients. Chest 1989; 96(4):729–37.

121. Sajkov D, Cowie R, Thornton A, et al. Pulmonary hypertension and hypoxemia in obstructive sleep apnea syndrome. Am J Respir Crit Care Med 1994;149(2 Pt 1):416–22.

122. Sanner B, Doberauer C, Konermann M, et al. Pulmonary hypertension in patients with obstructive sleep apnea syndrome. Arch Intern Med 1997;157(21):2483–7.

123. Yamakawa H, Shiomi T, Sasanabe R, et al. Pulmonary hypertension in patients with severe obstructive sleep apnea. Psychiatry Clin Neurosci 2002; 56(3):311–2.

124. Laks L. Pulmonary arterial pressure in sleep apnea. Sleep 1993;16(8 Suppl):S41–3.

125. Motta J, Guilleminault C, Schroeder J, et al. Tracheostomy and hemodynamic changes in sleep-inducing apnea. Ann Intern Med 1978; 89(4):454–8.

126. Tilkian A, Guilleminault C, Schroeder J, et al. Hemodynamics in sleep-induced apnea. Studies during wakefulness and sleep. Ann Intern Med 1976;85(6):714–9.

127. Alchanatis M, Tourkohoriti G, Kakouros S, et al. Daytime pulmonary hypertension in patients with obstructive sleep apnea: the effect of continuous positive airway pressure on pulmonary hemodynamics. Respiration 2001;68(6):566–72.

128. Sajkov D, Wang T, Saunders N, et al. Continuous positive airway pressure treatment improves pulmonary hemodynamics in patients with obstructive sleep apnea. Am J Respir Crit Care Med 2002; 165(2):152–8.

129. Arias M, García-Río F, Alonso-Fernández A, et al. Pulmonary hypertension in obstructive sleep

apnoea: effects of continuous positive airway pressure: a randomized, controlled cross-over study. Eur Heart J 2006;27(9):1106–13.

130. Chaouat A, Weitzenblum E, Kessler R, et al. Five-year effects of nasal continuous positive airway pressure in obstructive sleep apnoea syndrome. Eur Respir J 1997;10(11):2578–82.

131. Simonneau G, Galiè N, Rubin L, et al. Clinical classification of pulmonary hypertension. J Am Coll Cardiol 2004;43(12 Suppl S):5S–12S.

132. Taraseviciute A, Voelkel N. Severe pulmonary hypertension in postmenopausal obese women. Eur J Med Res 2006;11(5):198–202.

133. Kramer M, Lane D. Aminorex, dexfenfluramine, and primary pulmonary hypertension. J Clin Epidemiol 1998;51(4):361–4.

134. Blankfield R, Tapolyai A, Zyzanski S. Left ventricular dysfunction, pulmonary hypertension, obesity, and sleep apnea. Sleep Breath 2001; 5(2):57–62.

Medications for Obesity: Mechanisms and Applications

George A. Bray, MD

KEYWORDS

- Sympathomimetic drugs • Lipase inhibitor
- Cannabinoid receptor antagonists
- Glucagon-like peptide analogues
- Seratonin agonist • Multiple amine reuptake inhibitor

Obesity is often described as an epidemic.[1–4] In this context, it is essential to develop ways of preventing more people from becoming obese. When prevention fails, however, treatment may be necessary. Obesity results from a prolonged imbalance between energy intake and energy expenditure. All treatments must shift this balance to be effective. In a recent clinical trial, 811 individuals who were assigned to one of four diets with different levels of fat, protein, and carbohydrate all lost the same amount of weight over 6 and 24 months, showing again that calories do count and that the composition of the diet does not.[5]

Let's begin with a brief description of the techniques that are available for management of obesity. Obesity is the result of a long-term positive imbalance between energy intake and energy expenditure, which means that treatments can be focused on energy intake or energy expenditure. Changes in body weight are thus the difference between energy intake as food and energy expenditure for metabolism and physical activity. **Fig. 1** uses the energy-balance diagram as a basis for briefly reviewing therapeutic options. At the top is the energy-balance equation showing changes in body fat on the left and the energy intake and expenditure on the right. Underneath that are the various strategies that have been used to approach treatment of a disordered energy balance.

Eating is a target for behavior therapy, drugs, and bariatric surgery. Physical activity and energy expenditure are targets for behavioral change and drugs, and patients who lose weight after bariatric surgery are often more physically active. When any of these therapeutic approaches is used consistently, weight loss is the expected result. In this article, the author examines the drugs that affect this system. Several different strategies have been used to treat obesity, including diet, exercise, behavior therapy, medications, and surgery. Criteria for selecting among these treatments involve evaluating the risks to the individual from obesity and balancing those against any possible problems with the treatment. Because all medications inherently have more risks than diet and exercise, deciding to use medications should only be done for people when the benefit justifies the risk.[4,6]

If an individual is to lose weight, he or she must go into "negative" energy balance in which the energy taken in as food is less, on average, than the energy needed for daily activities. Thus, the current group of medications can be divided into two broad categories: (1) those that act primarily on the central nervous system to reduce food intake and (2) those that act primarily outside the brain. Wherever the primary site of action may be, however, the net effect must be a reduction in food intake or an increase in energy expenditure. There currently are several drugs available in the United States to treat obesity.[6–12] **Table 1** summarizes these drugs.

MECHANISMS ON WHICH MEDICATIONS TO TREAT OBESITY WORK

Currently available medications work on two mechanisms: monoamines in the central nervous system or blockade of lipase digestion in the

The author has served as a consultant to Amylin.
Pennington Biomedical Research Center, 6400 Perkins Road, Baton Rouge, LA 70808, USA
E-mail address: brayga@pbrc.edu

Clin Chest Med 30 (2009) 525–538
doi:10.1016/j.ccm.2009.05.014
0272-5231/09/$ – see front matter © 2009 Elsevier Inc. All rights reserved.

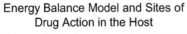

Energy Balance Model and Sites of
Drug Action in the Host

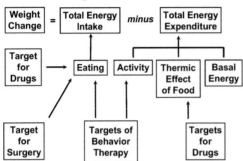

Fig. 1. Energy balance, body fat, and therapeutic options.

intestine. To give these and other potential medications a site for action, the following discussion focuses on central and peripheral mechanisms. It is clear that there are several different sites for action in each area.

The brain plays the central role in regulating food intake by receiving and processing information from the environment and internal milieu.[13] Several neurotransmitter systems, including monoamines, amino acids, and neuropeptides, are involved in modulating food intake. The monoamines include norepinephrine, serotonin, dopamine, and histamine, in addition to certain amino acids. The serotonin system has been one of the most extensively studied of the monoamine pathways. Its receptors modulate the quantity of food eaten and macronutrient selection. Stimulation of the serotonin receptors in the paraventricular nucleus reduces fat intake with little or no effect on the intake of protein or carbohydrate. This reduction in fat intake is probably mediated through 5-hydroxytryptophan (5-HT)-2C receptors because its effect is attenuated in mice that cannot express the 5-HT$_{2C}$ receptor.[14] Sibutramine blocks serotonin reuptake and norepinephrine reuptake. Lorcaserin is

Table 1
Drugs approved by the US Food and Drug Administration (FDA) for treatment of obesity

Generic Name	Trade Names	Status	Usual Dosage	Comments
Drugs approved by the FDA for long-term treatment of overweight patients				
Orlistat	Xenical	Not scheduled	120 mg three times a day	May have gastrointestinal side effects
Sibutramine	Meridia Reductil	DEA-IV	5–15 mg/d	Raises blood pressure
Drugs approved by the FDA for short-term treatment of overweight patients				
Benzphetamine	Didrex	DEA-III	25 mg/d in the morning	Short-term use only
Diethylpropion	Tenuate	DEA-IV	25 mg tid	Short-term use only
	Tepanil		25 mg tid	
	Tenuate dospan		75 mg in the morning	
Phendimetrazine	Standard release:	DEA-III	35-mg tid before meals	Short-term use only
	Bontril PDM			
	Plegine			
	Slow release:		105 mg in the morning	
	Bontril			
	Prelu-2			
	X-Trozine			
Phentermine	Standard release:	DEA-IV	18.75–37.5 mg tid	Short-term use only
	Adipex-P			
	Fastin			
	Obenix			
	Oby-Cap			
	Oby-Trim			
	Zantryl			
	Slow release:		15–30 mg/d in the morning of slow-release form	
	Ionamin			

Abbreviations: DEA, U.S. Drug Enforcement Agency; tid, three times daily.

an example of a drug in clinical trial that works by acting directly on serotonin receptors in the brain.

Stimulation of α_1-noradrenergic receptors decreases food intake. Phenylpropanolamine is an agonist acting on this receptor that has modest inhibition of food intake.[15] Some of the antagonists to the α_1-receptors that are used to treat hypertension produce weight gain, indicating that this receptor is also clinically important. In contrast, stimulation of α_2-receptors increases food intake in experimental animals, and a polymorphism in the α_{2a}-adrenoceptor has been associated with reduced metabolic rate in humans. In contrast, the activation of β_2-receptors in the brain reduces food intake. These receptors can be activated by agonist drugs, by releasing norepinephrine in the vicinity of these receptors, or by blocking the reuptake of norepinephrine. Sibutramine also uses this mechanism. Treatment with beta-blockers is associated with a small amount of weight gain.[16]

Histamine receptors can also modulate feeding. Stimulation of the H_1 receptor in the central nervous system reduces feeding, but this is not a practical strategy because these receptors are so widely distributed. Experimentally, this system has been attacked by modulating the H_3 autoreceptor, which controls histamine release.[17] When the autoreceptor is stimulated, histamine secretion is reduced and food intake increases. Blockade of this H_3 autoreceptor, conversely, decreases food intake. The histamine system is important in control of feeding because antipsychotic drugs that produce weight gain are modulators of histamine receptors.[18]

The endocannabinoid system is a recent addition to the list of central controllers of feeding.[19] Tetrahydrocannabinol, isolated from the marijuana plant, stimulates food intake. Isolation of the cannabinoid receptor was followed by identification of two fatty acids, anandamide and 2-arachidonylglycerol, which are endogenous ligands in the brain for this receptor. Infusion of anandamide or 2-arachidonylglycerol into the brain stimulates food intake. The cannabinoid-1 (CB-1) receptor is a preganglionic receptor, meaning that its activation inhibits synaptic transmission. Antagonists to this receptor have been shown to reduce food intake and lead to weight loss.

The opioid receptors were the first group of peptide receptors shown to modulate feeding.[20] They also modulate fat intake. The μ- and κ-opioid receptors can stimulate feeding. Stimulation of the μ-opioid receptors increases the intake of dietary fat in experimental animals. Corticotrophin-releasing hormone and the closely related urocortin

reduce food intake and body weight in experimental animals.

In addition to the drugs that act on the central nervous system, there are examples of drugs that act peripherally.[4] Blockade of intestinal lipase produces weight loss, and orlistat is an example of such a drug. A second drug in this class is in clinical trials. Pancreatic and intestinal peptides modulate food intake, and are thus candidates for treatment targets. Glucagon-like peptide-1 (GLP-1) from the L cells in the gut acts on the pancreas and brain to reduce food intake. Exenatide is a drug that works by this mechanism. Amylin is secreted from the pancreas and can reduce food intake. Pramlintide is an example of a drug that works by means of this mechanism.

DRUGS APPROVED BY THE US FOOD AND DRUG ADMINISTRATION THAT REDUCE FOOD INTAKE PRIMARILY BY ACTING ON THE CENTRAL NERVOUS SYSTEM

The drugs the author considers in this category are sibutramine, phentermine, and the other sympathomimetic drugs (see **Table 1**).

Sibutramine

Sibutramine is a serotonin-norepinephrine reuptake inhibitor that is approved by the US Food and Drug Administration (FDA) for long-term use.[9] Sibutramine has been evaluated extensively in several placebo-controlled, double-blind, multicenter clinical trials lasting 6 to 24 months and including men and women of all ethnic groups, with age ranging from 18 years to 65 years and body mass index (BMI) ranging from 27 kg/m^2 to 40 kg/m^2.[21–29] In a clinical trial lasting 8 weeks, sibutramine produced dose-dependent weight loss with dosages of 5 mg/d and 20 mg/d. In a 6-month dose-ranging study of 1047 patients, 67% treated with sibutramine achieved a 5% weight loss from baseline and 35% lost 10% or more.[21] There was a clear dose-response effect in this 24-week trial, and patients regained weight when the drug was stopped, indicating that the drug remained effective when used.

In a 1-year trial of 456 patients who received sibutramine (10 mg/d or 15 mg/d) or placebo, 56% of those who stayed in the trial for 12 months lost at least 5% of their initial body weight and 30% of the patients lost 10% of their initial body weight while taking the 10-mg dose.[22] In a third trial in patients who initially lost weight eating an extremely low-calorie diet before being randomized to sibutramine or placebo, sibutramine

(10 mg/d) produced additional weight loss, whereas the placebo-treated patients regained weight.[23] The Sibutramine Trial of Obesity Reduction and Maintenance (STORM) lasted 2 years and provided further evidence for weight maintenance.[24] Seven centers participated in this trial, in which patients were initially enrolled in a 6-month open-label phase and treated with sibutramine at a dosage of 10 mg/d. Of the patients who lost more than 8 kg, two thirds were then randomized to sibutramine and one third to placebo. During the 18-month double-blind phase of this trial, the placebo-treated patients steadily regained weight, maintaining only 20% of their weight loss at the end of the trial. In contrast, the subjects treated with sibutramine maintained their weight for 12 months and then regained an average of only 2 kg, thus maintaining 80% of their initial weight loss after 2 years. Despite the higher weight loss with sibutramine at the end of the 18 months of controlled observation, the blood pressure levels of the sibutramine-treated patients were still higher than in the patients treated with placebo.

The possibility of using sibutramine as intermittent therapy has been tested in a randomized placebo-controlled trial lasting 52 weeks.[25] The patients randomized to sibutramine received one of two regimens. One group received continuous treatment with 15 mg/d for 1 year, and the other had two 6-week periods when sibutramine was withdrawn. During these periods when the drug was replaced by placebo, there was a small regain in weight that was lost when the drug was again resumed. At the end of the trial, the continuous-therapy and intermittent-therapy groups had lost the same amount of weight.

Some trials have reported on the use of sibutramine to treat patients with hypertension.[26,27] In a 52-week trial involving patients with hypertension whose blood pressure levels were controlled with calcium channel blockers with or without beta-blockers or thiazides,[26] sibutramine dosages were increased from 5 mg/d to 20 mg/d during the first 6 weeks. Weight loss was significantly greater in the sibutramine-treated patients, averaging 4.4 kg (4.7%), as compared with 0.5 kg (0.7%) in the placebo-treated group. Diastolic blood pressure levels decreased 1.3 mm Hg in the placebo-treated group and increased 2 mm Hg in the sibutramine-treated group. The systolic blood pressure levels increased 1.5 mm Hg in the placebo-treated group and 2.7 mm Hg in the sibutramine-treated group. Heart rate was unchanged in the placebo-treated patients but increased by an average of 4.9 beats per minute in the sibutramine-treated patients.[27]

In two studies, patients with diabetes were treated for 12 weeks or 24 weeks with sibutramine.[28,29] In the 12-week trial, patients with diabetes treated with sibutramine at 15 mg/d lost 2.4 kg (2.8%), compared with 0.1 kg (0.12%) in the placebo group.[28] In this study, hemoglobin A1c levels decreased 0.3% in the drug-treated group and remained stable in the placebo group. Fasting glucose values decreased 0.3 mg/dL in the drug-treated patients and increased 1.4 mg/dL in the placebo-treated group. In the 24-week trial, the dosage of sibutramine was increased from 5 mg/d to 20 mg/d over 6 weeks.[29] Among those who completed the treatment, weight loss was 4.3 kg (4.3%) in the sibutramine-treated patients, compared with 0.3 kg (0.3%) in placebo-treated patients. Hemoglobin A1c levels decreased 1.67% in the drug-treated group, compared with 0.53% in the placebo-treated group. These changes in glucose and hemoglobin A1c levels were expected from the amount of weight loss associated with drug treatment.[29]

Sibutramine has also been used in children.[30–33] In a large 12-month multicenter trial, 498 adolescents aged 12 to 16 years were randomized to treatment with placebo or sibutramine, 10 mg/d, which could be increased to 15 mg/d in those who had not lost more than 10% of their body weight by 6 months.[32] After 12 months, the mean absolute change in BMI was -2.9 kg/m^2 (-8.2%) in the sibutramine-treated group compared with -0.3 kg/m^2 (-0.8%) in the placebo group ($P<.001$). Triglycerides, high-density lipoprotein (HDL) cholesterol, and insulin sensitivity improved, and there was no significant difference in the changes in systolic or diastolic blood pressure.

Sibutramine has also been studied as part of a behavioral weight-loss program. With sibutramine alone and minimal behavioral intervention, the weight loss over 12 months was approximately -5.0 ± 7.4 kg over 12 months. Behavior modification alone produced a weight loss of -6.7 ± 7.9 kg. Adding a brief behavioral therapy session in a group that also received sibutramine produced a slightly larger weight loss of -7.5 ± 8.0 kg. When the intensive lifestyle intervention was combined with sibutramine, the weight loss increased to -12.1 ± 9.8 kg.[34]

Sibutramine is available in 5-, 10-, and 15-mg doses; 10 mg/d as a single dosage is the recommended starting level, with titration up or down depending on response. Dosages higher than 15 mg/d are not recommended. Of the patients who lost 2 kg (4.4 lb) in the first 4 weeks of treatment, 60% achieved a weight loss of more than 5%, compared with less than 10% in those who did not lose 2 kg (4.4 lb) in 4 weeks. Combining data from the

11 studies on sibutramine showed a reduction in triglyceride, total cholesterol, and low-density lipoprotein cholesterol levels and an increase in HDL cholesterol levels that were related to the magnitude of the weight loss.

Safety

Sibutramine increases blood pressure levels in normotensive patients or prevents the decrease that might have occurred with weight loss. The magnitude of the change may be dose related; thus, lower doses are preferred. Systolic and diastolic blood pressure levels increased an average of +0.8 mm Hg and +0.6 mm Hg, and pulse increased approximately four to five beats per minute. Caution should be used when combining sibutramine with other drugs that may increase blood pressure levels. Sibutramine is contraindicated in patients with a history of coronary artery disease, congestive heart failure, cardiac arrhythmias, or stroke. Sibutramine should not be used with selective serotonin reuptake inhibitors or monoamine oxidase inhibitors, and there should be a 2-week interval between terminating monoamine oxidase inhibitors and beginning sibutramine. Because sibutramine is metabolized by the cytochrome P-450 enzyme system (isozyme CYP3A4), it may interfere with the metabolism of erythromycin and ketoconazole.

Sympathomimetic Drugs: Pharmacology and Efficacy

The sympathomimetic drugs benzphetamine, diethylpropion, phendimetrazine, and phentermine are grouped together because they act like norepinephrine.[4,9] Drugs in this group work by a variety of mechanisms, including the blockade of norepinephrine reuptake from synaptic granules.

All these drugs are absorbed orally and reach peak blood concentrations within a short period. The half-life in blood also is short for all except the metabolites of sibutramine, which have a long half-life. The two metabolites of sibutramine are active, but this is not true for the metabolites of other drugs in this group. Liver metabolism inactivates a large fraction of these drugs before excretion. Side effects include dry mouth, constipation, and insomnia. Food intake is suppressed by delaying the onset of a meal or by producing early satiety.

The efficacy of an appetite-suppressing drug can be established through randomized double-blind clinical trials that show a significantly greater weight loss than in the placebo group and a weight loss that is more than 5% greater than that with placebo.[4,9] Clinical trials of sympathomimetic drugs conducted before 1975 were generally short because it was widely believed that short-term treatment would "cure" obesity. This was unfounded optimism, and because the trials had a short duration and often used a crossover design, they provided few long-term data. The focus here is on longer term trials lasting 24 weeks or more that include an adequate control group.

One of the longest of these clinical trials of drugs in this group lasted 36 weeks and compared placebo treatment with continuous phentermine or intermittent phentermine.[35] Continuous and intermittent phentermine therapy produced more weight loss than placebo. In the drug-free periods, the patients treated intermittently slowed their weight loss, only to lose weight more rapidly when the drug was reinstituted. Phentermine and diethylpropion are classified by the US Drug Enforcement Agency as schedule IV drugs, and benzphetamine and phendimetrazine are schedule III drugs. This regulatory classification indicates the US Government's belief that they have the potential for abuse, although this potential seems to be low. Phentermine and diethylpropion are approved for only a "few weeks," which is usually interpreted as up to 12 weeks. Weight loss with phentermine and diethylpropion persists for the duration of treatment, suggesting that tolerance does not develop to these drugs. If tolerance were to develop, the drugs would be expected to lose their effectiveness and patients would require increased amounts of the drug to maintain weight loss. This does not occur.

Safety of sympathomimetic drugs

The side-effect profiles of sympathomimetic drugs are similar.[7,9] These agents produce insomnia, dry mouth, asthenia, and constipation. The safety of older sympathomimetic appetite suppressant drugs has been the subject of considerable controversy because dextroamphetamine is addictive. The sympathomimetic drugs phentermine, diethylpropion, benzphetamine, and phendimetrazine have little abuse potential, as assessed by the low rate of reinforcement when the drugs are self-injected intravenously by test animals.[7] Sympathomimetic drugs can also increase blood pressure levels.

DRUGS APPROVED BY THE US FOOD AND DRUG ADMINISTRATION THAT REDUCE FAT ABSORPTION
Orlistat: Pharmacology and Efficacy

Orlistat is a potent and selective inhibitor of pancreatic lipase that reduces the intestinal digestion of fat.[4,7] The drug has a dose-dependent effect on fecal fat loss, increasing it to approximately 30%

on a diet that has 30% of its energy as fat. Orlistat has little effect in subjects eating a low-fat diet, as might be anticipated from its mechanism of action.

The findings of several long-term clinical trials (1–4 years) with orlistat have been published.[36–40] The report of the first published trial consisted of two parts. In the first year, patients received a hypocaloric diet calculated to be 500 kcal/d less than the patient's requirements.[36] During the second year, the diet was calculated to maintain weight. By the end of year 1, the placebo-treated patients lost 6.1% of their initial body weight and the drug-treated patients lost 10.2%. The patients were randomized again at the end of year 1. Those switched from orlistat to placebo gained weight from−10% to−6% lower than baseline. Those switched from placebo to orlistat lost weight from−6% to−8.1% lower than baseline, which was essentially identical to the−7.9% loss in the patients treated with orlistat for the full 2 years.

In a second 2-year study, 892 patients were randomized.[37] One group remained on placebo throughout the 2 years (97 patients), and a second group remained on orlistat (120 mg three times per day) for 2 years (109 patients). At the end of 1 year, two thirds of the patients in the group treated with orlistat for 1 year (102 patients) were changed to orlistat (60 mg three times per day) and the others (95 patients) were switched to placebo. After 1 year, the weight loss was −8.7 kg in the orlistat-treated group and −5.8 kg in the placebo group (P<.001). During the second year, those switched to placebo after 1 year reached the same weight as those treated with placebo for 2 years (−4.5% in those treated with placebo for 2 years and −4.2% in those switched to placebo during year 2).

In a third 2-year study, 783 patients remained in the placebo- or orlistat-treated groups at 60 mg or 120 mg three times per day for the entire 2 years.[38] After 1 year with a weight-loss diet, the placebo group lost −7 kg, which was significantly less than the −9.6 kg lost by the group treated with orlistat at a dosage of 60 mg three times daily or the −9.8 kg lost by the group treated with orlistat at a dosage of 120 mg three times daily. During the second year, when the diet was liberalized to a "weight-maintenance" diet, all three groups regained some weight. At the end of 2 years, the patients in the placebo group weighed −4.3 kg lower than baseline, the patients treated with orlistat at a dosage of 60 mg three times per day weighed −6.8 kg lower than baseline, and the patients who took orlistat 120 mg three times per day weighed −7.6 kg lower than baseline.

The final 2-year trial evaluated 796 subjects in a general practice setting.[39] After 1 year of treatment with orlistat at a dosage of 120 mg three times per day, the orlistat-treated patients (n = 117) had lost −8.8 kg, compared with −4.3 kg in the placebo group (n = 91). During the second year, when the diet was liberalized to "maintain body weight," both groups regained some weight. At the end of 2 years, the orlistat group weighed −5.2 kg lower than their baseline weight, compared with −1.5 kg lower than baseline for the group treated with placebo.

A 4-year, double-blind, randomized, placebo-controlled trial with orlistat treated a total of 3304 overweight patients, 21% of whom had impaired glucose tolerance.[40] The lowest body weight was achieved during the first year and was more than −11% lower than baseline in the orlistat-treated group and 6% lower than baseline in the placebo-treated group. Over the remaining 3 years of the trial, there was a small regain in weight, such that by the end of 4 years, the orlistat-treated patients were −6.9% lower than baseline, compared with −4.1% for those receiving placebo. The trial also showed a 37% reduction in the conversion of patients from impaired glucose tolerance to diabetes. Essentially all this benefit occurred in the patients who had impaired glucose tolerance on enrollment into the trial.

Orlistat has also been used to treat obese children. A multicenter trial tested the effect of orlistat in 539 obese adolescents.[41] Subjects were randomized to placebo or orlistat at a dosage of 120 mg three times a day and a mildly hypocaloric diet containing 30% fat. By the end of the study, BMI had decreased by −0.55 kg/m^2 in the drug-treated group but had increased by +0.31 kg/m^2 in the placebo group. Also, at the end of the study, weight had increased by only +0.51 kg in the orlistat-treated group, compared with +3.14 kg in the placebo-treated group. This difference was attributable to differences in body fat. The side effects were gastrointestinal in origin, as expected from the mode of action of orlistat.

Weight maintenance with orlistat was evaluated in a 1-year study.[42] Patients were enrolled if they had lost more than 8% of their body weight over 6 months while eating a 1000-kcal/d (4180-kJ/d) diet. The 729 patients were randomized to receive placebo or orlistat at a dosage of 30 mg, 60 mg, or 120 mg three times per day for 12 months. At the end of this time, the placebo-treated patients had regained 56% of their body weight, compared with a 32.4% regain in the group treated with orlistat at a dosage of 120 mg three times per day. The other two dosages of orlistat were not different from placebo in preventing the regain of weight.

Three trials of orlistat have been conducted in patients with diabetes.[43–45] In one study, those treated with orlistat at a dosage of 120 mg three times daily for 1 year lost −6.5% of their body weight, compared with −4.2% in the placebo-treated group.[43] The subjects with diabetes also showed a significantly greater decrease in hemoglobin A1c levels. In another study of orlistat and weight loss, investigators pooled data on 675 subjects from three of the 2-year studies described previously in which glucose tolerance test results were available.[46] During treatment, 6.6% of the patients taking orlistat converted from a normal to an impaired glucose tolerance test result, compared with 10.8% in the placebo-treated group. None of the orlistat-treated patients who originally had normal glucose tolerance developed diabetes, compared with 1.2% in the placebo-treated group. Of those who initially had normal glucose tolerance, 7.6% in the placebo group but only 3% in the orlistat-treated group developed diabetes.

Safety of orlistat

Orlistat is not absorbed to any significant degree, and its side effects are thus related to the blockade of triglyceride digestion in the intestine.[47] Fecal fat loss and related gastrointestinal symptoms are common initially, but they subside as patients learn to use the drug. The quality of life in patients treated with orlistat may improve despite concerns about gastrointestinal symptoms. Orlistat can cause small but significant decreases in fat-soluble vitamins. Levels usually remain within the normal range, but a few patients may need vitamin supplementation. Because it is impossible to tell which patients need vitamins, it is wise to provide a multivitamin routinely with instructions to take it before bedtime. Orlistat does not seem to affect the absorption of other drugs, except acyclovir.

Combining orlistat and sibutramine

Because orlistat works peripherally to reduce triglyceride digestion in the gastrointestinal tract and sibutramine works on noradrenergic and serotonergic reuptake mechanisms in the brain, their mechanisms of action do not overlap and combining them might provide additive weight loss. To test this possibility, researchers randomly assigned patients to orlistat or placebo after 1 year of treatment with sibutramine.[48] During the additional 4 months of treatment, there was no further weight loss. Thus, we have no data indicating that adding orlistat and sibutramine is beneficial.

Rimonabant

Rimonabant, a cannabinoid receptor antagonist that blocks the CB-1 receptor, was approved by European regulatory authorities in 2006, but approval for marketing was withdrawn on October 23, 2008 because of increased risks for psychiatric side effects, including depression and anxiety. For details on the clinical trials with this drug, the reader is referred elsewhere.[4,9,12]

DRUGS THAT HAVE BEEN USED TO TREAT OBESITY BUT ARE NOT APPROVED BY THE US FOOD AND DRUG ADMINISTRATION FOR THAT PURPOSE
Fluoxetine

Fluoxetine is a selective serotonin-reuptake inhibitor that blocks serotonin transporters, thus prolonging the action of serotonin. It reduces food intake. In a 2-week placebo-controlled trial, fluoxetine at a dosage of 60 mg/d produced a 27% decrease in food intake.[49] Fluoxetine is approved by the FDA for treatment of depression. Fluoxetine at a dosage of 60 mg/d (three times the usual dosage for treatment of depression) was effective in reducing body weight in overweight patients. A meta-analysis of six studies using fluoxetine showed a wide range of results, with a mean weight loss in one study of −14.5 kg and a weight gain of +0.40 kg in another.[8] In the meta-analysis by Avenell and colleagues,[10] weight loss at 12 months was −0.33 kg (95% confidence interval [CI]: −1.49 to 0.82 kg). Goldstein and colleagues[50] reviewed the trials with fluoxetine, which included one 36-week trial in type 2 diabetic subjects; a 52-week trial in subjects with uncomplicated overweight; and two 60-week trials in subjects with dyslipidemia, diabetes, or both. A total of 719 subjects were randomized to fluoxetine, and 722 were randomized to placebo. Five hundred twenty-two subjects on fluoxetine and 504 subjects on placebo completed 6 months of treatment. Weight losses in the placebo and fluoxetine groups at 6 months and 1 year were −2.2 and −4.8 kg and −1.8 and −2.4 kg, respectively. The regain of 50% of the lost weight during the second 6 months of treatment with fluoxetine makes this drug inappropriate for the long-term treatment of obesity. Fluoxetine, although not a good drug for long-term treatment of obesity, may be preferred for the treatment of depressed obese patients over some of the tricyclic antidepressants that are associated with significant weight gain.

Bupropion

Bupropion is a norepinephrine- and dopamine-reuptake inhibitor that is approved for the treatment of depression and for help in smoking cessation. In one clinical trial, 50 overweight subjects were randomized to bupropion or placebo for 8 weeks with a blinded extension for responders to 24 weeks. The dosage of bupropion was increased to a maximum of 200 mg twice daily in conjunction with a calorie-restricted diet. At 8 weeks, 18 subjects in the bupropion group lost $-6.2 \pm 3.1\%$ of body weight compared with $-1.6 \pm 2.9\%$ of body weight by the 13 subjects in the placebo group ($P<.0001$). After 24 weeks, the 14 responders to bupropion lost $-12.9 \pm 5.6\%$ of their initial body weight, of which 75% was fat as determined by dual-energy x-ray absorptiometry.[51]

Two multicenter clinical trials, one in obese subjects with depressive symptoms and one in uncomplicated overweight patients, followed this study. In the study of overweight patients with depressive symptom ratings of 10 to 30 on a Beck Depression Inventory, 213 patients were randomized to 400 mg/d of bupropion and 209 subjects were assigned to placebo for 24 weeks. The 121 subjects in the bupropion group who completed the trial lost $-6.0 \pm 0.5\%$ of their initial body weight compared with $-2.8 \pm 0.5\%$ in the 108 subjects in the placebo group ($P<.0001$).[52] The study in uncomplicated overweight subjects randomized 327 subjects to bupropion at a dosage of 300 mg/d, bupropion at a dosage of 400 mg/d, or placebo in equal proportions. At 24 weeks, 69% of those randomized remained in the study and the percent losses of initial body weight were $-5 \pm 1\%$, minus;$7.2 \pm 1\%$, and $-10.1 \pm 1\%$ for the groups that received placebo, bupropion at a dose of 300 mg, and bupropion at a dose of 400 mg, respectively ($P<.0001$). The placebo group was randomized to the group receiving bupropion at a dose of 300 mg or the group receiving bupropion at a dose of 400 mg at 24 weeks, and the trial was extended to week 48. By the end of the trial, the dropout rate was 41% and the weight losses in the groups receiving bupropion at a dose of 300 mg and bupropion at a dose of 400 mg were $-6.2 \pm 1.25\%$ and $-7.2 \pm 1.5\%$ of initial body weight, respectively.[53] Thus, it seems that nondepressed subjects may respond to bupropion with weight loss to a greater extent than those with depressive symptoms.

Topiramate

Topiramate is approved for treatment of selected seizure disorders. It is a weak carbonic anhydrase inhibitor. Topiramate also modulates the effects at receptors for the γ-aminobutyric acid (GABA$_A$) receptor and the α-amino-3-hydroxy-5-methyl-4-isoxazolepropionic acid/kainate subtype of the glutamate receptor. This drug also exhibits state-dependent blockade of voltage-dependent Na$^+$ or Ca^{2+} channels. These mechanisms are believed to contribute to its antiepileptic properties. The modulation of GABA$_A$ receptors may provide one potential mechanism to reduce food intake, although other mechanisms, yet to be described, may be more important in defining its effects on body weight.[54] Topiramate is an antiepileptic drug that was discovered to lead to weight loss in the clinical trials for epilepsy. Weight losses of -3.9% of initial weight were seen at 3 months, and losses of -7.3% of initial weight were seen at 1 year.[55] Bray and colleagues[56] reported on a 6-month, placebo-controlled, dose-ranging study of topiramate. Three hundred eighty-five obese subjects were randomized to placebo or topiramate at 64 mg/d, 96 mg/d, 192 mg/d, or 384 mg/d. These dosages were gradually reached by a tapering increase and were reduced in a similar manner at the end of the trial. Weight loss from baseline to 24 weeks was -2.6%, -5%, -4.8%, -6.3%, and -6.3% in the placebo, 64-mg, 96-mg, 192-mg, and 384-mg groups, respectively. The most frequent adverse events were paresthesias; somnolence; and difficulty with concentration, memory, and attention.[56] This trial was followed by two other multicenter trials. The first trial randomized 1289 obese subjects to placebo or topiramate at a dosage of 89 mg/d, 192 mg/d, or 256 mg/d. This trial was terminated early because of the sponsor's decision to pursue a time-release form of the drug. The 854 subjects who completed 1 year of the trial before it was terminated lost -1.7%, -7%, -9.1%, and -9.7% of their initial body weight in the placebo, 89-mg, 192-mg, and 256-mg groups, respectively. Subjects in the topiramate groups had significant improvement in blood pressure and glucose tolerance.[57] The second trial enrolled 701 subjects who were treated with a very-low-calorie diet to induce an 8% loss of initial body weight. The 560 subjects who achieved an 8% weight loss were randomized to topiramate at a dosage of 96 mg/d or 192 mg/d or to placebo. This study was also terminated early. At the time of termination, 293 subjects had completed 44 weeks. The topiramate groups lost 15.4% and 16.5% of their baseline weight, whereas the placebo group lost 8.9%.[58] Although topiramate is still available as an antiepileptic drug, the development program to obtain an indication for overweight was terminated by the sponsor because of the associated adverse events.

Zonisamide

Zonisamide is an antiepileptic drug that has serotonergic and dopaminergic activity in addition to inhibiting sodium and calcium channels. Weight loss was noted in the clinical trials for the treatment of epilepsy, again suggesting a potential agent for weight loss. Gadde and colleagues[59] tested this possibility by performing a 16-week randomized controlled trial in 60 obese subjects. Subjects were placed on a calorie-restricted diet and randomized to zonisamide or placebo. The zonisamide was started at 100 mg/d and increased to 400 mg/d. At 12 weeks, those subjects who had not lost 5% of their initial body weight were increased to 600 mg/d. The zonisamide group lost −6.6% of their initial body weight at 16 weeks compared with −1% in the placebo group. Thirty-seven subjects completing the 16-week trial elected to continue for 32 weeks: 20 in the zonisamide group and 17 in the placebo group. At the end of 32 weeks, the 19 subjects in the zonisamide group lost −9.6% of their initial body weight compared with −1.6% for the 17 subjects in the placebo group.[59]

Metformin

Metformin is a biguanide that is approved for the treatment of diabetes mellitus. This drug reduces hepatic glucose production, decreases intestinal absorption from the gastrointestinal tract, and enhances insulin sensitivity. In clinical trials in which metformin was compared with sulfonylureas, it produced weight loss.[9] In one French trial, Biguanides in the Prevention of Obesity, metformin was compared with placebo in a 1-year multicenter study in 324 middle-aged subjects with upper body adiposity and the insulin resistance syndrome (metabolic syndrome). The subjects on metformin lost significantly more weight (1–2 kg) than the placebo group, and the study concluded that metformin may have a role in the primary prevention of type 2 diabetes.[60] In a meta-analysis of three of these studies, Avenell and colleagues[10] reported a weighted mean weight loss at 12 months of −1.09 kg (95% CI: −2.29 to 0.11 kg).

The best trial of metformin for obesity, however, is the Diabetes Prevention Program study of individuals with impaired glucose tolerance.[61] This study included a double-blind comparison of metformin at a dosage of 850 mg twice daily versus placebo. During the 2.8 years of this trial, the 1073 patients treated with metformin lost −2.5% of their body weight ($P<.001$) compared with the 1082 patients treated with placebo, and the conversion from impaired glucose tolerance to diabetes was reduced by 31% compared with placebo. In the Diabetes Prevention Program trial, metformin was more effective in reducing the development of diabetes in the subgroup that was most overweight and in the younger members

of the cohort. Although metformin does not produce enough weight loss (5%) to qualify as a "weight-loss drug" (FDA criteria require ≥5% weight loss), it would seem to be a useful choice for overweight individuals who have diabetes or are at high risk for diabetes. One area in which metformin has found use is in treating overweight women with the polycystic ovary syndrome, wherein the modest weight loss may contribute to increased fertility and reduced insulin resistance.[62]

Pramlintide

Amylin is a peptide found in the β-cell of the pancreas that is cosecreted along with insulin to circulate in the blood. Amylin and insulin are deficient in type 1 diabetics, in whom β-cells are immunologically destroyed. Pramlintide, a synthetic amylin analogue, has a prolonged biologic half-life.[63] Pramlintide is approved by the FDA for the treatment of diabetes. Unlike insulin and many other diabetic medications, pramlintide is associated with weight loss. In a study in which 651 subjects with type 1 diabetes were randomized to placebo or subcutaneous pramlintide at a dosage of 60 μg three or four times a day along with an insulin injection, the hemoglobin A1c decreased from 0.29% to 0.34% and weight decreased −1.2 kg relative to placebo.[64] Maggs and colleagues[65] analyzed the data from two 1-year studies in insulin-treated type 2 diabetic subjects randomized to pramlintide at a dosage of 120 μg twice a day or 150 μg three times a day. Weight decreased by −2.6 kg, and hemoglobin A1c decreased by 0.5%. When weight loss was then analyzed by ethnic group, African Americans lost −4 kg, whites lost −2.4 kg, and Hispanics lost −2.3 kg and the improvement in diabetes correlated with the weight loss, suggesting that pramlintide is effective in ethnic groups with the greatest burden from overweight. The most common adverse event was nausea, which was usually mild and confined to the first 4 weeks of therapy.

Exenatide

GLP-1 is derived from the processing of the proglucagon peptide, which is secreted by L cells in the terminal ileum in response to a meal. Increased GLP-1 inhibits glucagon secretion, stimulates insulin secretion, stimulates gluconeogenesis, and delays gastric emptying.[63,66] It has been postulated to be responsible for the superior weight loss and superior improvement in diabetes seen after gastric bypass surgery for overweight.[67,68] GLP-1 is rapidly degraded by dipeptidyl peptidase-4 (DPP-4), an enzyme that is elevated in the obese. Bypass operations for overweight increase GLP-1 but do not change the levels of DPP-4.[63,69]

Exenatide (exendin-4) is a 39–amino acid peptide that is produced in the salivary gland of the Gila monster lizard. It has 53% homology with GLP-1, but it has a much longer half-life. Exenatide is approved by the FDA for treatment of type 2 diabetics who are inadequately controlled while being treated with metformin or sulfonylureas.

In humans, exenatide reduces fasting and postprandial glucose levels, slows gastric emptying, and decreases food intake by 19%.[70] The side effects of exenatide in people are headache, nausea, and vomiting that are lessened by gradual dose escalation. Several clinical trials of 30-weeks' duration have been reported using exenatide at 10 μg/d administered subcutaneously or placebo.[71–73] In one trial with 377 type 2 diabetic subjects who were failing maximal sulfonylurea therapy, exenatide produced a decrease of 0.74% more in HgbA1c than placebo. Fasting glucose also decreased, and there was a progressive weight loss of 1.6 kg.[71] The interesting feature of this weight loss is that it occurred without lifestyle change, diet, or exercise. In a 26-week randomized controlled trial, exenatide produced a weight loss of −2.3 kg compared with a gain of +1.8 kg in the group receiving insulin glargine.[74]

DRUGS IN CLINICAL TRIAL
Serotonin 2C Receptor Agonists

Mice lacking the $5HT_{2C}$ receptor have increased food intake because they take longer to be satiated.[14] These mice also are resistant to fenfluramine, a serotonin agonist that causes weight loss. A human mutation of the $5HT_{2C}$ receptor is associated with early-onset increases in human body weight.[75,76] The precursor of serotonin, 5-HT, reduces food intake and body weight in clinical studies.[77,78] Fenfluramine[79,80] and dexfenfluramine,[81] two drugs that act on the serotonin system but were withdrawn from the market in 1997 because of cardiovascular side effects, also reduce food intake in human studies. Meta-chlorophenylpiperazine, a direct serotonin agonist, reduces food intake by 28% in women and 20% in men.[82] Another serotoninergic drug, sumatriptan, which acts on the $5\text{-}HT_{1B/1D}$ receptor, also reduced food intake in human subjects.[83]

The robust effects of agonists toward the HT_{2C} receptors in suppressing food intake have stimulated the development of several new compounds. Only one of these has advanced to formal clinical trials, however. The results of a phase II dose-ranging study for lorcaserin have been presented. A total of 459 male and female subjects with a BMI between 29 kg/m^2 and 46 kg/m^2 and with an average weight of 100 kg were enrolled in a randomized, double-blind, controlled trial comparing placebo with lorcaserin at dosages of 10 and 15 mg once daily and 10 mg twice daily (20 mg/d). During the 12 weeks of the trial, the placebo group lost −0.32 kg (n = 88 completers) tlsb -0.04ptcompared with −1.8 kg in those with the 10-mg/d dosage (N = 86 completers), −2.6 kg in those with the 15-mg/d dosage (N = 82 completers), and −3.6 kg in those with the 10-mg twice-daily dosage (20 mg total) (N = 77 completers). Side effects that were more frequent in the active treatment groups than in the placebo group were headache, nausea, dizziness, vomiting, and dry mouth. No cardiac valvular changes were noted.[84] Additional clinical trials are underway.

Multiple Monoamine-Reuptake Inhibitor

Tesofensine is a multiple monoamine-reuptake inhibitor reducing the reuptake of norepinephrine, serotonin, and dopamine. In clinical trials of neurologic disorders, it was found to produce weight loss. In preclinical trials, the drug was shown to be safe in animal models and to produce weight loss during clinical trials in patients who had Parkinson's disease or Alzheimer's disease.

A recent double-blind, randomized, placebo-controlled trial examined the effects of tesofensine at 0.25, 0.5, or 1.0 mg/d versus placebo in 203 obese patients given an energy-restricted diet. Of those randomized, 161 (79%) completed the study. From the end of the 2-week run-in period, during which there was a −1.1 kg weight loss, the mean weight loss was −2.2 kg in the placebo group, −6.7 kg in the low-dosage group, −11.3 kg in the intermediate-dosage group, and −12.8 kg in the high-dosage group. The most common adverse events caused by tesofensine were dry mouth, nausea, constipation, hard stools, diarrhea, and insomnia. After 24 weeks, the lower and intermediate dosages of tesofensine (0.25 mg/d and 0.5 mg/d) showed no significant increases in systolic or diastolic blood pressure compared with placebo, but there was a significant increase in blood pressure in the group receiving the highest dosage. Heart rate was increased by 0.4 beats per minute in the placebo group, 4.7 beats per minute in the low-dosage group, 7.8 beats per minute in the intermediate-dosage group, and 8.5 beats per minute in the high-dosage tesofensine group ($P = .0001$).[85]

Glucagon-Like Peptide-1 Agonist

Liraglutide is a second GLP-1 agonist that is in clinical trials. The rate of degradation of GLP-1 is delayed in this molecule by inserting a fatty acid residue onto one of the amino acids. This slows absorption and reduction. Liraglutide has been evaluated for diabetes and weight loss.[86]

COMBINATIONS OF DRUGS THAT PRODUCE WEIGHT LOSS

The first important clinical trial combining drugs that acted by separate mechanisms used phentermine and fenfluramine.[87] This trial showed a highly significant weight loss of nearly 15% lower than baseline with fewer side effects by using combination therapy. This combination became popular;[88] however, because of reports of aortic valvular regurgitation associated with its use, fenfluramine was withdrawn from the market worldwide on September 15, 1997.[89]

Several other combinations of existing drugs are now under development. One of these is the combination of phentermine with topiramate, in which weight losses greater than 10 kg have been reported. A second is a combination of phentermine with zonisamide. A third is the combination of naltrexone with bupropion, in which additive weight loss has been noted. Initial data have been published on all these combinations, but longer term studies are needed to evaluate the potential drug-drug interactions and side effects produced.

DRUGS THAT INCREASE ENERGY EXPENDITURE

There are no effective drugs in this class.

SUMMARY

There are presently comparatively few drugs available for the treatment of overweight patients, and their effectiveness is limited to palliation of the chronic disease of obesity. Drug development that is now underway is more rapid than in the past, however, and the author anticipates the discovery of safe and effective pharmacologic strategies for the management of obesity and its serious complications.

REFERENCES

1. World Health Organization. Obesity: preventing and managing the global epidemic. Geneva: World Health Organization; 1998.
2. NHLBI Obesity Education Initiative Expert Panel on the Identification, Evaluation, and Treatment of Overweight and Obesity in Adults. Clinical guidelines on the identification, evaluation, and treatment of overweight and obesity in adults—the evidence report. Obes Res 1998;6(Suppl 2):51S–209S.
3. Ogden CL, Yanovski SZ, Carroll MD, et al. The epidemiology of obesity. Gastroenterology 2007; 132(6):2087–102.
4. Bray GA. The metabolic syndrome and obesity. Totowa (NJ): Humana Press, Inc.; 2007.
5. Sacks FM, Bray GA, Carey V, et al. Comparison of weight-loss diets with different compositions of fat, carbohydrate and protein. N Engl J Med 2009;360: 859–73.
6. The practical guide. Identification, evaluation, and treatment of overweight and obesity in adults. National Heart, Lung, and Blood Institute; North American Association for the Study of Obesity. NIH Publication No. 00-4084. Washington, DC: US Department of Health and Human Services, Public Health Service; 2000.
7. Bray GA, Greenway FL. Current and potential drugs for treatment of obesity. Endocr Rev 1999;20(6):805–75.
8. Li Z, Maglione M, Tu W, et al. Meta-analysis: pharmacologic treatment of obesity. Ann Intern Med 2005; 142(7):532–46.
9. Bray GA, Greenway FL. Pharmacological treatment of the overweight patient. Pharmacol Rev 2007;59: 151–84.
10. Avenell A, Brown TJ, McGee MA, et al. What interventions should we add to weight reducing diets in adults with obesity? A systematic review of randomized controlled trials of adding drug therapy, exercise, behaviour therapy or combinations of these interventions. J Hum Nutr Diet 2004;17(4):293–316.
11. Bray GA, Ryan DH. Drug treatment of the overweight patient. Gastroenterology 2007;132(6):2239–52.
12. Rucker D, Padwal R, Li SK, et al. Long term pharmacotherapy for obesity and overweight: updated meta-analysis. BMJ 2007;335:1194–9.
13. Berthoud HR, Morrison C. The brain, appetite, and obesity. Annu Rev Psychol 2008;59:55–92.
14. Tecott LH, Sun LM, Akana SF, et al. Eating disorder and epilepsy in mice lacking 5-HT2C serotonin receptors. Nature 1995;374(6522):542–6.
15. Cheng JT, Kuo DY. Both alpha1-adrenergic and D(1)-dopaminergic neurotransmissions are involved in phenylpropanolamine-mediated feeding suppression in mice. Neurosci Lett 2003;347(2):136–8.
16. Rössner S, Taylor CL, Byington RP, et al. Long term propranolol treatment and changes in body weight after myocardial infarction. BMJ 1990;300(6729):902–3.
17. Sakata T. Histamine receptor and its regulation of energy metabolism. Obes Res 1995;3(Suppl 4): 541S–8S.
18. Kroeze WK, Hufeisen SJ, Popadak BA, et al. H1-histamine receptor affinity predicts short-term weight gain for typical and atypical antipsychotic drugs. Neuropsychopharmacology 2003;28:519–26.

19. Pagotto U, Marsicano G, Cota D, et al. The emerging role of the endocannabinoid system in endocrine regulation and energy balance. Endocr Rev 2006; 27:73–100.

20. Glass MJ, Billington CJ, Levine AS. Opioid and food intake: distributed functional neural pathways? Neuropeptides 1999;33:360–8.

21. Bray GA, Blackburn GL, Ferguson JM, et al. Sibutramine produces dose-related weight loss. Obes Res 1999;7:189–98.

22. Smith IG, Goulder MA. Randomized placebo-controlled trial of long-term treatment with sibutramine in mild to moderate obesity. J Fam Pract 2001;50(6):505–12.

23. Apfelbaum M, Vague P, Ziegler O, et al. Long-term maintenance of weight loss after a very-low-calorie diet: a randomized blinded trial of the efficacy and tolerability of sibutramine. Am J Med 1999;106(2):179–84.

24. James WP, Astrup A, Finer N, et al. Effect of sibutramine on weight maintenance after weight loss: a randomised trial. STORM Study Group. Sibutramine Trial of Obesity Reduction and Maintenance. Lancet 2000;356(9248):2119–25.

25. Wirth A, Krause J. Long-term weight loss with sibutramine: a randomized controlled trial. JAMA 2001; 286(11):1331–9.

26. McMahon FG, Fujioka K, Singh BN, et al. Efficacy and safety of sibutramine in obese white and African American patients with hypertension: a 1-year, double-blind, placebo-controlled, multicenter trial. Arch Intern Med 2000;160(14):2185–91.

27. McMahon FG, Weinstein SP, Rowe E, et al. Sibutramine is safe and effective for weight loss in obese patients whose hypertension is well controlled with angiotensin-converting enzyme inhibitors. J Hum Hypertens 2002;16(1):5–11.

28. Finer N, Bloom SR, Frost GS, et al. Sibutramine is effective for weight loss and diabetic control in obesity with type 2 diabetes: a randomised, double-blind, placebo-controlled study. Diabetes Obes Metab 2000;2(2):105–12.

29. Fujioka K, Seaton TB, Rowe E, et al. Weight loss with sibutramine improves glycaemic control and other metabolic parameters in obese patients with type 2 diabetes mellitus. Diabetes Obes Metab 2000;2(3): 175–87.

30. Berkowitz RI, Wadden TA, Tershakovec AM, et al. Behavior therapy and sibutramine for the treatment of adolescent obesity: a randomized controlled trial. JAMA 2003;289(14):1805–12.

31. Godoy-Matos A, Carraro L, Vieira A, et al. Treatment of obese adolescents with sibutramine: a randomized, double-blind, controlled study. J Clin Endocrinol Metab 2005;90(3):1460–5.

32. Berkowitz RI, Fujioka K, Daniels SR, et al. Effects of sibutramine treatment in obese adolescents: a randomized trial. Ann Intern Med 2006;145(2):81–90.

33. Daniels SR, Arnett DK, Eckel RH, et al. Overweight in children and adolescents: pathophysiology, consequences, prevention, and treatment. Circulation 2005;111(15):1999–2012.

34. Wadden TA, Berkowitz RI, Womble LG, et al. Randomized trial of lifestyle modification and pharmacotherapy for obesity. N Engl J Med 2005; 353(20):2111–20.

35. Munro J, MacCuish A, Wilson E, et al. Comparison of continuous and intermittent anorectic therapy in obesity. Br Med J 1968;1:352–4.

36. Sjostrom L, Rissanen A, Andersen T, et al. Randomised placebo-controlled trial of orlistat for weight loss and prevention of weight regain in obese patients. European Multicentre Orlistat Study Group. Lancet 1998;352(9123):167–72.

37. Davidson MH, Hauptman J, DiGirolamo M, et al. Weight control and risk factor reduction in obese subjects treated for 2 years with orlistat: a randomized controlled trial. JAMA 1999;281(3):235–42.

38. Rossner S, Sjostrom L, Noack R, et al. Weight loss, weight maintenance, and improved cardiovascular risk factors after 2 years treatment with orlistat for obesity. European Orlistat Obesity Study Group. Obes Res 2000;8(1):49–61.

39. Hauptman J. Orlistat: selective inhibition of caloric absorption can affect long-term body weight. Endocrine 2000;13:201–6.

40. Torgerson JS, Hauptman J, Boldrin MN, et al. XENical in the prevention of diabetes in obese subjects (XENDOS) study: a randomized study of orlistat as an adjunct to lifestyle changes for the prevention of type 2 diabetes in obese patients. Diabetes Care 2004;27(1):155–61.

41. Chanoine JP, Hampl S, Jensen C, et al. Effect of orlistat on weight and body composition in obese adolescents: a randomized controlled trial. JAMA 2005;293(23):2873–83.

42. Hill JO, Hauptman J, Anderson JW, et al. Orlistat, a lipase inhibitor, for weight maintenance after conventional dieting: a 1-y study. Am J Clin Nutr 1999;69(6):1108–16.

43. Hollander PA, Elbein SC, Hirsch IB, et al. Role of orlistat in the treatment of obese patients with type 2 diabetes. A 1-year randomized double-blind study. Diabetes Care 1998;21(8):1288–94.

44. Kelley DE, Bray GA, Pi-Sunyer FX, et al. Clinical efficacy of orlistat therapy in overweight and obese patients with insulin-treated type 2 diabetes: a 1-year randomized controlled trial. Diabetes Care 2002;25(6):1033–41.

45. Miles JM, Leiter L, Hollander P, et al. Effect of orlistat in overweight and obese patients with type 2 diabetes treated with metformin. Diabetes Care 2002; 25(7):1123–8.

46. Heymsfield SB, Segal KR, Hauptman J, et al. Effects of weight loss with orlistat on glucose tolerance and

progression to type 2 diabetes in obese adults. Arch Intern Med 2000;160(9):1321–6.

47. Zhi J, Mulligan TE, Hauptman JB. Long-term systemic exposure of orlistat, a lipase inhibitor, and its metabolites in obese patients. J Clin Pharmacol 1999;39(1):41–6.

48. Wadden TA, Berkowitz RI, Womble LG, et al. Effects of sibutramine plus orlistat in obese women following 1 year of treatment by sibutramine alone: a placebo-controlled trial. Obes Res 2000;8(6):431–7.

49. Lawton CL, Wales JK, Hill AJ, et al. Serotoninergic manipulation, meal-induced satiety and eating pattern: effect of fluoxetine in obese female subjects. Obes Res 1995;3(4):345–56.

50. Goldstein DJ, Rampey AH Jr, Roback PJ, et al. Efficacy and safety of long-term fluoxetine treatment of obesity—maximizing success. Obes Res 1995; 3(Suppl 4):481S–90S.

51. Gadde KM, Parker CB, Maner LG, et al. Bupropion for weight loss: an investigation of efficacy and tolerability in overweight and obese women. Obes Res 2001;9(9):544–51.

52. Jain AK, Kaplan RA, Gadde KM, et al. Bupropion SR vs. placebo for weight loss in obese patients with depressive symptoms. Obes Res 2002;10(10): 1049–56.

53. Anderson JW, Greenway FL, Fujioka K, et al. Bupropion SR enhances weight loss: a 48-week double-blind, placebo-controlled trial. Obes Res 2002;10(7):633–41.

54. Astrup A, Toubro S. Topiramate: a new potential pharmacological treatment for obesity. Obes Res 2004;12(Suppl):167S–73S.

55. Ben-Menachem E, Axelsen M, Johanson EH, et al. Predictors of weight loss in adults with topiramate-treated epilepsy. Obes Res 2003;11(4):556–62.

56. Bray GA, Hollander P, Klein S, et al. A 6-month randomized, placebo-controlled, dose-ranging trial of topiramate for weight loss in obesity. Obes Res 2003;11(6):722–33.

57. Wilding J, Van Gaal L, Rissanen A, et al. A randomized double-blind placebo-controlled study of the long-term efficacy and safety of topiramate in the treatment of obese subjects. Int J Obes Relat Metab Disord 2004;28(11):1399–410.

58. Astrup A, Caterson I, Zelissen P, et al. Topiramate: long-term maintenance of weight loss induced by a low-calorie diet in obese subjects. Obes Res 2004;12(10):1658–69.

59. Gadde KM, Franciscy DM, Wagner HR 2nd, et al. Zonisamide for weight loss in obese adults: a randomized controlled trial. JAMA 2003;289(14):1820–5.

60. Fontbonne A, Charles MA, Juhan-Vague I, et al. The effect of metformin on the metabolic abnormalities associated with upper-body fat distribution. BIGPRO Study Group. Diabetes Care 1996;19(9):920–6.

61. Knowler WC, Barrett-Connor E, Fowler SE, et al. Reduction in the incidence of type 2 diabetes with lifestyle intervention or metformin. N Engl J Med 2002;346(6):393–403.

62. Ortega-Gonzalez C, Luna S, Hernandez L, et al. Responses of serum androgen and insulin resistance to metformin and pioglitazone in obese, insulin-resistant women with polycystic ovary syndrome. J Clin Endocrinol Metab 2005;90(3):1360–5.

63. Riddle MC, Drucker DJ. Emerging therapies mimicking the effects of amylin and glucagon-like peptide 1. Diabetes Care 2006;29(2):435–49.

64. Ratner RE, Dickey R, Fineman M, et al. Amylin replacement with pramlintide as an adjunct to insulin therapy improves long-term glycaemic and weight control in Type 1 diabetes mellitus: a 1-year, randomized controlled trial. Diabet Med 2004; 21(11):1204–12.

65. Maggs D, Shen L, Strobel S, et al. Effect of pramlintide on A1C and body weight in insulin-treated African Americans and Hispanics with type 2 diabetes: a pooled post hoc analysis. Metabolism 2003;52(12):1638–42.

66. Patriti A, Facchiano E, Sanna A, et al. The enteroinsular axis and the recovery from type 2 diabetes after bariatric surgery. Obes Surg 2004;14(6):840–8.

67. Small CJ, Bloom SR. Gut hormones as peripheral anti obesity targets. Curr Drug Targets CNS Neurol Disord 2004;3(5):379–88.

68. Greenway SE, Greenway FL 3rd, Klein S. Effects of obesity surgery on non-insulin-dependent diabetes mellitus. Arch Surg 2002;137(10):1109–17.

69. Lugari R, Dei Cas A, Ugolotti D, et al. Glucagon-like peptide 1 (GLP-1) secretion and plasma dipeptidyl peptidase IV (DPP-IV) activity in morbidly obese patients undergoing biliopancreatic diversion. Horm Metab Res 2004;36(2):111–5.

70. Edwards CM, Stanley SA, Davis R, et al. Exendin-4 reduces fasting and postprandial glucose and decreases energy intake in healthy volunteers. Am J Physiol Endocrinol Metab 2001;281(1):E155–61.

71. Buse JB, Henry RR, Han J, et al. Effects of exenatide (exendin-4) on glycemic control over 30 weeks in sulfonylurea-treated patients with type 2 diabetes. Diabetes Care 2004;27(11):2628–35.

72. DeFronzo RA, Ratner RE, Han J, et al. Effects of exenatide (exendin-4) on glycemic control and weight over 30 weeks in metformin-treated patients with type 2 diabetes. Diabetes Care 2005;28(5): 1092–100.

73. Kendall DM, Riddle MC, Rosenstock J, et al. Effects of exenatide (exendin-4) on glycemic control over 30 weeks in patients with type 2 diabetes treated with metformin and a sulfonylurea. Diabetes Care 2005; 28(5):1083–91.

74. Heine RJ, Van Gaal LF, Johns D, et al. Exenatide versus insulin glargine in patients with suboptimally controlled type 2 diabetes: a randomized trial. Ann Intern Med 2005;143(8):559–69.

75. Gibson WT, Ebersole BJ, Bhattacharyya S, et al. Mutational analysis of the serotonin receptor 5HT2c in severe early-onset human obesity. Can J Physiol Pharmacol 2004;82(6):426–9.

76. Nilsson BM. 5-Hydroxytryptamine 2C (5-HT2C) receptor agonists as potential antiobesity agents. J Med Chem 2006;49(14):4023–34.

77. Cangiano C, Ceci F, Cascino A, et al. Eating behavior and adherence to dietary prescriptions in obese adult subjects treated with 5-hydroxytryptophan. Am J Clin Nutr 1992;56(5):863–7.

78. Cangiano C, Laviano A, Del Ben M, et al. Effects of oral 5-hydroxy-tryptophan on energy intake and macronutrient selection in non-insulin dependent diabetic patients. Int J Obes Relat Metab Disord 1998;22(7):648–54.

79. Rogers PJ, Blundell JE. Effect of anorexic drugs on food intake and the micro-structure of eating in human subjects. Psychopharmacology (Berl) 1979; 66(2):159–65.

80. Foltin RW, Haney M, Comer SD, et al. Effect of fenfluramine on food intake, mood, and performance of humans living in a residential laboratory. Physiol Behav 1996;59(2):295–305.

81. Drent ML, Zelissen PM, Koppeschaar HP, et al. The effect of dexfenfluramine on eating habits in a Dutch ambulatory android overweight population with an overconsumption of snacks. Int J Obes Relat Metab Disord 1995;19(5):299–304.

82. Walsh AE, Smith KA, Oldman AD, et al. m-Chlorophenylpiperazine decreases food intake in a test meal. Psychopharmacology (Berl) 1994;116: 120–2.

83. Boeles S, Williams C, Campling GM, et al. Sumatriptan decreases food intake and increases plasma growth hormone in healthy women. Psychopharmacology (Berl) 1997;129(2):179–82.

84. Smith SR, Prosser WA, Donahue DJ, et al. Lorcaserin (APD356), a selective 5-HT(2C) agonist, reduces body weight in obese men and women. Obesity 2008;17:494–503.

85. Astrup A, Madsbad S, Breum L, et al. Effect of tesofensine on bodyweight loss, body composition, and quality of life in obese patients: a randomised, double-blind, placebo-controlled trial. Lancet 2008; 372:1906–13.

86. Vilsbøll T, Zdravkovic M, Le-Thi T, et al. Liraglutide, a long-acting human glucagon-like peptide-1 analog, given as monotherapy significantly improves glycemic control and lowers body weight without risk of hypoglycemia in patients with type 2 diabetes. Diabetes Care 2007;30(6):1608–10.

87. Weintraub M. Long-term weight control: the National Heart, Lung, and Blood Institute funded multimodal intervention study. Clin Pharmacol Ther 1992;51(5): 581–5.

88. Stafford RS, Radley DC. National trends in antiobesity medication use. Arch Intern Med 2003;163(9): 1046–50.

89. Connolly HM, Crary JL, McGoon MD, et al. Valvular heart disease associated with fenfluramine-phentermine. N Engl J Med 1997;337(9):581–8.

Obesity and Bariatric Surgery

Basil M. Yurcisin, MD*, Moataz M. Gaddor, MD,
Eric J. DeMaria, MD

KEYWORDS

- Bariatric surgery • Obesity • Management

EPIDEMIOLOGY

Obesity has now reached epidemic proportions globally. Along with associated conditions, it represents one of the greatest worldwide health concerns. In the United States alone, according to the National Health and Nutrition Examination Survey (NHANES), from 2003 to 2004, obesity was present in 28.5% of adults aged 20 to 39 years, 36.8% of adults aged 40 to 59 years, and 31.0% of those aged 60 years or older.[1] The NHANES also indicated that more than 30% of children in the United States aged 12 to 19 years have a body mass index (BMI) greater than the 85th percentile for their age.[2] This crisis now involves the developing world, and the World Health Organization currently estimates that 1.7 billion individuals (approximately one fourth of the earth's population) on the planet are overweight or obese.[3] The prevalence of severe and morbid obesity is increasing more rapidly than other degrees of obesity.[4,5] Bariatric surgery has established itself as the only durable option for managing this epidemic, with a favorable impact on almost all related comorbidities.[6,7]

CLASSIFICATION

Categories of obesity and overweight are defined using BMI, which is calculated as weight in kilograms divided by the square of the height in meters. A person with a BMI of 25 to 29.9 kg/m^2 is considered overweight, a person with a BMI of 30 to 34.9 kg/m^2 is considered obese, a person with a BMI of 35 to 39.9 kg/m^2 is considered severely obese, and a person with a BMI greater than 40 kg/m^2 is considered morbidly obese.

This is a somewhat arbitrary classification system and is not without flaws. The BMI fails to recognize differences in body composition between genders, to separate persons with differing percentages of body fat (well-muscled athletes versus obese individuals), and to indicate risk profiles based on race (white women suffer similar comorbidities at a BMI of 35 kg/mg^2 as their African-American and Asian counterparts do at a BMI of 32 kg/m^2).[8] The impact of these discrepancies is seen when BMI is used as a tool to determine candidates for bariatric surgery.

The distribution of body fat has an important influence on the severity of comorbidities. Android or visceral obesity has been linked to significantly worse long-term health compared with gynoid or subcutaneous obesity.[9] Anthropomorphic measurements, such as waist-to-hip ratio, have been used to quantify central obesity; however, CT scans have shown that abdominal circumference is a more accurate measurement of visceral fat distribution.[10] An abdominal circumference of 35 in or greater in women and 40 in or greater in men is related to an increased risk for comorbid conditions.[11] Visceral obesity has been linked to metabolic syndrome, hypertension (HTN), type 2 diabetes mellitus (DM2), increased systemic inflammation, and hypercoagulability. Subcutaneous obesity is not as strongly associated with comorbidities.[12]

Because of gender and body habitus differences, many studies quantify weight loss in terms of excess weight loss (current weight − ideal body weight = excess weight). Comparison of the amount of excess body weight (EBW) loss allows comparison of outcomes among the various bariatric procedures. Buchwald and colleagues[6]

Department of Surgery, Duke University Medical Center, DUMC Box 3288, Durham, NC 27710, USA
* Corresponding author.
E-mail address: basil.yurcisin@duke.edu (B.M. Yurcisin).

Clin Chest Med 30 (2009) 539–553
doi:10.1016/j.ccm.2009.05.013

used this measurement when performing a meta-analysis of bariatric surgery outcomes from 1990 to 2002 involving more than 22,000 patients.

ETIOLOGY

Obesity is multifactorial in origin, and the exact mechanism for development of morbid obesity is not entirely known. Causes likely include a combination of genetic, endocrine, behavioral, socio-economic, psychologic, and environmental factors. Multiple studies have identified a genetic predisposition to obesity, and several genetic markers have been described. In adoption studies, severity of obesity was found to be more concordant with natural rather than adoptive parents.[13,14] Furthermore, monozygotic twins have more similar BMIs than dizygotic twins, even given different rearing environments.[10,15]

Gastrointestinal and neuroendocrine peptides are involved in weight homeostasis. Ghrelin, a potent orexigenic peptide mainly secreted by gastric fundus A cells, increases in response to fasting and decreases postprandially.[16] Ghrelin levels are low in obese individuals[17] because it decreases in response to increased intake. The adipocyte hormone leptin stimulates anorexigenic neuropeptides in the hypothalamus to increase satiety; obese individuals often have increased serum levels of leptin and may be resistant to this hormone's effect.[18]

Gender and ethnicity differences manifest wide variations in the magnitude of obesity. An estimated 33% of American men are obese as compared with 35% of American women.[19] In 2006, the NHANES reported that 58% of non-Hispanic black women aged 40 to 59 years old in the United States are obese compared with only 38% non-Hispanic white women. The prevalence of overweight in Mexican-American male children and adolescents is significantly greater than in non-Hispanic white male children and adolescents. Mexican-American and non-Hispanic black female children and adolescents are significantly more likely to be overweight compared with non-Hispanic white female children and adolescents.[1]

COMORBIDITIES

Obesity is rapidly becoming the most prevalent modifiable risk factor for coronary artery disease (CAD),[20] the leading cause of death among American adults.[21] Concurrent with the exponential growth of obesity worldwide is the increase in obesity-related comorbidities. Many of these conditions (**Box 1**) carry an increased risk for mortality and include but are not limited to metabolic syndrome, CAD, HTN, congestive heart

---

Box 1
Conditions associated with obesity

CAD

DM2

Cancers (endometrial, breast, and colon)

HTN

Dyslipidemia (eg, high total cholesterol, high triglycerides)

Stroke

Liver and gallbladder disease

Sleep apnea and respiratory disorders

Osteoarthritis

Gynecologic problems (infertility, abnormal menses, and polycystic ovary)

Pseudotumor cerebri

---

failure, DM2, dyslipidemia, arthritis, infertility, pseudotumor cerebri, obesity hypoventilation syndrome (OHS), obstructive sleep apnea (OSA), chronic obstructive pulmonary disease, gastroesophageal (GE) reflux disease, hypercoagulability and venous thromboembolism (VTE), and certain types of cancer (colon, breast, prostate, and ovary). It is estimated that these associated conditions are responsible for more than 2.5 million deaths per year worldwide.[6]

WEIGHT LOSS STRATEGIES

Intentional weight loss, even to a modest degree (5%–10%), has a significant impact on the morbidity and mortality associated with obesity.[22] Current management strategies for weight loss attempt to create a negative energy balance through diet, exercise, behavior modification, pharmacotherapy, and surgery. The method of weight loss does not seem to affect the level of benefit obtained; however, surgery has established itself as the most durable. Benefits of weight loss in regard to the cardiovascular system are outlined in **Box 2**.

There are many strategies for weight reduction, including hospital-supervised, commercially available, and psychiatric-behavior modification programs and medications. Unfortunately, although many people can lose weight successfully through dietary manipulation, only 5% to 10% of patients with extreme obesity are able to sustain significant weight reduction.[23] The National Institutes of Health (NIH) Technology Assessment Conference in 1992 concluded that dietary management of severe obesity, with or without behavioral modification, failed to provide acceptable evidence of long-term efficacy.[24]

Box 2
Cardiovascular benefits of weight loss

Decreased blood volume

Decreased stroke volume

Decreased cardiac output

Decreased pulmonary capillary wedge pressure

Decreased left ventricular mass

Decreased resting oxygen consumption

Decreased systemic arterial pressure

Decreased resting heart rate

Decreased filling pressures both sides of heart

Decreased QT_C interval

Data from Poirier P, Giles TD, Bray GA, et al. Obesity and cardiovascular disease: pathophysiology, evaluation, and effect of weight loss an update of the 1997 American Heart Association Scientific Statement on Obesity and Heart Disease from the Obesity Committee of the Council on Nutrition, Physical Activity, and Metabolism. Circulation 2006;113: 898–918.

Current pharmacotherapy includes orlistat, a pancreatic lipase inhibitor that blocks fat absorption, and sibutramine, which works as an appetite suppressant through blockage of norepinephrine and dopamine reuptake. These agents provide only modest weight loss and are inadequate monotherapy for the morbidly obese patient.[6] The sustainability of all forms of weight loss is enhanced by the inclusion of an exercise regimen to the weight reduction approach (see the article by Bray in this issue).[11]

Bariatric surgery is the best current treatment for morbid obesity, providing the only mechanism for effective and sustained weight reduction, especially for those who have not experienced long-term success through other means.[25] Obesity surgery is able to produce durable weight loss and remission of DM2, in addition to having a similar effect on other comorbidities and all-cause mortality. These benefits can be achieved in centers of excellence (COEs) with an associated 90-day mortality rate of less than 1% (similar to cholecystectomy complication rates).[8]

EVOLUTION OF BARIATRIC SURGERY

The evolution of bariatric surgery began in the 1950s when two surgeons at the University of Minnesota developed the intestinal bypass operation after observing the effects of short-gut syndrome. In this procedure, an end-to-end anastomosis was created between the proximal jejunum and the distal ileum. The bypassed small bowel was drained into the colon. Although this procedure did produce significant weight loss, it was wrought with complications, including electrolyte imbalance, intractable diarrhea, blind-loop syndrome, autoimmune disease, cirrhosis, and liver failure.[26]

The development of gastric bypass in the 1960s and gastric banding in the 1980s by Mason and his colleagues[27,28] proved that effective weight loss could be achieved surgically with a much improved safety profile.[29] It was observed that patients who had undergone subtotal gastrectomy for peptic ulcer disease tended to remain underweight and had difficulty in gaining weight. Gastric bypass involved creating a small gastric pouch that was connected to a segment of jejunum, achieving restriction of oral intake and malabsorption. Originally, a Billroth II connection to the small bowel was used. This was modified over subsequent decades to a Roux-en-Y configuration.

The vertical banded gastroplasty (VBG) and subsequent invention of the adjustable gastric band gave bariatric surgeons a set of purely restrictive procedures to add to their armamentarium. Hess and colleagues[30] and Scopinaro and colleagues[31] used biliopancreatic diversion with duodenal switch (BP-DS) to increase the malabsorption achieved with gastric bypass. Currently, gastric bypass (~70%) and gastric banding (~20%) are the two most common bariatric procedures performed in the United States. MacDonald and colleagues[32] and Pories and colleagues[33] individually reported the efficacy of gastric bypass by proving durable weight loss, resolution of comorbidities, and decreased mortality in 608 patients with up to 16 years of follow-up, cementing the use of this modality to achieve weight loss.

The laparoscopic revolution had an immense impact on the growth of bariatric surgery. Laparoscopic Roux-en-Y gastric bypass (LRYGB) and laparoscopic adjustable gastric banding (LAGB) have been shown to be safe and effective procedures.[34,35] Patients are seeking laparoscopic surgery in increasing numbers because of the fact that it is less invasive, is associated with less pain, and has quicker recovery times.[36] At present, almost all bariatric procedures are performed laparoscopically unless body habitus, previous or revisional surgery status, or technical difficulty prevents accomplishment.

Further advances in outcomes assessment and quality control continue to advance the practice of bariatric surgery. Reports of serious complications and deaths along with skyrocketing malpractice claims raised concerns that many hospitals were performing too few bariatric procedures and were ill equipped to accomplish these complex procedures safely.[37,38] In response to these reports, the American Society for Bariatric and Metabolic Surgery (ASMBS) created the COE classification for hospitals performing bariatric surgery. The ASMBS also formed the independent nonprofit Surgical Review Corporation (SRC) to manage the COE program; currently 365 sites have this designation. As a result of more stringent quality control, recent data have shown an almost 80% reduction in inpatient mortality rates from 1988 to 2004 (0.89% to 0.19%).[39]

The NIH's Longitudinal Assessment of Bariatric Surgery (LABS) and the SRC's Bariatric Outcomes Longitudinal Database (BOLD) have been established to help centralize obesity surgery statistics. With an expected annual addition of more than 100,000 patients, the primary goals of the BOLD are to (1) allow real-time monitoring of compliance with COE requirements; (2) provide the SRC with credible data that can be used to demonstrate to consumers, employers, medical professionals, and payers the value and efficacy of bariatric surgery; and (3) collect information needed to improve patient outcomes.[40] Continued participation in large national databases should allow the bariatric surgical community to provide better definitions of success and failure for obesity surgery. Also, it may help to determine which patients are likely to benefit the most from each of the available operative procedures.

INDICATIONS AND CONTRAINDICATIONS

Although badly in need of updating in light of modern data, the 1991 NIH Consensus Panel established eligibility criteria for surgical management. In general, candidates for bariatric surgery have a BMI of 40 kg/m² or greater or 35 kg/m² or greater with an established comorbidity and documented failure of nonsurgical methods of weight loss.[25] Contraindications for bariatric surgery include patients who are unable to understand the nature of bariatric surgery or to make the necessary postoperative lifestyle changes (eg, vitamin supplementation, diet, and follow-up) and those with current substance abuse, untreated psychiatric or eating disorders, and noncompliance with previous medical care. Patients with illnesses that greatly reduce life expectancy or their ability to undergo general anesthesia, such as cancer and end-stage renal, hepatic, or cardiopulmonary disease, are poor candidates (**Box 3**).[41] Bariatric surgery in adolescent (< 18 years old) and geriatric (> 65 years old) populations is

---

> **Box 3**
> **NIH guidelines for candidates for bariatric surgery**
>
> - BMI of 40 kg/m² or greater
> - BMI of 35 to 39.9 kg/m² with severe comorbid conditions, such as life-threatening cardiopulmonary problems (eg, severe sleep apnea, obesity-related cardiomyopathy) or diabetes
> - Documented failure of nonsurgical weight loss
> - BMI of 35 to 39.9 kg/m² with obesity-induced physical problems interfering with lifestyle (eg, joint disease treatable but for the obesity, body size problems precluding or severely interfering with employment and family activities)
> - Not have an underlying endocrine abnormality that can contribute to obesity, ongoing substance abuse, or uncontrolled psychiatric disorders
> - Be able to understand the surgery and consequences of treatment and be compliant with follow-up and vitamin supplementation guidelines
> - Not have an illness that greatly reduces life expectancy (eg, cancer, end-stage renal disease, end-stage hepatic disease, end-stage cardiopulmonary disease)

controversial but is gaining acceptance and is discussed elsewhere in this article.

PATIENT EVALUATION AND WORKUP

Preoperative assessment of candidates for bariatric procedures is based on the principle of identifying modifiable health concerns and implementing risk-reducing treatments to have an impact on perioperative morbidity and mortality. The initial evaluation of the patient who is to undergo bariatric surgery should begin with a candid discussion. Bariatric surgery carries significant risks and can fail in its attempt to improve the health and reduce the weight of the patient. Patients should take part in a preoperative seminar outlining expectations in regard to postoperative recovery, diet alteration, activity, and clinical outcomes.[41] Beneficial outcomes are only achieved consistently with careful patient selection and preoperative planning.[42,43] To evaluate the potential patient properly, surgeons should ideally employ the assistance of a multidisciplinary team, including nutritionists, psychologists or psychiatrists, and appropriate medical specialty consultants as needed.[41] Appropriate laboratory testing is driven by findings within the history and physical examination (**Box 4**).

> **Box 4**
> **Recommended preoperative testing**
>
> Complete blood cell count
> Comprehensive metabolic panel
> Hemoglobin A1c
> Ferritin
> Thyroid-stimulating hormone
> Lipid profile
> Barium swallow or endoscopy
> Electrocardiogram

Patients with significant medical comorbidities identified during the history and physical examination should receive subspecialty consultation. Morbidly obese patients are at an increased risk for having HTN, dyslipidemia, and diabetes, all of which are risk factors for CAD.[44,45] A reliable assessment tool for cardiac function is estimation of exercise tolerance; those not able to walk four blocks or climb two flights of stairs without symptoms have twice the risk for serious postoperative complications compared with those who have unlimited exercise tolerance.[46] A preoperative electrocardiogram (ECG) should be obtained for all obese patients 30 years of age or older and for those with evidence of underlying cardiac disease. Patients with known cardiovascular disease, poor exercise tolerance, or ECG changes should have a preoperative evaluation by a cardiologist. Echocardiography, stress testing, and cardiac catheterization may be indicated in these patients.

The two components of respiratory dysfunction in obesity, OSA and OHS, are collectively known as Pickwickian syndrome. Patients with a history of snoring or daytime somnolence or who have a large neck circumference may need polysomnography to rule out OSA. OHS is characterized by hypoxemia (partial pressure of arterial oxygen < 55 mm Hg) and hypercarbia (partial pressure of carbon dioxide > 47 mm Hg) found on arterial blood gas analysis. Pickwickian syndrome is frequently complicated by severe pulmonary HTN, right heart failure, and polycythemia. Patients diagnosed with OSA or OHS should have a preoperative evaluation conducted by a pulmonologist. It is important to identify these patients and institute pre- and perioperative continuous positive airway pressure (CPAP) therapy to avoid lethal apnea.[47]

Patients with chronic severe hypoxemia may manifest polycythemia and pulmonary HTN. Polycythemia further increases an already significant risk for deep venous thrombosis and pulmonary embolism (PE). In the periprocedural setting, obese patients are most at risk for thromboembolic events because of immobilization, interoperative pneumoperitoneum, and increased postoperative circulating levels of procoagulable factors. Preoperative heparin, early ambulation, and postoperative enoxaparin should be standard to minimize VTE. Intermittent venous compression boots are useful in counteracting increased venous stasis and the propensity for clotting. Consideration should be given to prophylactic insertion of an inferior vena cava filter in patients who are at high risk for VTE (venous stasis, BMI ≥ 60 kg/m^2, truncal obesity, prior VTE, and known hypercoagulable state).[48]

Airway management in the obese population presents a critical concern. Before surgery, it is frequently necessary to oxygenate and intubate obese patients, who are positioned in the 25° reverse-Trendelenburg position. Dixon and colleagues[49] reported that this position was associated with greater lung volumes and mean arterial oxygen tensions and with less atelectasis and pulmonary shunting when compared with these parameters in supine patients before intubation. During surgical procedures, patients who have OSA are at significant risk for acute upper airway obstruction and respiratory arrest. An oral airway is strongly recommended after muscle paralysis because of the redundant tissue of the soft palate. It can be useful if one anesthetist is responsible for airway positioning, including two-handed seal of the mask, and a second anesthetist is responsible for adequate ventilation. If the patient has severe pulmonary disease and CPAP is ineffective or cannot be tolerated, prophylactic tracheostomy should be considered.

The use of preoperative endoscopy is reserved for patients with complaints of reflux, dyspepsia, or dysphagia. Obesity is known to be associated with a higher risk for reflux, erosive esophagitis, and esophageal adenocarcinoma.[50] Many bariatric procedures render the remnant stomach inaccessible to traditional endoscopy; thus, the threshold for investigating the upper gastrointestinal (UGI) system should be low. Contrast-enhanced radiologic studies may provide an alternative approach to investigation.[51] The American Society for Gastrointestinal Endoscopy has recommended *Helicobacter pylori* screening and treatment of individuals with positive test results before bariatric surgery to reduce the incidence of marginal ulcer as a complication of gastric bypass.[52] This recommendation is often viewed as controversial in bariatric surgery circles.

The most common cause of elevated liver function test (LFT) results in patients being considered for bariatric surgery is nonalcoholic fatty liver disease, which can progress to cirrhosis. Elevated LFT results may be investigated with ultrasound or CT to determine presence of cirrhosis or portal HTN.[53] Bariatric surgery may have a favorable effect on steatosis, but the value is not definitive.[54,55] Rapid weight loss after bariatric surgery is associated with up to a 35% incidence of gallstone formation and need for subsequent cholecystectomy. Preoperative workup with ultrasound may be warranted in this population, although controversy exists as to the need for prophylactic cholecystectomy.[56] If the gallbladder is not removed, postoperative treatment for 6 months with ursodiol may prevent symptomatic events and reduces the risk for gallstone formation to 2%.[57] Compliance with this medication can be difficult secondary to adverse side effects (nausea, diarrhea, and pruritus).

Psychologic screening ensures the absence of severe untreated psychologic or psychosocial issues and determination that the patient has realistic expectations and a fundamental understanding of the operation. Currently, there is a lack of consensus as to how to proceed with evaluating the psychiatric state of these patients. Within many centers, however, the interview is quite standardized. Binge eating, personality disorders, and untreated or undertreated depression warrant delay for treatment before surgery.[58] Personality disorders and severe psychiatric disorders requiring admission for inpatient treatment are predictors of poor outcome.[59] The appropriately managed patient who is undergoing psychiatric treatment can have an acceptable outcome.[60]

According to the ASMBS position statement, the preoperative nutritional assessment should be conducted by a qualified professional so as to identify the patient's nutritional and educational needs.[61] Adherence to outlined preoperative behavioral changes, especially with respect to exercise and dietary restrictions, has been shown to improve long-term outcomes.[62] Participation and success (5%–10% weight loss) in a preoperative weight loss program may be associated with a less technically difficult operation and better postoperative weight loss at 3 months. Preoperative weight loss has not been shown to have an impact on the incidence of complications and resolution of comorbidities, and mandating it may cause an unnecessary delay in surgery.[63]

RISK ASSESSMENT

In 2007, DeMaria and colleagues[64] suggested a clinically useful risk stratification tool for application in patients being considered for bariatric surgery. The obesity surgery mortality risk score assigns one point to each of five preoperative variables: BMI of 50 kg/m² or greater, male gender, HTN, pulmonary embolic risk factors, and age of 45 years or older. A score of 0 to 1 was classified as class A, a score of 2 to 3 as class B, and a score of 4 to 5 as class C, with associated mortality risks of 0.2%, 1.1%, and 2.4%, respectively (**Table 1**). This system was later validated by a multicenter

Table 1
Obesity surgery mortality risk score

Variables[a]		
BMI >50 kg/m²		
Male gender		
HTN		
Increased risk for pulmonary embolism		
Previous VTE		
Inferior vena cava filter		
Pulmonary HTN		
Age ≥45 years		

Mortality Assessment		
Score	Class	Mortality Risk
0–1	A	0.2%
2–3	B	1.1%
4–5	C	2.4%

[a] Presence of each variable is equal to one point, resulting in a score of 0 to 5.

study in more than 4000 patients.[65] Use of this scoring system can guide preoperative discussion while obtaining informed consent and can aid in standardization and assessment of outcomes.

Risk for complications and death has further been linked to surgeon expertise in some studies. Among them, Fernandez and colleagues[66] reported an overall leak rate of 6.8% in their first 102 LRYGBs, followed by a reduction to 1.8% over the next 164 patients. Maher and colleagues[67] recently reported continued reduction in adverse outcomes for experienced surgeons performing LRYGBs in a series of 450 consecutive laparoscopic procedures, with no leak or mortality over the final year of their study. To minimize perioperative risk, obesity surgery should be performed in a COE by an experienced bariatric surgeon.

PROCEDURES

Bariatric surgical procedures can be classified into three categories: (1) malabsorptive, producing weight loss by interfering with caloric digestion and absorption; (2) restrictive, producing weight loss by limiting caloric intake; and (3) mixed, producing weight loss through both mechanisms. The only truly malabsorptive procedure was the intestinal bypass, and, as discussed earlier, it has been abandoned secondary to poor outcomes. Although many procedures exist, most have been relegated to the historical perspective. A discussion of the most commonly performed operations follows. **Table 2** compares EBW lost and perioperative mortality rates for the different bariatric procedures.

Restrictive Procedures

Vertical banded gastroplasty
The VBG, considered a restrictive procedure, is performed by creating a small gastric pouch along the lesser curvature of the stomach near the GE junction. This pouch empties into the rest of the stomach by means of a 1-cm prosthetic banded outlet stoma (**Fig. 1**). This operation has largely been abandoned because of its inferior results and complication profile. Randomized controlled trials of gastric bypass versus VBG have shown the superiority of the bypass procedure. Gastric bypass achieves better resolution of diabetes and EBW when compared with VBG (60%–70% versus 40%–50%).[68,69] Early complications of VBG include outlet stenosis and leak at the staple line, whereas late complications encompass staple-line fistula, band erosion, stoma stenosis, food intolerance, and pouch dilation. In a Spanish study, 100 patients undergoing VBG were followed over a minimum of 5 years; 25% required reoperation for problems related to the technique.[70] VBG has essentially been replaced by LAGB, an easier and safer operation.

Laparoscopic adjustable gastric banding
In 2001, the US Food and Drug Administration approved LAGB for use in the United States. Two approved silicone bands are on the market. The band is placed around the proximal stomach, the circumference of which can be changed by accessing a subcutaneous port percutaneously and altering the amount of saline in the bladder (**Fig. 2**). Percutaneous access allows manipulation of the band after surgery in response to weight loss and patient complaints. Weight loss after LAGB has been reported to be between 56% and 59% of EBW.[71,72] American trials, however, have yielded varied results.[73,74] Long-term studies validating LAGB safety and efficacy are needed. Perioperative complications include gastric or esophageal perforation and bleeding. Late complications include band slippage, gastric obstruction, port malfunction or infection, and band erosion.

Sleeve gastrectomy
Sleeve gastrectomy (SG) represents a bariatric surgical option that is gaining significant

Table 2
Comparison of excess body weight lost and operative mortality rates in bariatric procedures

Procedure	Mean Excess Body Weight Lost (%)	Mortality ($\leq$ 30 Days)
Gastric banding	47.5	0.1%
Gastroplasty	68.2	(mortality of gastric banding and VBG is combined)
Gastric bypass	61.6	0.5%
Biliopancreatic diversion $\pm$ switch	70.1	1.1%
All patients undergoing bariatric surgery	61.2	

Data from Buchwald H, Avidor Y, Braunwald E, et al. Bariatric surgery: a systematic review and meta-analysis. JAMA 2004;292:1724–37.

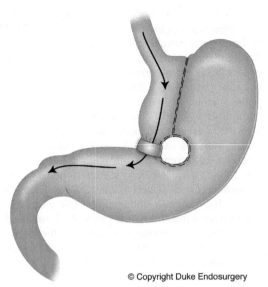

© Copyright Duke Endosurgery

Fig. 1. Vertical banded gastroplasty. (*Courtesy of* Duke Endosurgery Center, Durham, NC; with permission.)

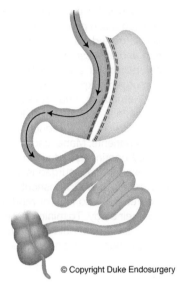

© Copyright Duke Endosurgery

Fig. 3. Sleeve gastrectomy. (*Courtesy of* Duke Endosurgery Center, Durham, NC; with permission.)

momentum. Originally a component of the BP-DS operation, SG has evolved through use as a staging procedure for superobese or high-risk patients to a stand-alone operation. During SG, the stomach is freed from its lateral attachments and the greater curvature of the stomach is removed. This effectively creates a tubular "sleeve" of remaining gastric tissue (**Fig. 3**). Complications include leak, nausea and vomiting,

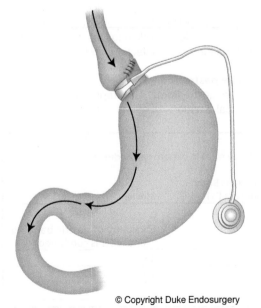

© Copyright Duke Endosurgery

Fig. 2. Adjustable gastric band. (*Courtesy of* Duke Endosurgery Center, Durham, NC; with permission.)

PE, and hemorrhage. One year after surgery, loss of 59% of EBW has been reported.[75] Long-term results for this procedure are pending, but a growing body of evidence suggests 3- to 5-year weight loss results similar to other bariatric procedures.

Mixed Procedures

Biliopancreatic diversion with duodenal switch

The BP-DS involves removal of most of the greater curvature by tubularizing the stomach as described with the SG and transection of the duodenum 2 cm distal to the pylorus. A Roux-en-Y anastomosis is created to the distal jejunum, achieving more bypassed bowel than the gastric bypass (**Fig. 4**). This mixed but predominantly malabsorptive procedure is reserved for the extremely obese (BMI $\geq$60 kg/m^2) and those who have experienced failure with other bariatric operations. Reduction of EBW can approximate 70% to 90%.[76] Treated patients usually pass four to six stools per day, which are foul smelling and float, reflecting inefficient fat absorption. After BP-DS, patients are at risk for iron deficiency anemia and vitamin B_{12} deficiency. Additionally, protein deficiency, osteoporosis secondary to calcium and vitamin D malabsorption, night blindness and skin eruptions secondary to vitamin A deficiency, and problems with fat-soluble vitamins E and K may occur.[30]

Roux-en-Y gastric bypass

LRYGB, a technically demanding procedure with a steep learning curve,[77] combines restriction

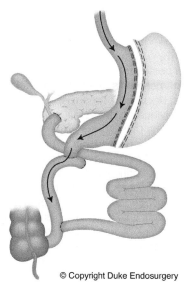

© Copyright Duke Endosurgery

Fig. 4. Biliopancreatic diversion with duodenal switch. (*Courtesy of* Duke Endosurgery Center, Durham, NC; with permission.)

and malabsorption to assist weight loss. A small 15- to 30-mL gastric pouch is created along the lesser curve of the stomach near the GE junction, followed by construction of a gastrojejunostomy (GJ) with a 1-cm stoma to drain the pouch (**Fig. 5**). A 50-cm jejunal limb provides moderate malabsorption and limits bile reflux. This alimentary limb can be tunneled through the mesocolon (retrocolic) or allowed to pass anterior to the colon and stomach (antecolic). Significantly improved

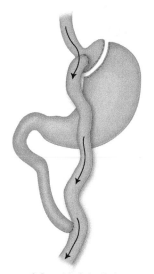

© Copyright Duke Endosurgery

Fig. 5. Roux-en-Y gastric bypass. (*Courtesy of* Duke Endosurgery Center, Durham, NC; with permission.)

weight loss has been achieved in the superobese population (BMI ≥ 50 kg/m^2) with a 150-cm Roux limb, referred to as long-limb gastric bypass.[78]

LRYGB is the most common bariatric surgical procedure performed in the United States. The laparoscopic technique is associated with increases in operative time, cost, and incidence of gastrojejunal stricture. Advantages include decreases in hospital length of stay, incidence of wound infection, incisional hernia, and perioperative blood transfusions. Internal hernias may increase in frequency with the laparoscopic technique as a result of decreased severity of adhesions. At 2 years, patients undergoing successful gastric bypass can expect between 69% and 82% of EBW loss.[35,79]

COMPLICATIONS OF BARIATRIC SURGERY

The most feared complication of gastric surgery for morbid obesity is gastrointestinal leak. Risk factors for leak include increasing age, revisional surgery, male gender, and sleep apnea.[80] After gastric bypass, the excluded stomach can perforate because of marked dilatation resulting from biliopancreatic limb obstruction. This complication is often heralded by frequent hiccups and can be diagnosed by noting a large gastric bubble on abdominal radiographs. Impending gastric perforation requires urgent percutaneous or operative decompression. In patients undergoing revisional gastric surgery for obesity, a gastrostomy tube should be inserted prophylactically for decompression.

The most common site of leak after gastric bypass is at the GJ anastomosis, followed by the jejunojejunal (JJ) anastomosis and excluded stomach. Leaks can occur at any staple line or site of serosal injury. A leak occurring at the JJ anastomosis is more ominous than a leak at the GJ anastomosis, with an associated mortality rate of 40%.[80] Even for the most vigilant surgeons, leaks occur, and the most important risk reduction strategy is early detection. Symptoms of leak can include back or shoulder pain, anxiety, or the feeling of impending doom. Signs that may indicate leak include tachycardia ($P \geq 125$), tachypnea, hypoxemia, hypotension, and oliguria. In any patient with persistent signs or symptoms, the choice of a contrast enhanced UGI series versus repeat laparoscopy should be entertained. Even in the face of a negative UGI series, continued suspicion of leak, nonimprovement, or instability should prompt re-exploration.

Once a leak is identified, management proceeds according to the status of the patient. In the clinically stable patient with a contained leak, management with closed-suction drainage, broad-spectrum antibiotics, nil per os, and total parenteral nutrition has been shown to be safe, especially when presentation is delayed.[80] The stable early postoperative patient with a leak may be better served with laparoscopy for minimal indications. Early re-exploration offers the advantage of diagnosis and treatment with a high level of accuracy. The use of CT or UGI series may be of more use in the patient with delayed presentation. In an unstable patient with a high index of suspicion for a leak, immediate return to the operating room should not be delayed for UGI series or CT.

Marginal ulcers develop in 1% to 16% of patients after gastric bypass,[81] even when they are treated with postoperative acid suppression. This complication usually responds to medical therapy with proton pump inhibitors with or without sucralfate and discontinuation of nonsteroidal anti-inflammatory drugs. The incidence of ulcers is higher in smokers, which serves as yet another reason to encourage cessation. Surgical management may be necessary in those who have persistent pain or recurrent bleeding despite maximal medical management. Stomal stenosis can occur after gastric bypass or VBG. Outpatient endoscopic dilatation is usually successful in resolving stenosis, although more than one treatment may be necessary.[82]

Revision of failed gastroplasty is often unsuccessful secondary to recurrence of stomal dilation and problems with gastric emptying; conversion to gastric bypass provides better results.[83] Laparoscopic gastric banding with ineffective weight loss can likewise be converted to gastric bypass, but the complication rate with this and any revision is higher than for primary gastric bypass. Revision of a dilated GJ stoma has not been effective, but application of an adjustable band to the pouch above the stoma has been suggested as an option for this problem. Less invasive endoscopic procedures aimed at suture reduction of the pouch size or tightening of the stoma have been successful, at least with short-term follow-up.[82] The long-term efficacy of these therapies is not known and is being formally assessed as part of a clinical trial.

Nutritional follow-up is mandatory after gastric bypass because these patients are at risk for deficiency states and their sequelae. Vitamin B_{12}, iron, and calcium supplements are often necessary, along with routine administration of multivitamins. A high-protein diet (50 g/d for women and 65 g/d for men) is required to avoid protein malnutrition.

The operative mortality rate after gastric bypass surgery has been reduced to approximately 0.5%

in most series. Independent risk factors associated with increased risk for death include gastrointestinal leak, pulmonary embolus, HTN, and preoperative weight.[84] The two most common causes of postoperative mortality are anastomotic leak and peritonitis (~75%) and lethal PE (~25%).[85] Despite the prophylactic measures discussed previously, the overall incidence of postoperative PE is 0.9%.

Failure to lose weight after gastric bypass is rare. Significant regaining of the lost weight occurs in 5% to 10% of patients.[8] It is often attributable to progressive noncompliant eating and other poor behavioral habits, development of a functional gastrogastric fistula, gradual enlargement of the gastric pouch, or dilation of the gastrojejunal anastomosis. If a patient has significant obesity-related comorbidities that have failed to resolve or have returned with weight gain, conversion to long-limb gastric bypass or BP-DS can be performed. These modifications can be associated with steatorrhea, fat-soluble vitamin deficiency, and osteoporosis.

RESULTS
Weight Loss

Weight loss after bariatric surgery is mostly attributed to malabsorption or restriction, but other mechanisms, such as dumping syndrome, Roux limb length, and gut hormones, may have a role. The surgical approach used (open versus laparoscopic) does not affect weight loss achieved,[86,87] but there can be wide variation in the weight lost among the available procedures.[6] Postoperative recovery and length of hospital stay are much shorter in the patient undergoing laparoscopy. Postoperative weight loss is greatest at 2 years, with the most pronounced velocity of weight loss in the first 6 to 12 months.[88] Younger, female, white, muscular, and highly motivated individuals who demonstrate compliance with the treatment regimen tend to lose the most weight.[8,89]

Failure of bariatric surgery is not adequately defined at present. Use of the large databases discussed previously (LABS and BOLD) should help to develop this definition. Currently, some surgeons define success by reduction of BMI (< 35 kg/m^2), whereas others define success by degree of EBW lost (≥40%). Also of major importance in evaluating outcome is the documentation of comorbidity resolution. With the new understanding that weight loss surgery is, in fact, metabolic surgery, nonresolution of significant comorbidities should be considered failure.

Comorbidity Resolution

In addition to sustained weight loss, bariatric surgery has been shown to have a significant and initially unexpected impact on almost all comorbidities of obesity. The effect that is perhaps most surprising and discussed is on DM2. Bariatric surgery has the ability to cause diabetes remission in 75% to 80% of those with the disease undergoing obesity surgery. In patients without complete remission, half show significant improvement.[6,33] Multiple meta-analyses have confirmed rates of diabetes remission in 83% to 86% of patients.[6,89,90] The effect is rapid and pronounced; many patients are discharged from the hospital without hypoglycemic medication.[33] The landmark Swedish Obesity Study (SOS) followed 2010 patients who underwent bariatric surgery in comparison to 2037 matched-pair control patients managed medically. At 2 and 10 years, the surgical arm of the population showed reduction in hypertriglyceridemia, hyperuricemia, and diabetes.[91] The immensity of the problem of DM2 in regard to health care cost and associated morbidity (ie, blindness, renal failure, amputations, stroke, CAD) demands continued investigation of bariatric surgery's effect on diabetes.

Similarly, hyperlipidemia and HTN have been shown to resolve or improve after bariatric surgery. In a study of 400 patients, Peluso and Vanek[92] documented resolution of hyperlipidemia in 80% to 100% of patients after bariatric surgery. A study of 1025 patients after gastric bypass showed a 66% reduction in EBW and a 69% remission in HTN at 1 year; at the 5-year follow-up, this effect was 66%.[90] Weight loss has a significant impact on HTN; in general, a decrease of 1% in body weight lowers systolic pressure by 1 mm Hg and diastolic pressure by 2 mm Hg.[93] The amelioration of dyslipidemia seems to have a stronger association with the more malabsorptive procedures. Reduction in HTN seems to be independent of the type of surgery performed.[6]

Cancer and OSA are influenced by weight reduction procedures. Patients who have undergone bariatric surgery show a greater than 80% improvement in cancer[94] and OSA.[6] After surgery, patients show arterial increases in oxygen concentration and decreases in carbon dioxide concentration.[95] Bariatric surgery has also been shown to improve sleep efficiency, the Epworth Sleepiness Scale score, and the need for CPAP after surgery.[96] The literature is replete with reports documenting resolution or improvement of virtually every comorbidity of obesity. It is not uncommon for the patient to have an increased quality of life, an enhanced self-image, a reduced number of prescribed medications, and a significantly improved 5-year mortality risk after bariatric surgery.

Mortality Reduction

With the significant decrease in weight and comorbidities, the risk for obesity-related mortality improves. A large, prospective, observational study in more than 43,000 US women with a 12-year follow-up showed that a 9-kg decrease in weight was associated with a 53% decrease in all obesity-related deaths.[97] The SOS reported an 80% drop in the annual mortality rate in its surgically treated arm versus its medically managed arm.[91] In another study of more than 6000 patients, the cohort that had bariatric surgery (n = 1035) had a 5-year mortality rate of 0.68% compared with 6.17% in the age- and gender-matched controls (n = 5746) who did not have surgery.[98] The evidence supporting the benefit of weight loss is staggering. Bariatric surgery is the most effective method of achieving sustained weight loss in obese patients.

SPECIAL POPULATIONS

In general, extremely old (> 65 years) and extremely young (< 18 years) individuals may not be considered good candidates for surgery, although such arbitrary barriers to treatment are being eroded over time. In particular, barriers to adolescent gastric bypass are rapidly lessening in the face of studies showing sustained weight loss, comorbidity resolution, and improved self-image.[99] Many case reports and anecdotal accounts of treatment, with benefit, of patients upward of 78 years old exist. Current research is attempting to establish the role of bariatric surgery in these populations, especially in regard to the use of reversible procedures with better safety profiles.

Maternal obesity represents a growing concern in the United States. Some estimate that as many as 80% of patients undergoing LRYGB are women, most of whom are of child-bearing age.[100,101] Many reports have documented the safety of modern bariatric surgery in this population, especially when performed at a COE.[102–104] The current recommendation is to delay pregnancy after bariatric surgery for 2 years, because this is the time when weight loss and complication rates are the highest.[105]

SUMMARY

The growth of bariatric surgery has paralleled the explosion of overweight and obesity on a global scale. Weight loss in overweight individuals has been documented to have a favorable impact on morbidity and mortality. Bariatric surgery has established itself as the most reliable way to achieve significant weight loss in overweight and obese populations. Surgical procedures to reduce EBW have evolved and are now considered safe, especially when performed by experienced surgeons in a COE. Bariatric surgery not only causes weight loss but has a significant impact on comorbidities and the overall mortality of obesity. The indications for, and populations benefited by, bariatric surgery continue to expand. The new designation, metabolic surgery, carries a significance that can have an impact on how some of the most devastating diseases faced by medicine today are managed.

REFERENCES

1. Ogden CL, Carroll MD, Curtin LR, et al. Prevalence of overweight and obesity in the United States, 1999–2004. JAMA 2006;295(13):1549–55.
2. Ogden CL, Flegal KM, Carroll MD, et al. Prevalence and trends in overweight among US children and adolescents, 1999–2000. JAMA 2002;288(14): 1728–32.
3. Deitel M. Overweight and obesity worldwide now estimated to involve 1.7 billion people. Obes Surg 2003;13(3):329–30.
4. Flegal KM, Carroll MD, Ogden CL, et al. Prevalence and trends in obesity among US adults, 1999–2000. JAMA 2002;288(14):1723–7.
5. Sturm R. Increases in clinically severe obesity in the United States, 1986–2000. Arch Intern Med 2003; 163(18):2146–8.
6. Buchwald H, Avidor Y, Braunwald E, et al. Bariatric surgery: a systematic review and meta-analysis. JAMA 2004;292(14):1724–37.
7. Sjostrom L, Lindroos AK, Peltonen M, et al. Lifestyle, diabetes, and cardiovascular risk factors 10 years after bariatric surgery. N Engl J Med 2004; 351(26):2683–93.
8. Pories WJ. Bariatric surgery: risks and rewards. J Clin Endocrinol Metab 2008;93(11 Suppl 1): S89–96.
9. Canoy D, Boekholdt SM, Wareham N, et al. Body fat distribution and risk of coronary heart disease in men and women in the European Prospective Investigation into Cancer and Nutrition in Norfolk cohort: a population-based prospective study. Circulation 2007;116(25):2933–43.
10. Austin MA, Friedlander Y, Newman B, et al. Genetic influences on changes in body mass index: a longitudinal analysis of women twins. Obes Res 1997; 5(4):326–31.
11. Klein S, Burke LE, Bray GA, et al. Clinical implications of obesity with specific focus on cardiovascular disease: a statement for professionals from the American Heart Association Council on Nutrition, Physical Activity, and Metabolism: endorsed by the American College of Cardiology Foundation. Circulation 2004;110(18):2952–67.
12. Fox CS, Massaro JM, Hoffmann U, et al. Abdominal visceral and subcutaneous adipose tissue compartments: association with metabolic risk factors in the Framingham Heart Study. Circulation 2007;116(1):39–48.
13. Vogler GP, Sorensen TI, Stunkard AJ, et al. Influences of genes and shared family environment on adult body mass index assessed in an adoption study by a comprehensive path model. Int J Obes Relat Metab Disord 1995;19(1):40–5.
14. Stunkard AJ, Sorensen TI, Hanis C, et al. An adoption study of human obesity. N Engl J Med 1986; 314(4):193–8.
15. Stunkard AJ, Harris JR, Pedersen NL, et al. The body-mass index of twins who have been reared apart. N Engl J Med 1990;322(21):1483–7.
16. Korner J, Bessler M, Cirilo LJ, et al. Effects of Roux-en-Y gastric bypass surgery on fasting and postprandial concentrations of plasma ghrelin, peptide YY, and insulin. J Clin Endocrinol Metab 2005;90(1): 359–65.
17. Neary NM, Small CJ, Bloom SR. Gut and mind. Gut 2003;52(7):918–21.
18. Jequier E. Leptin signaling, adiposity, and energy balance. Ann N Y Acad Sci 2002;967:379–88.
19. Ogden CL, Yanovski SZ, Carroll MD, et al. The epidemiology of obesity. Gastroenterology 2007; 132(6):2087–102.
20. Kligman MD, Dexter DJ, Omer S, et al. Shrinking cardiovascular risk through bariatric surgery: application of Framingham risk score in gastric bypass. Surgery 2008;143(4):533–8.
21. Anderson RN, Smith BL. Deaths: leading causes for 2002. Natl Vital Stat Rep 2005;53(17):1–89.
22. Goldstein DJ. Beneficial health effects of modest weight loss. Int J Obes Relat Metab Disord 1992; 16(6):397–415.
23. Fisher BL, Schauer P. Medical and surgical options in the treatment of severe obesity. Am J Surg 2002; 184(6B):9S–16S.
24. NIH Technology Assessment Conference Panel. Methods for voluntary weight loss and control. Ann Intern Med 1992;116(11):942–9.
25. NIH Conference. Gastrointestinal surgery for severe obesity. Consensus Development Conference Panel. Ann Intern Med 1991;115(12): 956–61.
26. Hocking MP, Duerson MC, O'Leary JP, et al. Jejunoileal bypass for morbid obesity. Late follow-up in 100 cases. N Engl J Med 1983;308(17):995–9.
27. Mason EE. Vertical banded gastroplasty for obesity. Arch Surg 1982;117(5):701–6.
28. Mason EE, Ito C. Gastric bypass in obesity. Surg Clin North Am 1967;47(6):1345–51.

29. Griffen WO Jr, Young VL, Stevenson CC. A prospective comparison of gastric and jejunoileal bypass procedures for morbid obesity. Ann Surg 1977;186(4):500–9.

30. Hess DS, Hess DW, Oakley RS. The biliopancreatic diversion with the duodenal switch: results beyond 10 years. Obes Surg 2005;15(3):408–16.

31. Scopinaro N, Papadia F, Camerini G, et al. A comparison of a personal series of biliopancreatic diversion and literature data on gastric bypass helps to explain the mechanisms of resolution of type 2 diabetes by the two operations. Obes Surg 2008;18(8):1035–8.

32. MacDonald KG Jr, Long SD, Swanson MS, et al. The gastric bypass operation reduces the progression and mortality of non-insulin-dependent diabetes mellitus. J Gastrointest Surg 1997;1(3):213–20 [discussion: 220].

33. Pories WJ, Swanson MS, MacDonald KG, et al. Who would have thought it? An operation proves to be the most effective therapy for adult-onset diabetes mellitus. Ann Surg 1995;222(3):339–50 [discussion: 350–2].

34. O'Brien PE, Dixon JB, Brown W, et al. The laparoscopic adjustable gastric band (Lap-Band): a prospective study of medium-term effects on weight, health and quality of life. Obes Surg 2002;12(5):652–60.

35. Wittgrove AC, Clark GW. Laparoscopic gastric bypass, Roux-en-Y—500 patients: technique and results, with 3–60 month follow-up. Obes Surg 2000;10(3):233–9.

36. Nguyen NT, Goldman C, Rosenquist CJ, et al. Laparoscopic versus open gastric bypass: a randomized study of outcomes, quality of life, and costs. Ann Surg 2001;234(3):279–89 [discussion: 289–91].

37. Birkmeyer NJ, Wei Y, Goldfaden A, et al. Characteristics of hospitals performing bariatric surgery. JAMA 2006;295(3):282–4.

38. Kelly J, Tarnoff M, Shikora S, et al. Best practice recommendations for surgical care in weight loss surgery. Obes Res 2005;13(2):227–33.

39. Smith BR, Schauer P, Nguyen NT. Surgical approaches to the treatment of obesity: bariatric surgery. Endocrinol Metab Clin North Am 2008;37(4):943–64.

40. Available at: http://www.surgicalreview.org. Accessed May 20, 2009.

41. Buchwald H. Bariatric surgery for morbid obesity: health implications for patients, health professionals, and third-party payers. J Am Coll Surg 2005;200(4):593–604.

42. Collazo-Clavell ML. Safe and effective management of the obese patient. Mayo Clin Proc 1999;74(12):1255–9 [quiz 1259–60].

43. Cowan GS Jr, Hiler ML, Buffington C. Criteria for selection of patients for bariatric surgery. Eur J Gastroenterol Hepatol 1999;11(2):69–75.

44. Fox CS, Pencina MJ, Meigs JB, et al. Trends in the incidence of type 2 diabetes mellitus from the 1970s to the 1990s: the Framingham Heart Study. Circulation 2006;113(25):2914–8.

45. Gregg EW, Cheng YJ, Cadwell BL, et al. Secular trends in cardiovascular disease risk factors according to body mass index in US adults. JAMA 2005;293(15):1868–74.

46. Reilly DF, McNeely MJ, Doerner D, et al. Self-reported exercise tolerance and the risk of serious perioperative complications. Arch Intern Med 1999;159(18):2185–92.

47. Qaseem A, Snow V, Fitterman N, et al. Risk assessment for and strategies to reduce perioperative pulmonary complications for patients undergoing noncardiothoracic surgery: a guideline from the American College of Physicians. Ann Intern Med 2006;144(8):575–80.

48. Keeling WB, Haines K, Stone PA, et al. Current indications for preoperative inferior vena cava filter insertion in patients undergoing surgery for morbid obesity. Obes Surg 2005;15(7):1009–12.

49. Dixon BJ, Dixon JB, Carden JR, et al. Preoxygenation is more effective in the 25 degrees head-up position than in the supine position in severely obese patients: a randomized controlled study. Anesthesiology 2005;102(6):1110–5 [discussion: 1115A].

50. Hampel H, Abraham NS, El-Serag HB. Meta-analysis: obesity and the risk for gastroesophageal reflux disease and its complications. Ann Intern Med 2005;143(3):199–211.

51. Frigg A, Peterli R, Zynamon A, et al. Radiologic and endoscopic evaluation for laparoscopic adjustable gastric banding: preoperative and follow-up. Obes Surg 2001;11(5):594–9.

52. Anderson MA, Gan SI, Fanelli RD, et al. Role of endoscopy in the bariatric surgery patient. Gastrointest Endosc 2008;68(1):1–10.

53. Siegelman ES, Rosen MA. Imaging of hepatic steatosis. Semin Liver Dis 2001;21(1):71–80.

54. Dallal RM, Mattar SG, Lord JL, et al. Results of laparoscopic gastric bypass in patients with cirrhosis. Obes Surg 2004;14(1):47–53.

55. Kral JG, Thung SN, Biron S, et al. Effects of surgical treatment of the metabolic syndrome on liver fibrosis and cirrhosis. Surgery 2004;135(1):48–58.

56. Villegas L, Schneider B, Provost D, et al. Is routine cholecystectomy required during laparoscopic gastric bypass? Obes Surg 2004;14(2):206–11.

57. Sugerman HJ, Brewer WH, Shiffman ML, et al. A multicenter, placebo-controlled, randomized, double-blind, prospective trial of prophylactic ursodiol for the prevention of gallstone formation following gastric-bypass-induced rapid weight

loss. Am J Surg 1995;169(1):91–6 [discussion: 96–7].

58. van Hout GC, Verschure SK, van Heck GL. Psychosocial predictors of success following bariatric surgery. Obes Surg 2005;15(4):552–60.

59. Herpertz S, Kielmann R, Wolf AM, et al. Do psychosocial variables predict weight loss or mental health after obesity surgery? A systematic review. Obes Res 2004;12(10):1554–69.

60. Clark MM, Balsiger BM, Sletten CD, et al. Psychosocial factors and 2-year outcome following bariatric surgery for weight loss. Obes Surg 2003;13(5): 739–45.

61. Aills L, Blankenship J, Buffington C, et al. ASMBS allied health nutritional guidelines for the surgical weight loss patient. Surg Obes Relat Dis 2008; 4(Suppl 5):S73–108.

62. Cottam DR, Atkinson J, Anderson A, et al. A case-controlled matched-pair cohort study of laparoscopic Roux-en-Y gastric bypass and Lap-Band patients in a single US center with three-year follow-up. Obes Surg 2006;16(5):534–40.

63. Tarnoff M, Kaplan LM, Shikora S. An evidenced-based assessment of preoperative weight loss in bariatric surgery. Obes Surg 2008;18(9):1059–61.

64. DeMaria EJ, Portenier D, Wolfe L. Obesity surgery mortality risk score: proposal for a clinically useful score to predict mortality risk in patients undergoing gastric bypass. Surg Obes Relat Dis 2007; 3(2):134–40.

65. DeMaria EJ, Murr M, Byrne TK, et al. Validation of the obesity surgery mortality risk score in a multicenter study proves it stratifies mortality risk in patients undergoing gastric bypass for morbid obesity. Ann Surg 2007;246(4):578–82 [discussion: 583–4].

66. Fernandez AZ Jr, DeMaria EJ, Tichansky DS, et al. Experience with over 3,000 open and laparoscopic bariatric procedures: multivariate analysis of factors related to leak and resultant mortality. Surg Endosc 2004;18(2):193–7.

67. Maher JW, Martin Hawver L, Pucci A, et al. Four hundred fifty consecutive laparoscopic Roux-en-Y gastric bypasses with no mortality and declining leak rates and lengths of stay in a bariatric training program. J Am Coll Surg 2008;206(5):940–4 [discussion: 944–5].

68. Howard L, Malone M, Michalek A, et al. A prospective randomized comparison and 5-year follow-up. Obes Surg 1995;5(1):55–60.

69. Sugerman HJ, Starkey JV, Birkenhauer R. A randomized prospective trial of gastric bypass versus vertical banded gastroplasty for morbid obesity and their effects on sweets versus non-sweets eaters. Ann Surg 1987;205(6):613–24.

70. Baltasar A, Bou R, Arlandis F, et al. Vertical banded gastroplasty at more than 5 years. Obes Surg 1998;8(1):29–34.

71. Ceelen W, Walder J, Cardon A, et al. Surgical treatment of severe obesity with a low-pressure adjustable gastric band: experimental data and clinical results in 625 patients. Ann Surg 2003;237(1):10–6.

72. Dargent J. Laparoscopic adjustable gastric banding: lessons from the first 500 patients in a single institution. Obes Surg 1999;9(5):446–52.

73. DeMaria EJ, Sugerman HJ, Meador JG, et al. High failure rate after laparoscopic adjustable silicone gastric banding for treatment of morbid obesity. Ann Surg 2001;233(6):809–18.

74. Ren CJ, Weiner M, Allen JW. Favorable early results of gastric banding for morbid obesity: the American experience. Surg Endosc 2004;18(3):543–6.

75. Lee CM, Cirangle PT, Jossart GH. Vertical gastrectomy for morbid obesity in 216 patients: report of two-year results. Surg Endosc 2007;21(10):1810–6.

76. Rabkin RA, Rabkin JM, Metcalf B, et al. Laparoscopic technique for performing duodenal switch with gastric reduction. Obes Surg 2003;13(2):263–8.

77. Schauer P, Ikramuddin S, Hamad G, et al. The learning curve for laparoscopic Roux-en-Y gastric bypass is 100 cases. Surg Endosc 2003;17(2): 212–5.

78. Brolin RE, Kenler HA, Gorman JH, et al. Long-limb gastric bypass in the superobese. A prospective randomized study. Ann Surg 1992;215(4):387–95.

79. Schauer PR, Ikramuddin S, Gourash W, et al. Outcomes after laparoscopic Roux-en-Y gastric bypass for morbid obesity. Ann Surg 2000;232(4): 515–29.

80. Lee S, Carmody B, Wolfe L, et al. Effect of location and speed of diagnosis on anastomotic leak outcomes in 3828 gastric bypass cases. J Gastrointest Surg 2007;11(6):708–13.

81. Rasmussen JJ, Fuller W, Ali MR. Marginal ulceration after laparoscopic gastric bypass: an analysis of predisposing factors in 260 patients. Surg Endosc 2007;21(7):1090–4.

82. Go MR, Muscarella P 2nd, Needleman BJ, et al. Endoscopic management of stomal stenosis after Roux-en-Y gastric bypass. Surg Endosc 2004; 18(1):56–9.

83. Sugerman HJ, Kellum JM Jr, DeMaria EJ, et al. Conversion of failed or complicated vertical banded gastroplasty to gastric bypass in morbid obesity. Am J Surg 1996;171(2):263–9.

84. Fernandez AZ Jr, Demaria EJ, Tichansky DS, et al. Multivariate analysis of risk factors for death following gastric bypass for treatment of morbid obesity. Ann Surg 2004;239(5):698–702 [discussion: 702–3].

85. Podnos YD, Jimenez JC, Wilson SE, et al. Complications after laparoscopic gastric bypass: a review of 3464 cases. Arch Surg 2003;138(9):957–61.

86. Evans RK, Bond DS, Demaria EJ, et al. Initiation and progression of physical activity after

laparoscopic and open gastric bypass surgery. Surg Innov 2004;11(4):235–9.

87. van Dielen FM, Soeters PB, de Brauw LM, et al. Laparoscopic adjustable gastric banding versus open vertical banded gastroplasty: a prospective randomized trial. Obes Surg 2005;15(9):1292–8.

88. Magro DO, Geloneze B, Delfini R, et al. Long-term weight regain after gastric bypass: a 5-year prospective study. Obes Surg 2008;18(6):648–51.

89. Schauer PR, Burguera B, Ikramuddin S, et al. Effect of laparoscopic Roux-en Y gastric bypass on type 2 diabetes mellitus. Ann Surg 2003;238(4):467–84 [discussion: 484–5].

90. Sugerman HJ, Wolfe LG, Sica DA, et al. Diabetes and hypertension in severe obesity and effects of gastric bypass-induced weight loss. Ann Surg 2003;237(6):751–6 [discussion: 757–8].

91. Sjostrom CD, Lissner L, Wedel H, et al. Reduction in incidence of diabetes, hypertension and lipid disturbances after intentional weight loss induced by bariatric surgery: the SOS Intervention Study. Obes Res 1999;7(5):477–84.

92. Peluso L, Vanek VW. Efficacy of gastric bypass in the treatment of obesity-related comorbidities. Nutr Clin Pract 2007;22(1):22–8.

93. Hypertension Prevention Trial. Three-year effects of dietary changes on blood pressure. Hypertension Prevention Trial Research Group. Arch Intern Med 1990;150(1):153–62.

94. Christou NV, Sampalis JS, Liberman M, et al. Surgery decreases long-term mortality, morbidity, and health care use in morbidly obese patients. Ann Surg 2004;240(3):416–23 [discussion: 423–4].

95. Rasheid S, Banasiak M, Gallagher SF, et al. Gastric bypass is an effective treatment for obstructive sleep apnea in patients with clinically significant obesity. Obes Surg 2003;13(1):58–61.

96. Varela JE, Hinojosa MW, Nguyen NT. Resolution of obstructive sleep apnea after laparoscopic gastric bypass. Obes Surg 2007;17(10):1279–82.

97. Williamson DF, Pamuk E, Thun M, et al. Prospective study of intentional weight loss and mortality in never-smoking overweight US white women aged 40–64 years. Am J Epidemiol 1995;141(12):1128–41.

98. Christou NV, MacLean LD. Effect of bariatric surgery on long-term mortality. Adv Surg 2005;39:165–79.

99. Treadwell JR, Sun F, Schoelles K. Systematic review and meta-analysis of bariatric surgery for pediatric obesity. Ann Surg 2008;248(5):763–76.

100. Kakarla N, Dailey C, Marino T, et al. Pregnancy after gastric bypass surgery and internal hernia formation. Obstet Gynecol 2005;105(5 Pt 2):1195–8.

101. Pope GD, Birkmeyer JD, Finlayson SR. National trends in utilization and in-hospital outcomes of bariatric surgery. J Gastrointest Surg 2002;6(6):855–60 [discussion: 861].

102. Bar-Zohar D, Azem F, Klausner J, et al. Pregnancy after laparoscopic adjustable gastric banding: perinatal outcome is favorable also for women with relatively high gestational weight gain. Surg Endosc 2006;20(10):1580–3.

103. Sheiner E, Levy A, Silverberg D, et al. Pregnancy after bariatric surgery is not associated with adverse perinatal outcome. Am J Obstet Gynecol 2004;190(5):1335–40.

104. Wittgrove AC, Jester L, Wittgrove P, et al. Pregnancy following gastric bypass for morbid obesity. Obes Surg 1998;8(4):461–4 [discussion: 465–6].

105. Patel JA, Colella JJ, Esaka E, et al. Improvement in infertility and pregnancy outcomes after weight loss surgery. Med Clin North Am 2007;91(3):515–28, xiii.

Airway Management in the Obese Patient

Ali A. El Solh, MD, MPH[a,b,c],*

KEYWORDS

- Obesity • Airway management • Noninvasive ventilation
- Tracheostomy • Intubation

Obesity is a serious disorder and an increasing problem all over the world.[1] During the past several decades, the worldwide prevalence of obesity has steadily risen, with the greatest increase occurring in the United States.[2] The incidence of obesity has doubled in adults and tripled in children in the United States over the past 30 years; more than 60 million adults and 9 million children aged 6 to 19 years are obese or overweight.[3] Furthermore, the prevalence of extreme obesity (body mass index [BMI] >40) has seen the greatest growth this past decade.[4] This increase was seen in both sexes, all racial/ethnic groups, all age groups, and all education levels.[5] With such global epidemic, the presentation of an acutely ill or injured morbidly obese patient is currently a common occurrence. Obese patients may present also for an elective procedure, for bariatric surgery, or for obstetric anesthesia or analgesia. Expertise in airway management becomes an important skill for any health care provider involved in the care of these patients. The main body of this review will discuss strategies for airway assessment before intubation, controversies surrounding airway management, and approach to safe extubation in this population. The article will also address the role of noninvasive ventilation in the management of obese patients (other than sleep apnea) and practiced techniques for temporary tracheostomy placement in critically ill obese patients.

AIRWAY MANAGEMENT

A number of studies have suggested that obesity increases the risk of perioperative respiratory complications and complicates airway management.[6] A BMI greater than 26 kg/m^2 results in a 3-fold increase in difficult ventilation via a mask[7] and in a 10-fold increased incidence of difficult endotracheal intubation.[8] Despite the lack of outcome data, a thorough preoperative assessment has been strongly recommended before any elective procedure in a morbidly obese patient. Review of medical records for coexisting comorbidities (including hypertension and cardiovascular disease, type 2 diabetes, and osteoarthritis) and previous anesthesia reports for evidence of difficulty with tracheal intubation is now considered a routine preoperative assessment. Questions relating to symptoms of daytime drowsiness, snoring, frequent awakenings, and periods of apnea during sleep are sought for the presence of sleep apnea. When present, these patients may have a diminution of the pharyngeal space secondary to fat deposition in the pharyngeal wall,[9] which can make airway access and mask ventilation difficult. In addition, obstructive sleep apnea (OSA) has important implications for use of sedatives and opiates in the perioperative period.[10] Unfortunately, most morbidly obese surgical patients have not had a polysomnographic study to confirm the diagnosis.[11]

a Veterans Affairs Western New York Healthcare System, Medical Research Building (20), 3495 Bailey Avenue, Buffalo, NY 14215-1199, USA
b The Western New York Respiratory Research Center, Department of Medicine, School of Medicine and Biomedical Sciences, State University of New York at Buffalo, Buffalo, NY 14214-3005, USA
c Department of Social and Preventive Medicine, School of Public Health, State University of New York at Buffalo, Buffalo, NY 14214-3005, USA
* Veterans Affairs Western New York Healthcare System, Medical Research Building (20), 3495 Bailey Avenue, Buffalo, NY 14215-1199.
E-mail address: solh@buffalo.edu

Clin Chest Med 30 (2009) 555–568
doi:10.1016/j.ccm.2009.05.005
0272-5231/09/$ – see front matter. Published by Elsevier Inc.

chestmed.theclinics.com

The key to proper airway management in obese patients is anticipation of difficulty, adequate preparation (patient and equipment), and a detailed plan of action should problems arise. Various factors should be optimized including positioning of the obese patient, preoxygenation, intubating devices, and knowledge of alternate airway tools.

Positioning the Morbidly Obese Patient

Because repositioning a morbidly obese patient may be impossible if difficulties during laryngoscopy and/or intubation are encountered, careful patient positioning and choice of airway management are vitally important. Classic teaching has been to position the patient in the "sniffing" position, or supine with moderate head elevation and atlanto-occipital extension.[12] The sniffing position was first described by Jackson[13] and is believed to align the oral, pharyngeal, and laryngeal axes for a direct view of the glottic opening. Although the sniffing position is advantageous not only for laryngoscopy but also for mask ventilating the patient's lungs before tracheal intubation, morbidly obese patients are more prone to hypoxemia in the supine position than individuals of normal weight owing to reduction in expiratory reserve volume. This is attributed to the mechanical effect of increased fat within the chest wall, abdominal wall, and abdomen, which combine to compress the thoracic cage, diaphragm, and lungs. The resultant impairment of diaphragmatic descent reduces functional residual capacity (FRC), which in turn increases airway resistance and worsens ventilation perfusion mismatch.[14] An alternative approach is to place the obese patient in the "ramped position" by using folded blankets, stacked under the patient's upper body, neck, and head, to elevate the head. According to Collins and coworkers,[15] the "ramped" position improved the laryngeal view when compared with a standard "sniff" position in morbidly obese patients undergoing elective bariatric surgery. Furthermore, Dixon and colleagues[16] noted 23% improvement in mean arterial oxygen tension when these patients were placed in a 25° reverse Trendelenburg position. However, attaining the optimum position in each patient can be tedious, as it requires adding or removing blankets while repositioning the patient each time. Use of other devices including a commercially available foam pillow (Troop Elevation Pillow, Mercury Medical, Clearwater, Florida) to achieve this position has been described in recent literature.[17,18] Head-up position also can be achieved by a simple maneuver of configuring the operating room table, similar to a reclining chair with the back or trunk portion of the table up.[19]

With the patient lying on the table, the electronic table controls can be used to flex the table at the trunk-thigh hinge and raise the "back" or "trunk" section of the table up as necessary to achieve the optimum position. This can be done with or without the headpiece at the head end of the table.

Preoxygenation

In patients of normal weight, a forced vital capacity ventilation for eight breaths during 60 seconds with high flows of oxygen 100% was shown to achieve adequate denitrogenation and slower desaturation during apnea compared with the usual 3 minutes tidal-volume ventilation technique.[20] Obesity, however, impairs seriously the effectiveness of preoxygenation because of a decrease in FRC secondary to cephalad diaphragmatic displacement.[21] The adoption of the sitting position for preoxygenation with eight deep breaths of ventilation over 60 seconds can increase the apnea tolerance by almost 1 minute compared with the same maneuver performed with the patient in the supine position.[22] Obviously, the utility of this approach is limited to patients who are scheduled for elective surgery. Other studies have examined the impact of different strategies known to increase the FRC on the effectiveness of preoxygenation.[23] Cressey and colleagues[23] found a non–statistically significant increase of 37 seconds in the time to desaturate to 90% when 7.5 cm H_2O continuous positive airway pressure (CPAP) was applied during preoxygenation to morbidly obese women. Although this level of CPAP might be insufficient to effectively shift the abdominal content, the application of CPAP at 10 cm H_2O for 5 minutes during the administration of oxygen followed by ventilation via face mask with positive end-expiratory pressure at 10 cm H_2O for 5 minutes was effective in improving oxygenation and in reducing atelectasis as assessed by CT scan.[24] Similar findings were reported by Gander and coworkers[25] who randomized 30 morbidly obese patients to receive positive end expiratory pressure (PEEP) during induction or to no PEEP. The group who received 100% O_2 through a CPAP (10 cm H_2O) for 5 minutes followed by pressure control ventilation for another 5 minutes until tracheal intubation had longer nonhypoxic apnea and less atelectasis formation. More recently, El-Khatib and colleagues[26] confirmed these observations by showing that the application of noninvasive bilevel positive airway pressure (BiPAP) (17/7 cm H_2O) in morbidly obese patients undergoing urgent surgery improved oxygenation significantly before rapid sequence induction of anesthesia.

Mask Ventilation and Tracheal Intubation

In an attempt to standardize airway management, the American Society of Anesthesiology issued a consensus in 1993 that was updated in 2003 in which the Society defines difficult airway as "the clinical situation in which a conventionally trained anesthesiologist experiences difficulty with face mask ventilation of the upper airway, difficulty with tracheal intubation or both."[3,27] Difficult mask ventilation is defined as the inability of an unassisted anesthesiologist to maintain the measured oxygen saturation as measured by pulse oximetry greater than 92% or to prevent or reverse signs of inadequate ventilation during positive-pressure mask ventilation under general anesthesia. Difficult intubation has been defined by the need for more than three intubation attempts or attempts at intubation that last more than 10 minutes.

While the rate of difficult mask ventilation (DMV) in the general population ranges from 0.07% to 15.00%,[8,28,29] the incidence of DMV in obese patients has been rarely assessed in studies related to airway management, and no previous specific studies regarding difficulty with mask ventilation alone have been performed. Hence, an initial step in the management of the obese patient requiring invasive ventilation is to determine the risk for difficult mask ventilation. Difficult mask ventilation may occur before attempting intubation or may occur after intubation failure.[30] Five criteria have been identified as independent risk factors for DMV: age older than 55 years, body mass index greater than 26 kg/m², lack of teeth, presence of beard, and history of snoring.[7] The presence of obesity plus another risk factor indicates a high likelihood of DMV. Similar predictors are provided by the mnemonic MOANS (mask seal, obesity, age >55 years, no teeth, and stiffness),[31] although there is no clear correlation between each of these attributes and the degree of difficulty.

By the same token, the predictive role of obesity as an independent risk factor for difficult intubation remains controversial. Part of the problem in determining the incidence of airway difficulty stems from the various ways of defining what constitutes a "difficult intubation." In two series of morbidly obese patients undergoing upper abdominal surgery, the incidence of difficult intubation was 13% and 24% respectively.[32,33] Another study examining 1833 intubations among all patients undergoing general anesthesia revealed that obesity provided a 20.2% predictive value of difficult intubation compared with patients with normal body mass index.[34] Additionally,

a threefold increase in difficult laryngoscopy has been reported among obese patients compared with patients with normal BMI. In the Australian Incident Monitoring Study, limited neck mobility and mouth opening accounted for most cases of difficult intubation in obese subjects.[29] Naguib and colleagues[35] added to the preceding list a short sternomental distance, a receding mandible, and prominent teeth as potential causes for difficult intubation. Others identified neck circumference greater than 40 cm and a Mallampati score of 3 or more as sole predictors of difficult intubation in morbidly obese patients.[36] However, the magnitude of obesity does not always correlate with difficulty in managing the airway. Preoperative bedside screening tests including the Mallampati oropharyngeal classification,[37] as well as thyromental and sternomental distances,[38] have been shown to be neither sensitive nor specific enough for routine clinical use.[34] Gaszynski[39] was unable to validate any of these characteristics in a group of 87 morbidly obese patients undergoing elective surgery. In fact, all morbidly obese patients with BMI greater than 50 kg/m² were intubated by first attempt. Furthermore, OSA, a well-known risk factor for difficult laryngoscopy in lean individuals,[40,41] was not associated with difficult intubation in the obese patients. A recent study[42] found that the Extended Mallampati Score[43] and the diagnosis of diabetes mellitus may prove superior to the modified Mallampati classification in the prediction of difficult laryngoscopy in the morbidly obese population (**Box 1**). Glycosylation of joints owing to chronic hyperglycemia can result in limited mobility, which may also affect the cervical and laryngeal areas.[44] The study was limited however by the heterogeneity of examiners and laryngoscopists and the subjective assessment of airway examinations.

It was suggested that the poor predictability of neck circumference in estimating difficult intubation in obese subjects might be related to the unequal distribution of fat and soft tissue at various topographic regions within the neck.[45] The use of MRI or CT scans to quantify the amount of soft tissue at the level of the vocal cords and suprasternal notch has been proposed as a possible diagnostic imaging to predict difficult laryngoscopy.[46] However, MRI and CT scans are costly and may not be always be practical in this population. In the past few years, several studies have relied on ultrasound to predict difficult intubation.[47] Ezri and colleagues[48] suggested that abundance of fat tissue at the anterior neck region, as measured by ultrasound, was indicative of difficult laryngoscopy, but Komatsu and coworkers[49] could not substantiate these findings when tested on 64 obese patients (BMI >35 kg/m^2) undergoing elective surgery. Because of a low predictive power of these constructed models and techniques, preplanned strategy remains central to safe and successful intubation.

Awake Intubation and Videolaryngoscope

Awake intubation using a flexible fiber-optic bronchoscope is considered the method of choice when treating an obese patient with an anticipated difficult airway;[50] however, the significant equipment costs and skill maintenance issues have limited the widespread adoption of this approach. One recent survey reported that only 59% of US anesthesiologists are proficient in fiber-optic intubation.[51] Various rigid indirect fiber-optic and video-based intubation devices have been developed as alternatives to flexible fiber-optic bronchoscope intubation and direct laryngoscopy in the difficult airway. Although the application of these devices has yet to be determined in the overall airway management of the obese patient, the use of a videolaryngoscope for intubation may allow a better visualization of the glottic anatomy, thereby improving the intubation conditions. In a randomized study of 80 morbidly obese patients undergoing bariatric surgery, Marrel and coworkers[52] reported that the grade of laryngoscopy, as assessed by the Cormack and Lehane scale, was significantly lower compared with the direct vision. The minimal arterial oxygen saturation (SpO2) reached during the intubation was also higher with the videolaryngoscope but it did not attain statistical significance. Hirabayashi and colleagues[53] demonstrated similar improvement in glottic opening in four morbidly obese patients using GlideScope in comparison with the Macintosh direct laryngoscope. Recently, a large study consisting of 318 morbidly obese patients scheduled for elective surgery confirmed that video-assisted tracheal intubation devices (LMCA CTrach and the Airtraq laryngoscope) allowed optimization of arterial oxygenation, and early definitive airway as compared with the conventional Macintosh laryngoscope.[54]

Rapid Sequence Intubation

Rapid sequence induction with cricoid pressure remains one of the most common intubation techniques for morbidly obese patients.[55] An early form of rapid sequence induction and intubation (RSI) was described in the early 1950s.[56] The technique was subsequently modified and the most noticeable being the introduction of cricoid pressure by Barry Sellick in 1961.[57] The technique consists of seven distinct steps designed to minimize the risk of regurgitation of gastric contents into the lungs (**Box 2**). During the procedure, cricoid pressure is applied immediately after loss of consciousness and no bag or mask ventilation is performed before the first laryngoscopy. Although these actions seem simple and easy to follow, there has been no randomized trial assessing the efficacy of RSI in morbidly obese patients.

The widespread application of RSI has pushed some critics to question its safety in the obese patients. First, there is a continuous debate about whether obese patients are at increased risk for acid aspiration syndrome. Available data on gastric pH, volume, and barrier pressure in morbidly obese patients are conflicting. A gastric pH less than 2.5 and a residual gastric fluid volume of 25 mL or higher are critical factors in the risk for aspiration-induced lung injury. Vaughan and colleagues[58] found that more than 70% of obese patients had a combination of gastric volumes 25 mL or more and pH 2.5 or lower compared with only 5% in nonobese individuals. Similar observations were noted by Fisher and colleagues.[59] Of 30 morbidly obese patients presenting for bariatric surgery evaluation, 11 had prolonged esophageal acid exposure with pH 4 or lower for more than 5% of observed time. Zacchi and coworkers[60] have challenged these contentions, showing that obese patients without symptoms of gastro-esophageal reflux have a resistance gradient between the stomach and the gastro-esophageal junction similar to that in nonobese subjects. The rate of gastric emptying was also no different in obese and nonobese patients.[61] In addition, no correlation could be established between gastric volume and fasting duration.[62] If any, a substantially *lower* incidence of combined high gastric volume and low pH was found in fasted, obese patients compared with lean patients.[63] Second, the use of cricoid pressure as a measure against passive regurgitation did not prevent aspiration completely[64,65] and there is little evidence that it improved patient outcome.[66] Garrard and colleagues[67] reported a reduction in lower esophageal sphincter pressure during the application of cricoid pressure in anesthetized patients. Moreover, CT and MRI studies on nonanesthetized volunteers have shown that in up to 50% of the subjects the esophagus was viewed lateral to the cricoid ring and that cricoid pressure displaced it more laterally.[68,69] Cricoid pressure can also have negative hemodynamic consequences. The application of cricoid pressure in healthy adult patients has been shown to increase systolic arterial blood pressure and to cause a significant rise in heart rate.[70] Even when performed correctly, cricoid pressure may interfere with laryngeal mask airway insertion, laryngoscopy, and success in intubation.[71] Haslam and colleagues[72] studied the effect of gradual increment of cricoid pressure on laryngoscopy on 40 patients undergoing elective surgery including obese individuals. Five subjects with a good initial view (anteroposterior length of the rima glottidis >5 mm) showed a marked deterioration in laryngoscopic view as cricoid pressure increased; in three of these subjects laryngoscopic view progressed to obscure the larynx completely at a force of 30 N, 40 N, and 60 N, respectively. Third, the process of protecting the lungs by doing a rapid sequence induction adds risk to the airway management of the morbidly obese patient. Because of the speed and commitment associated with this technique, a failed intubation offers no opportunity for the morbidly obese patient to resume spontaneous ventilation for anywhere from 5 to 15 minutes, depending on the choice of neuromuscular blocking drug. In addition, if ventilation via the face mask after anesthetic induction proves to be difficult, it is common for the morbidly obese patient to have rapid arterial oxygen desaturation of blood oxygen content as detailed previously. Thus, avoiding a rapid sequence induction technique affords additional time to use maneuvers such as sedated fiber-optic intubation while maintaining spontaneous ventilation, or induction of anesthesia, and establishing ventilation via mask before administering any neuromuscular drug.

The optical stylet combined with RSI laryngoscopy is a novel fiber-optic technique for the potentially difficult laryngoscope obese patient. Although RSI flexible fiber-optic intubation has been described, it requires significant expertise and working at arm's length with a 60 cm-flexible instrument.[73] By comparison, the optical stylet is shaped and positioned as a standard stylet, and its use fiber-optically involves minimal movement to switch from a direct view of its distal tip to a fiber-optic view through the eyepiece.[74] It offers the option of transitioning to fiber-optic intubation within the insertion time frame of a standard stylet on the first laryngoscopy.

Extraglottic Devices

Many different devices for airway management have been recommended by the American Society of Anesthesiologists (ASA) difficult airway algorithm.[75] The standard laryngeal mask airway (LMA) has been used to facilitate blind endotracheal intubation in numerous situations where laryngoscope and conventional intubations have been difficult (**Fig. 1**). Because of the reduced chest compliance and sheer mass of the chest wall in obese patients, higher inflation pressures are required to ventilate such patients. Such high pressures may preclude the use of the LMA for ventilation. Instead, the intubating laryngeal airway mask (ILMA) is considered a superior alternative. In 118 consecutive morbidly obese patients, Frappier and coworkers[76] achieved successful

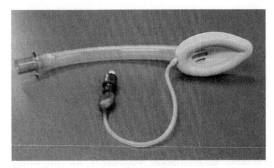

Fig. 1. The laryngeal mask airway.

tracheal intubation of 96.3% with the ILMA. These results were later duplicated in 50 morbidly obese with a comparable success rate of 96%.[77] There was also lower overall difficulty airway management scores as measured by the visual analog scale in obese patients as compared with lean patients. The preponderance of adipose tissue, predominantly in the lateral pharyngeal walls, is thought to guide the ILMA into place during its descent into the pharynx and stabilize its position after cuff inflation.

The esophageal tracheal combitube (ETC) is another alternative for rescue ventilation in the patients with difficult airway (**Fig. 2**). Two case reports reported successful ventilation with the ETC in grossly obese patients with bull neck.[78,79] The importance of the ETC in the field of airway management is that it represents one of the few extraglottic devices, which may provide effective protection to those at risk for aspiration.[80] However, the use of ETC can be associated with serious complications, including esophageal laceration, pneumomediastinum, and pneumoperitoneum.[81]

New extraglottic devices have been introduced in recent years, many of which may also play an important role in rescuing a failed airway. Several recent reports have detailed successful use of the Laryngeal Tube (VBM Medizintechnik, Sulz, Germany),[82] the CobraPLA (Engineered Medical System, Indianapolis, Indiana)[83] and the PAx-pressTM (Vital Signs Inc., Totowa, New Jersey)[84] in providing effective ventilation and oxygenation in patients under a variety of difficult circumstances. Whether these devices will receive acceptance equal to that of the ILMA and ETC in the obese patient with difficult airway is unknown. The choice of devices will ultimately depend on experience and clinical judgment.

EXTUBATION

The process of extubating a morbidly obese patient can be a daunting task. In normal-weight patients, the practice of extubating the trachea soon after surgery followed by assisted mask ventilation until the patient is fully awake may not be practical in an obese patient. If the obese patient was difficult to intubate, extreme care should be taken at extubation, as reintubation may be more difficult than the original procedure. Because patients with morbid obesity are at higher risk for postextubation stridor,[85] the cuff leak test has been suggested as a tool for identifying laryngeal edema. Initial inconsistencies in the reproducibility of this technique have cast doubts on its utility.[86,87] With the widespread use of ultrasonographic imaging in the management of critically ill patients, noninvasive examination of the vocal cords and the larynx became more accessible. The use of laryngeal ultrasound to detect patients at risk of postextubation stridor, by evaluating peri-cuff airflow has been recently described. Using real time laryngeal ultrasonography, Ding and colleagues[88] showed that a lower air column width during balloon deflation was a good predictor of postextubation stridor. Although the study did not include the BMI of patients who participated in the trial, the noninvasive nature of the test may still prove of utility in this population pending validation of the data in obese patients.

Ultrasound imaging has been advocated also as a novel technique for predicting extubation outcome. Because there is a direct correlation between respiratory muscle endurance and excursions of the diaphragm, liver, and spleen, measurement of liver and spleen displacement (MLSD) during spontaneous breathing trial may prove useful in assessing extubation readiness.

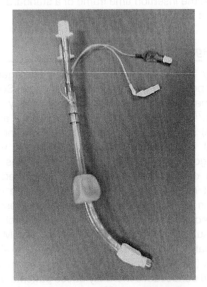

Fig. 2. The esophageal tracheal combitube.

Using a cutoff value of 1.1 cm for MLSD between the end of inspiration and the end of expiration, the sensitivity and specificity to predict successful extubation were 84.4% and 82.6%, respectively.[89] Whether these parameters hold true for patients who are obese remains to be seen.

In approaching tracheal extubation in obese patients, a reverse Trendelenburg position is recommended to optimize ventilation, decrease the risk of reflux, and access to the airway if reintubation becomes necessary. Placement of an airway exchange catheter[90] to retain a conduit for possible reintubation may prove to be useful for obese patients at risk for difficult intubation. The catheter allows for gas exchange either by jet ventilation or oxygen insufflation until the patient is deemed stable. Although the utility of this catheter has yet to be proven in obese patients, the airway exchange catheter is considered effective and safe with low risk of aspiration or barotrauma and may obviate the need for nasal cannula or facemask following tracheal extubation.[91]

After full recovery, patients should be informed and counseled regarding problems encountered and its relevance to further airway management. Clear description regarding the problem and subsequent solution should also be kept in the hospital records.

NONINVASIVE VENTILATION

Treatment of acute hypercapnic respiratory failure with noninvasive ventilation (NIV) has been proposed as a means of avoiding invasive mechanical ventilation and the associated complications. Although two consensus conferences pointed out that the use of NIV for treatment of acute respiratory failure in the morbidly obese is a relative contraindication,[92,93] earlier studies reported successful application of NIV in morbidly obese patients with hypercapnic respiratory failure.[94–96] A more recent investigation reviewed the outcome of 50 morbidly obese patients admitted to a medical intensive care unit with acute respiratory failure requiring ventilatory assistance.[97] A total of 33 patients were treated with NIV of whom 64% avoided invasive mechanical ventilation. Patients successfully treated with NIV had a significantly lower BMI, demonstrated improvement in gas exchange, and had a shorter hospital stay and a lower mortality. In contrast, patients who failed a trial of NIV and those who required invasive mechanical ventilation demonstrated a longer intensive care unit and hospital length of stay and higher mortality (31%). In the absence of randomized controlled trials, these case series have shown that NIV is safe in this

population and may be associated with improvements in arterial blood gas measurements, thereby providing support for its application. The benefit of NIV in morbidly obese patients stems from the significant unloading of inspiratory muscles. Using a full face mask with the application of bilevel ventilation in 18 subjects with a BMI of 40 kg/m^2 or higher, Pankow and colleagues[98] showed a drop of 46% in diaphragmatic activity. Subsequently, Rabec and colleagues[99] successfully treated 39 of 41 morbidly obese patients with acute respiratory failure using BiPAP. All 39 patients were discharged home without need for tracheal intubation. Of note, the application of NIV in these patients required inspiratory pressures in excess of 15 cm H_2O owing to the reduced lung volumes and increased airway resistance.[100,101]

Numerous studies have highlighted the complexity of respiratory management of critically ill obese patients during the period following liberation from mechanical ventilation.[102,103] The development of respiratory instability, episodic desaturation in the supine position, and the respiratory depressant effects of sedatives and opioid analgesia predispose these patients to prolonged periods of apneas, hypoxemia, and severe hypercapnia culminating in respiratory failure. Review of the literature puts the rate of reintubation postextubation in severely obese patients at 8% to 14% among patients undergoing mechanical ventilation for more than 48 hours.[104,105] Earlier investigations suggested that the prophylactic use of NIV in morbidly obese patients during the first 24 hours postoperatively reduced pulmonary dysfunction after gastroplasty and accelerated reestablishment of preoperative pulmonary function. Joris and colleagues[106] demonstrated that the application of BiPAP set at 12 and 4 cm H_2O improved significantly the peak expiratory flow rate, the forced vital capacity, and the oxygen saturation on the first postoperative day. These improvements are attributed to a combined effect of improved lung inflation, prevention of alveolar collapse, and reduced inspiratory threshold load. Similar physiologic effects are thought to be responsible for the reduced rate of respiratory failure postextubation. In a nonrandomized concurrent prospective study of 62 morbidly obese patients treated in a medical ICU, El Solh and colleagues[107] reported a 16% absolute risk reduction in the rate of respiratory failure when NIV was instituted immediately postextubation. Subgroup analysis of hypercapnic patients showed reduced hospital mortality in the NIV group compared with historic controls matched for age, BMI, and Acute Physiologic and Chronic Health Evaluation II score. Hence, early intervention with noninvasive ventilation may be effective in averting respiratory failure before the development of respiratory distress and may be responsible for decreasing mortality in selected patients with chronic hypercapnia.

TRACHEOSTOMY

Tracheostomy continues to be the standard procedure for management of long-term ventilator-dependent patients. It presents several advantages over endotracheal intubation, including lower airway resistance, smaller dead space, less movement of the tube within the trachea, greater patient comfort, and more efficient suction.[108,109] Despite the controversy as to the proper time to perform tracheostomy, prospective studies suggest that there may be a benefit to early tracheostomy.[110] Yet, in the absence of valid evidence that is based on randomized controlled trials, the decision to place a tracheostomy is made on the consideration of the benefits versus risks of the procedure.

Surgical Tracheostomy

The overall complication rate of surgical tracheostomy in obese patients is estimated at 25%, most of which are minor.[111] Serious complications occur in 10% and are usually life threatening.[111] In patients who require tracheostomy, morbidly obese patients present a unique surgical challenge because of increased submental and anterior cervical adipose tissue. The initial goal of securing a stable airway can be compromised by the size discrepancy and curvature mismatch between a standard-size tracheostomy tube and the increased distance between skin and trachea. Standard tracheotomy tubes are typically too short and angulated. Consequently, they are more likely to get occluded or dislodged. When obstruction of the tracheotomy tube occurs in the first 24 hours postoperatively, it is usually the result of tube impingement on the posterior tracheal wall, partial displacement into the mediastinum, a blood clot, or a mucous plug. When one of these complications occurs in the morbidly obese patient who is lying supine and partially sedated, hypoxemia develops rapidly as a consequence of reduced expiratory reserve volume.[112] To avert anoxic encephalopathy, immediate resuscitation is required. As a result, it is recommended that morbidly obese patients be monitored in an ICU setting for at least 72 hours following a surgical tracheostomy. Nonetheless, the risk of developing this complication persists beyond this time frame. Submental fat deposition that may reach below the sternal notch could

also occlude the outer opening of the standard tracheostomy, rendering any oxygenation extremely limited or nonexistent. Simmons[113] recommended the application of an elastic bandage or a Barton bandage to move the chin out of the way. Others have considered the use of an extension attached to the outer opening.[114]

Accidental decannulation of tracheostomy tube in morbidly obese patients can be also life threatening in the setting of critical care illness. Morbidly obese patients with short, thick necks usually have too much soft tissue between the trachea and the skin. Unsuccessful blinded reinsertion attempts may cause tube misplacement in the pretracheal fascia with resultant tracheal compression and respiratory arrest. Some surgeons advocate performing a Björk flap at the time of surgery to prevent tube misplacement in the pretracheal fascia; however, this technique may be associated with higher incidence of tracheal stenosis postdecannulation.[115] Others prefer[116] a cervical lipectomy in combination with tracheostomy. Whether morbidly obese patients will benefit from the application of these techniques to reduce the rate of extratracheal placement of tracheostomy tube is unclear because there are no studies to date providing a conclusive answer.

Percutaneous Dilatation Tracheostomy

Percutaneous dilatation tracheostomy (PDT) is a widely used and accepted method in ICUs for long-term ventilation of critically ill patients. The technique was first described in 1985 by Ciaglia and colleagues[117] as an alternative to standard tracheostomy. The perceived advantages of PDT include its speed, simplicity, and cost, plus the fact that PDT obviates the need to transport critically ill patients outside of the ICU.[118] Traditionally, obesity has been considered a relative contraindication to the performance of PDT because, in these patients, conditions in the neck can make it difficult to properly identify anatomic landmarks.[119] Complications were related to imprecise paramedian puncture of the trachea or the formation of a paramedian stoma with potential lesions of the lateral tracheal wall.[120] However, there is also no concrete evidence supporting the superiority of standard tracheostomy in this patient group. A recent retrospective study that analyzed perioperative complications of standard tracheostomy in 427 critically ill patients found that morbidly obese patients were 4.4 times more likely than nonobese patients to suffer complications associated with standard tracheostomy (25% versus 14%, $P = .03$).[111] In comparison, the rate of PDT complications in morbidly obese patients

Table 1
Studies evaluating percutaneous dilatation tracheostomy in obese patients

Authors	Year of Publication	Study Design	No. Obese Patients	Mean BMI or BMI range, kg/m^2	PDT	Complication Rate, %
Aldawood et al.[121]	2008	Prospective	50	30	50	12.0
Heyrosa et al.[122]	2006	Retrospective	143	35–105	89	5.6
Byhahn et al.[123]	2005	Case control	73	27.5–64.3	73	43.8
Mansharamani et al.[124]	2000	Case series	13	28.1–67.0	13	7.7
Scott and Leigh[125]	2000	Case report	3	43.0–48.1	3	Not stated
Unwin et al.[126]	2000	Case report	1	58	1	Not stated

Abbreviations: BMI, body mass index; PDT, percutaneous dilational tracheostomy.

ranged from 5.6% to 43.8% (**Table 1**). Recently, a meta-analysis of 23 studies that included 2237 patients who had PDT examined the incidence of complications of PDT with and without fiber-optic bronchoscopy assistance.[127] In the blind-PDT group, the incidence of complications was 16.8%, whereas in the fiber-optic bronchoscopy–assisted PDT group, the incidence of complications was 8.3% (P<.001). Various authors[128,129] have proposed the use of ultrasonography as an alternative to fiber-optic bronchoscopy support to guide the procedure in real time or as a complementary tool to evaluate the cervical anatomy before the puncture. Kollig and colleagues[130] found that ultrasound examination of the neck changed the puncture site in 24% of their patients. One case report of a morbidly obese patient reiterated the safety of ultrasound in localizing the site for PDT.[120] Neck thickness had no influence on ultrasonographic findings. Notwithstanding, PDT should be postponed in obese patients who are dependent on high positive end-expired pressure or who require an FIO_2 greater than 0.6 to maintain their oxygen saturation. In such cases, accidental endotracheal tube cuff rupture could result in grave hypoxemia before airtight ventilation is reestablished.

SUMMARY

Airway management of the obese patient represents a daunting task for health care practitioners. There are no reliable methods so far for determining in advance which patients may require alternative rescue devices for assisted intubation. A thorough evaluation and preparation for anticipated difficult airway including proper positioning, preoxygenation, and the immediate readiness of rescue ventilation devices are critical. Although laryngoscopy can be associated with a high degree of success, there is little margin for failure. Critical desaturation will be precipitous, and repeat laryngoscopy efforts carry significant risks. Early application of noninvasive ventilation in the postoperative period particularly in those with documented sleep apnea improves respiratory physiology and may prevent reintubation. For those patients with prolonged mechanical ventilation, percutaneous dilatation tracheostomy is safe and well tolerated when performed by experienced personnel.

REFERENCES

1. Organization WH. Obesity: preventing and managing the global epidemic. Report of a WHO consultation on obesity 1998.

2. Mokdad AH, Ford ES, Bowman BA, et al. Prevalence of obesity, diabetes, and obesity-related health risk factors, 2001. JAMA 2003;289:76–9.

3. Ogden CL, Carroll MD, McDowell MA, et al. Obesity among adults in the United States—no change since 2003–2004. NCHS data brief no 1. Hyattsville (MD): National Center for Health Statistics; 2007.

4. Vallejo M. Anesthetic management of the morbidly obese parturient. Curr Opin Anaesthesiol 2007; 20(3):175–80.

5. Freedman DS, Khan LK, Serdula MK, et al. Trends and correlates of class 3 obesity in the United States from 1990 through 2000. JAMA 2002;288: 1758–61.

6. Chung F, Mezei G, Tong D. Pre-existing medical conditions as predictors of adverse events in day-case surgery. Br J Anaesth 1999;83:262–70.

7. Langeron O, Masso E, Huraux C, et al. Prediction of difficult mask ventilation. Anesthesiology 2000;92: 1229–36.

8. El-Ganzouri AR, McCarthy RJ, Tuman KJ, et al. Preoperative airway assessment: predictive value of a multivariate risk index. Anesth Analg 1996;82: 1197–204.

9. Busetto L, Enzi G, Inelmen EM, et al. Obstructive sleep apnea syndrome in morbid obesity: effects of intragastric balloon. Chest 2005;128:618–23.

10. Gross JB, Bachenberg KL, Benumof JL, et al. American Society of Anesthesiologists Task Force on Perioperative Management. Practice guidelines for the perioperative management of patients with obstructive sleep apnea: a report by the American Society of Anesthesiologists Task Force on Perioperative Management of patients with obstructive sleep apnea. Anesthesiology 2006; 104:1081–93.

11. Kaw R, Michota F, Jaffer A, et al. Unrecognized sleep apnea in the surgical patient: implications for the perioperative setting. Chest 2006;129: 198–205.

12. Bannister FB, Macbeth RG. Direct laryngoscopy and tracheal intubation. Lancet 1944;244:651–4.

13. Jackson C. The technique of insertion of intratracheal insufflation tubes. Surg Gynecol Obstet 1913;17:507–9.

14. Yap JC, Watson RA, Gilbey S, et al. Effects of posture on respiratory mechanics in obesity. J Appl Physiol 1995;79:1199–205.

15. Collins JS, Lemmens HJ, Brodsky JB, et al. Laryngoscopy and morbid obesity: a comparison of the "sniff" and "ramped" positions. Obes Surg 2004; 14:1171–5.

16. Dixon BJ, Dixon JB, Carden JR, et al. Preoxygenation is more effective in the 25 degrees head-up position than in the supine position in severely obese patients: a randomized controlled study. Anesthesiology 2005;102:1110–5.

17. Nissen MD, Gayes JM. An inflatable, multichambered upper body support for the placement of the obese patient in the head-elevated laryngoscopy position. Anesth Analg 2007;104:1305–6.

18. Wong AB, Moore MS. Positioning of obese patients in out-of-operating room locations. Anesth Analg 2007;104:1306.

19. Rao SL, Kunselman AR, Schuler HG, et al. Laryngoscopy and tracheal intubation in the head-elevated position in obese patients: a randomized, controlled, equivalence trial. Anesth Analg 2008; 107(6):1912–8.

20. Baraka AS, Taha SK, Aouad MT, et al. Preoxygenation: comparison of maximal breathing and tidal volume breathing techniques. Anesthesiology 1999;91:612–6.

21. Berthoud MC, Peacock JE, Reilly CS. Effectiveness of preoxygenation in morbidly obese patients. Br J Anaesth 1991;67:464–6.

22. Altermatt FR, Muñoz HR, Delfino AE, et al. Pre-oxygenation in the obese patient: effects of position on tolerance to apnoea. Br J Anaesth 2005;95(5): 706–9.

23. Cressey DM, Berthoud MC, Reilly CS. Effectiveness of continuous positive airway pressure to enhance pre-oxygenation in morbidly obese women. Anaesthesia 2001;56:680–4.

24. Coussa M, Proietti S, Schnyder P, et al. Prevention of atelectasis formation during the inducation of general anesthesia in morbidly obese patients. Anesth Analg 2004;98:1491–5.

25. Gander S, Frascarolo P, Suter M, et al. Positive end-expiratory pressure during induction of general anesthesia increases duration of nonhypoxic apnea in morbidly obese patients. Anesth Analg 2005;100:580–4.

26. El-Khatib MF, Kanazi G, Baraka AS. Noninvasive bi-level positive airway pressure for preoxygenation of the critically ill morbidly obese patient. Can J Anaesth 2007;54(9):744–7.

27. Caplan RA, Benumof J, Berry F. Practice guidelines for management of the difficult airway: an updated report by the American Society of Anesthesiologists Task Force on Management of the Difficult Airway. Anesthesiology 2003;98:1269–77.

28. Asai T, Koga K, Vaughan RS. Respiratory complications associated with tracheal intubation and extubation. Br J Anaesth 1998;80:767–75.

29. Williamson JA, Webb RK, Szekely S, et al. Australian incident monitoring study: difficult intubation: an analysis of 2,000 incident reports. Anaesth Intensive Care 1993;21:602–7.

30. Crosby ET, Cooper RM, Douglas MJ, et al. The unanticipated difficult airway with recommendations for management. Can J Anaesth 1998;45:757–76.

31. Murphy M, Walls RM. Identification of the difficult and failed airway. In: Walls RM, Murphy MF, Luten RC, editors. Manual of emergency airway management. Philadelphia: Lippincott Williams and Wilkins; 2004. p. 70–2.

32. Buckley F, Robinson N, Simonowitz D, et al. Anesthesia in the morbidly obese patient: a comparison of anaesthetic and analgesic regimens for upper abdominal surgery. Anaesthesia 1983;38:840–51.

33. Cherit G, Gonzalez R, Borunda D, et al. Anesthesia for morbidly obese patients. World J Surg 1998;22: 969–73.

34. Voyagis G, Kyriakis K, Dimitriou V, et al. Value of oropharyngeal Mallampati classification in predicting difficult laryngoscopy among obese patients. Eur J Anaesthesiol 1998;15:330–4.

35. Naguib M, Malabarey T, Alsatli RA, et al. Predictive models for difficult laryngoscopy and intubation: a clinical, radiographic and three-dimensional computer imaging study. Can J Anaesth 1999;46:748–59.

36. Brodsky JB, Lemmens HJ, Brock-Utne JG, et al. Morbid obesity and tracheal intubation. Anesth Analg 2002;94:732–6.

37. Mallampati SR, Gatt SP, Gugino LD, et al. A clinical sign to predict difficult tracheal intubation: a prospective study. Can Anaesth Soc J 1985;32: 429–34.

38. Butler PJ, Dhata SS. Prediction of difficult laryngoscopy: an assessment of the thyromental distance and Mallampati predictive tests. Anaesth Intensive Care 1992;20:139–42.

39. Gaszynski T. Standard clinical tests for predicting difficult intubation are not useful among morbidly obese patients. Anesth Analg 2004;99:956.

40. Hiremath AS, Hillman DR, James AL, et al. Relationship between difficult tracheal intubation and obstructive sleep apnoea. Br J Anaesth 1998;80: 606–11.

41. Benumof JL. Obstructive sleep apnea in the adult obese patient: implications for airway management. J Clin Anesth 2001;13:144–56.

42. Mashour GA, Kheterpal S, Vanaharam V, et al. The extended Mallampati score and a diagnosis of diabetes mellitus are predictors of difficult laryngoscopy in the morbidly obese. Anesth Analg 2008; 107(6):1919–23.

43. Mashour GA, Sandberg WS. Craniocervical extension improves the specificity and predictive value of the Mallampati airway evaluation. Anesth Analg 2006;103:1256–9.

44. Riessell E, Orko R, Maunuksela EL, et al. Predictability of difficult laryngoscopy in patients with long-term diabetes mellitus. Anaesthesia 1990;45: 1024–7.

45. Gonzalez H, Minville V, Delanoue K, et al. The importance of increased neck circumference to intubation difficulties in obese patients. Anesth Analg 2008;106(4):1132–6.

46. Caballero P, Alvarez-Sala R, Garcia-Rio F, et al. CT in the evaluation of the upper airway in healthy subjects and in patients with obstructive sleep apnea syndrome. Chest 1998;113:111–6.

47. Hatfield A, Bodenham A. Ultrasound: an emerging role in anaesthesia and intensive care. Br J Anaesth 1999;83:789–800.

48. Ezri T, Gewurtz G, Sessler DI, et al. Prediction of difficult laryngoscopy in obese patients by ultrasound quantification of anterior neck soft tissue. Anaesthesia 2003;58:1111–4.

49. Komatsu R, Sengupta P, Wadhwa A, et al. Ultrasound quantification of anterior soft tissue thickness fails to predict difficult laryngoscopy in obese patients. Anaesth Intensive Care 2007; 35(1):32–7.

50. Murphy M, et al. Flexible fiberoptic intubation. In: Walls R, Murphy M, Luten R, et al, editors. Manual of emergency airway management. 2nd edition. Philadelphia: Lippincott Williams & Wilkins; 2004. p. 127–34.

51. Ezri T, Szmuk P, Warters R, et al. Difficult airway management practice patterns among anesthesiologists practicing in the United States: have we made any progress? J Clin Anesth 2003;15:418–22.

52. Marrel J, Blanc C, Frascarolo P, et al. Videolaryngoscopy improves intubation condition in morbidly obese patients. Eur J Anaesthesiol 2007;24(12): 1045–9.

53. Hirabayashi Y, Hakozaki T, Fujisawa K, et al. Use of a new video-laryngoscope (GlideScope) in patients with a difficult airway. Masui 2007;56(7):854–7.

54. Dhonneur G, Abdi W, Ndoko SK, et al. Video-assisted versus conventional tracheal intubation in morbidly obese patients. Obes Surg 2008, in press.

55. Reed A, Kramer D. Airway management. In: Alvarez A, Brodsky J, Alpert M, et al, editors. Morbid obesity: peri-operative management. Cambridge, UK: Cambridge University Press; 2005. p. 287–95.

56. Salem MR. Rapid sequence induction and intubation: fact and fiction. In: proceedings of the 2nd Annual Scientific Meeting of the Society for Airway Management. Newport Beach, California, September 5–7, 1997.

57. Sellick BA. Cricoid pressure to control regurgitation of stomach contents during induction of anaesthesia. Lancet 1961;2:404–6.

58. Vaughan RW, Bauer S, Wise L. Volume and pH of gastric juice in obese patients. Anesthesiology 1975;43:686–9.

59. Fisher BL, Pennathur A, Mutnick JL, et al. Obesity correlates with gastroesophageal reflux. Dig Dis Sci 1999;44(11):2290–4.

60. Zacchi P, Mearin F, Humbert P, et al. Effect of obesity on gastroesophageal resistance to flow in man. Dig Dis Sci 1991;36:1473–80.

61. Maddox A, Horowitz M, Wishart J, et al. Gastric and esophageal emptying in obesity. Scand J Gastroenterol 1989;24:593–8.

62. Hartsilver E, Vanner R, Bewley J, et al. Gastric pressure during emergency Caesarean section under general anaesthesia. Br J Anaesth 1999;82:752–4.

63. Harter RL, Kelly WB, Kramer MG, et al. A comparison of the volume and pH of gastric contents of obese and lean surgical patients. Anesth Analg 1998;86:147–52.

64. Kluger MT, Short TG. Aspiration during anaesthesia: a review of 133 cases from the Australian Anaesthetic Incident Monitoring Study (AIMS). Anaesthesia 1999;54(1):19–26.

65. Warner MA, Warner ME, Webber JG. Clinical significance of pulmonary aspiration during the perioperative period. Anesthesiology 1993;78:56–62.

66. Neilipovitz DT, Crosby ET. No evidence for decreased incidence of aspiration after rapid sequence induction. Can J Anaesth 2007;54: 748–64.

67. Garrard A, Campbell AE, Turley A, et al. The effect of mechanically induced cricoid force on lower oesophageal sphincter pressure in anesthetized patients. Anaesthesia 2004;59:435–9.

68. Smith KJ, Ladak S, Choi PTL, et al. The cricoid cartilage and the esophagus are not aligned in close to half of adult patients. Can J Anaesth 2002;49:503–7.

69. Smith KJ, Dobranowski J, Yip G, et al. Cricoid pressure displaces the esophagus: an observational study using magnetic resonance imaging. Anesthesiology 2003;99:60–4.

70. Saghaei M, Masoodifar M. The pressor response and airway effects of cricoid pressure during induction of general anesthesia. Anesth Analg 2001;93(3):787–90.

71. Freid E. The rapid sequence induction revisited: obesity and sleep apnea syndrome. Anesthesiol Clin North America 2005;23:551–64.

72. Haslam N, Parker L, Duggan JE. Effect of cricoid pressure on the view at laryngoscopy. Anaesthesia 2005;60(1):41–7.

73. Li J, Murphy-Lavoie H, Bugas C, et al. Complications of emergency intubation with and without paralysis. Am J Emerg Med 1999;17:141–3.

74. Bozeman WP, Kleiner DM, Huggett V. A comparison of rapid-sequence intubation and etomidate-only intubation in the prehospital air medical setting. Prehosp Emerg Care 2006;10:8–13.

75. Benumof JL. Laryngeal mask airway and the ASA difficult airway algorithm. Anesthesiology 1996;84: 686–99.

76. Frappier J, Guenoun T, Journois D, et al. Airway management using the intubating laryngeal mask airway for morbidly obese patients. Anesth Analg 2003;96:1510–5.

77. Combes X, Sauvat S, Leroux B, et al. Intubating laryngeal mask airway in morbidly obese and lean patients. Anesthesiology 2005;102:1106–9.

78. Banyai M, Falger S, Roggla M, et al. Emergency intubation with the Combitube in a grossly obese patient with bull neck. Resuscitation 1993;26:271–6.

79. Della Puppa A, Pittoni G, Frass M. Tracheal esophageal Combitube: a useful airway for morbidly obese patients who cannot intubate or ventilate. Acta Anaesthesiol Scand 2002;46:911–3.

80. Urtabia R, Aguila C, Cumsille M. Combitube: a study for proper use. Anesth Analg 2000;90:958–62.

81. Vezina D, Lessard M, Bussieres J, et al. Complications associated with the use of the esophageal tracheal Combitube. Can J Anaesth 1998;45:823–4.

82. Matioc AA, Olson J. Use of the Laryngeal Tube™ in two unexpected difficult airway situations: lingual tonsillar hyperplasia and morbid obesity. Can J Anesth 2004;51:1018–21.

83. Agro F, Carassiti M, Magnani C, et al. Airway control via the CobraPLA during percutaneous dilatational tracheotomy in five patients. Can J Anaesth 2005;52:418–20.

84. Dimitriou V, Voyagis GS, Iatrou C, et al. The PAxpressTM is an effective ventilatory device but has an 18% failure rate for flexible lightwand-guided tracheal intubation in anesthetized paralyzed patients. Can J Anaesth 2003;50:495–500.

85. Frat JP, Gissot V, Ragot S, et al. for the Association des Réanimateurs du Centre-Ouest (ARCO) study group. Impact of obesity in mechanically ventilated patients: a prospective study. Intensive Care Med 2008;34(11):1991–8.

86. Engoren M. Evaluation of the cuff-leak test in a cardiac surgery population. Chest 1999;116:1029–31.

87. Kriner EJ, Shafazand S, Colice GL. The endotracheal tube cuff-leak test as a predictor for postextubation stridor. Respir Care 2005;50(12):1617–8.

88. Ding LW, Wang HC, Wu HD, et al. Laryngeal ultrasound: a useful method in predicting post-extubation stridor. A pilot study. Eur Respir J 2006;27(2):384–9.

89. Jiang JR, Tsai TH, Jerng JS, et al. Ultrasonographic evaluation of liver/spleen movements and extubation outcome. Chest 2004;126(1):179–85.

90. Benumof JL. Additional safety measures when changing endotracheal tubes. Anesthesiology 1991;75:921–2.

91. Loudermilk EP, Hartmannsgruber M, Stoltzfus DP, et al. A prospective study of the safety of tracheal extubation using a pediatric airway exchange catheter for patients with a known difficult airway. Chest 1997;111(6):1660–5.

92. Noninvasive positive pressure ventilation consensus statement: Consensus Conference on Noninvasive Positive Pressure Ventilation. Respir Care 1997;42:364–9.

93. Pauwels R, Buist AS, Calverley PMA, et al. Global strategy for the diagnosis, management and prevention of chronic obstructive pulmonary disease. Am J Respir Crit Care Med 2001;163:1256–76.

94. Shivaram U, Cash ME, Beal A. Nasal continuous positive airway pressure in decompensated hypercapnic respiratory failure as a complication of sleep apnea. Chest 1993;104:770–4.

95. Sturani C, Galavotti V, Scarduelli C, et al. Acute respiratory failure due to severe obstructive sleep apnoea syndrome, managed with nasal positive pressure ventilation. Monaldi Arch Chest Dis 1994;49:558–60.

96. Muir JF, Cuvelier A, Bota S, et al. Modalities of ventilation in obesity. Monaldi Arch Chest Dis 1998;53:560–3.

97. Duarte A, Justino E, Bigler T, et al. Outcomes of morbidly obese patients requiring mechanical ventilation for acute respiratory failure. Crit Care Med 2007;35:732–7.

98. Pankow W, Hijjeh N, Schuttler F, et al. Influence of noninvasive positive pressure ventilation on inspiratory muscle activity in obese subjects. Eur Respir J 1997;10:2847–52.

99. Rabec C, Merati M, Baudouin N, et al. Management of obesity and respiratory insufficiency: the value of dual-level pressure nasal ventilation. Rev Mal Respir 1998;15:269–78.

100. Pelosi P, Croci M, Ravagnan I, et al. Total respiratory system, lung, and chest wall mechanics in sedated paralyzed postoperative morbidly obese patients. Chest 1996;109:144–51.

101. Perez de Llano LA, Golpe R, Piquer MO, et al. Short and long term effects of nasal intermittent positive pressure ventilation in patients with obesity-hypoventilation syndrome. Chest 2005;128:587–94.

102. Taylor RR, Kelly TM, Elliott CG, et al. Hypoxemia after gastric bypass surgery for morbid obesity. Arch Surg 1985;120:1298–302.

103. El Solh A, Sikka P, Bozkanat E, et al. Morbid obesity in the medical ICU. Chest 2001;120:1989–97.

104. Gaszynski T, Gaszynski W, Strzelczyk J. Critical respiratory events in morbidly obese. Twoj Magazyn Medyczny Chirurgia 2003;3:55–8.

105. Blouw E, Rudolph A, Narr B, et al. The frequency of respiratory failure in patients with morbid obesity undergoing gastric bypass. AANA J 2003;71:45–50.

106. Joris JL, Sottiaux TM, Chiche JD, et al. Effect of bi-level positive airway pressure (BiPAP) nasal ventilation on the postoperative pulmonary restrictive syndrome in obese patients undergoing gastroplasty. Chest 1997;111:665–70.

107. El Solh A, Aquilina A, Pineda L, et al. Noninvasive ventilation for prevention of post extubation respiratory failure in obese patients. Eur Respir J 2006;28:588–95.

108. Astrachan DI, Kirchner JC, Goodwin WJ Jr. Prolonged intubation vs. tracheotomy: complications, practical and psychological considerations. Laryngoscope 1988;98:1165–9.

109. Diehl JL, El Atrous S, Touchard D, et al. Changes in the work of breathing induced by tracheotomy in ventilator-dependent patients. Am J Respir Crit Care Med 1999;159:383–8.

110. Rumbak M, Newton M, Truncale T, et al. A prospective, randomized study comparing early percutaneous dilational tracheostomy to prolonged translaryngeal intubation (delayed tracheotomy) in critically ill medical patients. Crit Care Med 2004;32:1689–93.

111. El Solh A, Jaafar W. A comparative study of the complications of surgical tracheostomy in morbidly obese critically ill patients. Crit Care 2007;11:R3.

112. Thomas PS, Cowen ERT, Hulands G, et al. Respiratory function in the morbidly obese before and after weight loss. Thorax 1989;44:382–6.

113. Simmons B. Tracheotomy in sleep apnea syndrome. Ear Nose Throat J 1984;63:222–6.

114. Ghorayeb B. Tracheotomy in the morbidly obese patient. Arch Otolaryngol Head Neck Surg 1987;113:556–8.

115. Tommerup B, Borgeskov S. Endoscopic evaluation at follow up after Bjork tracheostomy. Scand J Thorac Cardiovasc Surg 1983;17:181–4.

116. Gross ND, Cohen JI, Andersen PE, et al. 'Defatting' tracheotomy in morbidly obese patients. Laryngoscope 2002;112:1940–4.

117. Ciaglia P, Firsching R, Syniec C. Elective percutaneous dilatational tracheostomy. A new simple bedside procedure; preliminary report. Chest 1985;87:715–9.

118. Freeman BD, Isabella K, Cobb JP, et al. A prospective, randomized study comparing percutaneous with surgical tracheostomy in critically ill patients. Crit Care Med 2001;29:926–30.

119. Moe KS, Stoeckli SJ, Schmid S, et al. Percutaneous tracheostomy: a comprehensive evaluation. Ann Otol Rhinol Laryngol 1999;108:384–91.

120. Sustić A, Zupan Z, Antoncić I. Ultrasound-guided percutaneous dilatational tracheostomy with laryngeal mask airway control in a morbidly obese patient. J Clin Anesth. 2004;16(2):121–3.

121. Aldawood AS, Arabi YM, Haddad S. Safety of percutaneous tracheostomy in obese critically ill patients: a prospective cohort study. Anaesth Intensive Care 2008;36(1):69–73.

122. Heyrosa MG, Melniczek DM, Rovito P, et al. Percutaneous tracheostomy: a safe procedure in the morbidly obese. J Am Coll Surg 2006;202:618–22.

123. Byhahn C, Lischke V, Meininger D, et al. Peri-operative complications during percutaneous tracheostomy in obese patients. Anaesthesia 2005;60:12–5.

124. Mansharamani NG, Koziel H, Garland R, et al. Safety of bedside percutaneous dilatational tracheostomy in obese patients in the ICU. Chest 2000;117:1426–9.

125. Scott MJ, Leigh J. Percutaneous tracheostomy in three morbidly obese patients using the "Blue Rhino technique." Anaesthesia 2000;55:917–9.

126. Unwin S, Short S, Hunt P. Percutaneous dilational tracheostomy in the morbidly obese. Anaesthesia 2000;55:393–4.

127. Kost KM. Endoscopic percutaneous dilatational tracheostomy: a prospective evaluation of 500 consecutive cases. Laryngoscope 2007;115:1–30.

128. Hatfield A, Bodenham A. Portable ultrasonic scanning of the anterior neck before percutaneous dilatational tracheostomy. Anaesthesia 1999;54:660–3.

129. Sustic A. Role of ultrasound in the airway management of critically ill patients. Crit Care Med 2007;35:S173–7.

130. Kollig E, Heydenreich U, Roetman B, et al. Ultrasound and bronchoscopic controlled percutaneous tracheostomy on trauma UCI. Injury 2000;31:663–8.

Anesthetic Management of Patients with Obesity with and Without Sleep Apnea

Anthony N. Passannante, MD*, Michael Tielborg, MD

KEYWORDS

- Obesity • Sleep apnea • Anesthetic
- Management • Complications

Over the past few decades, obesity has become one of the most pressing global public health problems. The World Health Organization estimates that in 2006 there were 1.6 billion overweight adults (aged 15 years or older); at least 300 million of those were obese.[1] Some areas of North America, Eastern Europe, the United Kingdom, the Middle East, the Pacific Islands, China, and Australia have seen a tripling of obesity rates since 1980. Recent data demonstrate that more than 30% of the US population is obese (body mass index [BMI] 30 or greater), and 4.9% of the population is morbidly obese (BMI 40 or greater). The data regarding children is even more sobering. Worldwide, a staggering 22 million children younger than 5 years are thought to be obese.[2] In the United States, the trend among children and adolescents has paralleled the alarming trends observed in the adult population.

Obesity is most commonly discussed in the modern medical literature in terms of BMI. BMI, calculated by the formula: weight (kg)/height (m^2), functions well as an assessment tool for most adults. The formula has limitations, however, when applied to heavily muscled individuals, or to the pediatric population, which generally requires classification based on percentiles referencing established height/weight growth curves. As BMI increases, an impact on nearly every organ system can be anticipated: the heart may become enlarged, fat may infiltrate the myocardium; chronic hypoxemia from obstructive sleep apnea may lead to pulmonary hypertension and right ventricular dilation; lung volumes are affected by decreases in functional residual capacity, diminished expiratory reserve volumes, and total lung capacity. Oxygen consumption is increased and metabolic rate is elevated. Metabolic disturbances are more common, with type 2 diabetes mellitus affecting these individuals at higher rates than their lean cohorts. Orthopedic problems involving the hips, shoulders, and knees are also common. All of these factors combine to make the perioperative care of these patients substantially more challenging.

Given the constellation of comorbidities associated with excess body weight, it is surprising to find a paucity of literature revealing a definitive increase in overall operative risk. Aside from some evidence of increases in sternal wound infections after coronary bypass surgery[3] and an increased incidence of arterial hypoxemia in the recovery room, even in the absence of sleep apnea, surgical interventions do not seem to present obese patients with substantial additional danger.[4,5] With the accumulation of data indicating bariatric surgery offers sustained reductions in body weight, reductions in cardiovascular risk factors, and a reduction in all-cause mortality,[6] it is likely that laparoscopic gastric bypass surgery will bring an increasing number of obese patients to the operating

Department of Anesthesiology, University of North Carolina Hospitals, N2201 West Wing UNC Hospitals, Campus Box 7010, Chapel Hill, NC 27599-7010, USA
* Corresponding author.
E-mail address: apassannante@aims.unc.edu (A.N. Passannante).

Clin Chest Med 30 (2009) 569–579
doi:10.1016/j.ccm.2009.05.009
0272-5231/09/$ – see front matter © 2009 Elsevier Inc. All rights reserved.

room.[7] This section will concentrate on intraoperative issues important to the care of patients with obesity. The specific challenges of airway management in this population will be addressed only in passing, as this topic is covered in depth elsewhere in the monograph (see article by Solh in this issue). In order, the major topics to be covered are the pharmacokinetics of obesity, positioning of obese patients, regional anesthesia in obese patients, the intensity of monitoring required, laparoscopy in obese patients, and minimizing hypoxemia during anesthesia.

PHARMACOKINETICS OF OBESITY

As with normal weight patients, the main factors that affect tissue drug distribution in obese patients are plasma protein binding, body composition, and regional blood flow. Changes in any of these factors may alter the volume of distribution of a drug. Although not extensively studied, plasma protein binding does not appear to be significantly different in obese individuals. Obese patients do have both an increased lean body mass (LBM), and an increased fat mass, but the percentage increase in fat mass is greater than the percentage increase in lean body mass.[8] Simple arithmetic leads to the conclusion that obese patients will thus have less lean body mass per kilogram, and more fat body mass per kilogram, than normal weight individuals. In general terms, blood flow to fat is poor, accounting for perhaps 5% of cardiac output, compared with roughly 73% to viscera and 22% to lean tissue.[9] As blood volume increases directly with body weight, and many obese individuals will have an increased cardiac output, the vessel-rich group of organs is very well perfused in obese individuals.[10,11] This has implications for both injected and inhaled anesthetics. Unfortunately, the obesity pandemic has not given rise to an increase in pharmacokinetic studies in obese patients. Data regarding four classes of anesthetic drugs will be summarized: induction drugs (unfortunately only propofol [Diprivan]), opioids, neuromuscular blockers, and volatile anesthetics.

Induction Drugs

To date, pharmacokinetic studies of induction drugs have concentrated on propofol. A comparison study with normal weight controls showed that dosing propofol on the basis of total body weight (TBW) gave acceptable clinical results, unchanged initial volume of distribution, clearance was related to body weight, and volume of distribution at steady state was correlated with body weight. There was no evidence of propofol

accumulation when dosing schemes based on mg/kg of total body weight were used.[12]

Opioids

The situation is somewhat more complicated with opioids. Remifentanil (Ultiva) pharmacokinetics has been compared in 12 obese and 12 normal weight controls. The obese subjects reached significantly higher plasma concentrations after a loading dose than the control group, suggesting that, to avoid overdosage, remifentanil should be dosed on the basis of ideal body weight (IBW) or LBM.[13] While sufentanil (Sufenta) is not extensively used in current clinical practice, a recent study measured plasma sufentanil levels during and after an infusion directed by parameters derived from a normal weight population (as virtually all of our drug dosage recommendations are derived), and found that actual plasma concentrations of sufentanil were accurately predicted when dosing was based on TBW.[14] With the more commonly administered opioid, fentanyl, a different relationship exists. Another recent study compared measured plasma fentanyl concentrations in normal weight (BMI <30) and obese (BMI >30) subjects undergoing major surgery with a fentanyl infusion based on TBW, and found that such an infusion led to an overestimation of fentanyl dose requirements in obese patients. The authors derived a parameter they refer to as pharmacokinetic mass, which could be used to linearly predict fentanyl clearance, and thus accurately guide fentanyl infusions. For patients weighing 140 to 200 kg the pharmacokinetic mass was 100 to 108 kg, which illustrates the magnitude of dosing error that using TBW can lead to with fentanyl.[15]

Neuromuscular Blockers

The dosing of neuromuscular blockers is somewhat more predictable. The polar, hydrophilic nature of nondepolarizing neuromuscular blockers tends to limit their volume of distribution, creating a more reliable clinical effect when based on IBW. Vecuronium (Norcuron), for instance, will have a prolonged duration of action if it is administered on the basis of TBW. If dosed based on IBW, volume of distribution, total clearance, and elimination half-life were equivalent between obese and normal subjects.[16] A small study comparing the effects of rocuronium (Zemuron) dosed by TBW with rocuronium dosed by IBW also concludes that rocuronium dosage in obese patients should be guided by IBW to avoid significant prolongation of the duration of action (55 minutes versus 22 minutes until 25% twitch tension return).[17] The same authors used a similar model to study the effects of cisatracurium (Nimbex) in obese patients, and found comparable results, with dosage guided by TBW leading to a prolonged duration of action.[18] Thus, based on available data, nondepolarizing neuromuscular blockers should be dosed based on IBW to avoid prolonged duration of action.

Volatile Anesthetic Agents

Volatile anesthetic agents are commonly used in clinical practice, with two new drugs becoming widely used over the past decade. These newer agents, sevoflurane (Ultane) and desflurane (Suprane), offer lower blood solubility, quicker anesthetic uptake, distribution, and also recovery after drug delivery is terminated. Anesthetic vapors less likely to get widely distributed in fat, and more likely to leave the body quickly after cessation of delivery, would be expected to offer clinical advantages when caring for morbidly obese patients.

Two comparison studies between isoflurane (Forane) and sevoflurane in morbidly obese patients showed faster emergence after surgery with sevoflurane.[19,20] A comparison study between sevoflurane and desflurane in obese patients showed faster emergence and marginally higher oxygen saturation in patients treated with desflurane.[21] A third study compared recovery profiles after desflurane, isoflurane, and propofol, and concluded that immediate and intermediate recovery is quicker in patients when desflurane is used for maintenance of anesthesia.[22]

Although the pharmacokinetic characteristics of the newer volatile anesthetic drugs do offer the possibility of a more rapid emergence and quicker recovery, it is clear that all of the modern anesthetic vapors are safe to use in obese patients. If rapid initial emergence is of paramount importance, desflurane may be the best choice, whereas sevoflurane offers clinical advantages in certain situations (mask induction), and isoflurane offers a long record of safety and low administration costs.

POSITIONING OBESE PATIENTS FOR SURGERY

There is no definitive body of literature suggesting that obese patients have more frequent complications from positioning during anesthesia than normal weight patients. Practicing clinicians know well, however, that standard protective strategies may not work well in obese patients. Even the supine position may offer difficulty, as some patients are so large that standard operating room tables are either too small, or not engineered to bear the weight. Despite what would normally be regarded as adequate padding for surgery, complications have nevertheless occurred. A recent report describes rhabdomyolysis of the gluteal muscles leading to renal failure in several morbidly obese patients who were supine for 5-hour gastric bypass operations.[23] Another case report describes rhabdomyolysis leading to renal failure and death after bariatric surgery.[6]

The prone position can also present unique challenges, as obese patients' bodies may not fit well into frames designed for normal weight individuals, and alternatives such as gel rolls are subject to excessive compression from the excess weight placed on them. Even after the patient is positioned, it is not uncommon for some shifting to occur as the procedure progresses. Given the fact that pressure points well protected at the beginning of the case may not be adequately protected at the end, it is essential that all pressure points be carefully and regularly checked.

The lateral position offers its own challenges, with the patient's downward hip subject to substantial pressure regardless of the type of padding placed under it. The patient's nondependent arm must be well padded and supported, and it may or may not be necessary to use a traditional axillary roll support, depending on the amount of soft tissue present under the patient.

The lithotomy position may be difficult as the weight of the patient's legs may exceed the capacity of the standard stirrups. Compartment syndrome has been reported as a complication of this position.[24]

As the obesity pandemic spreads, health care organizations must appropriately plan for the care of morbidly obese patients while at the same time taking into account the health and safety of the providers involved in caring for these patients. Institutions, particularly those with busy bariatric surgery programs, might consider the purchase of special operating room tables, and perhaps even motorized hospital beds to facilitate transport of morbidly obese patients to and from the operating room. When it is necessary to move an anesthetized morbidly obese patient, adequate staffing and equipment, such as rollers or sliding boards should be immediately and easily available to minimize the risk of injury to those moving the patient.

REGIONAL ANESTHESIA IN OBESE PATIENTS

There is extensive experience with regional anesthesia in morbidly obese patients, much of which comes from modern obstetric anesthetic practice. It is clear that spinal and epidural anesthesia are technically feasible and safe in this population. It is also clear that regional techniques are more technically difficult, that indwelling catheters are more likely to migrate, and that specially designed equipment may be necessary.[25] Continuous techniques such as indwelling spinal anesthetic catheters and spinal-epidural anesthesia have become more popular, and may offer specific advantages when maternal cardiovascular disease make a gradual onset of sympathetic block desirable.[26,27] Regardless of whether or not spinal or epidural techniques are used, special care may need to be taken in dosing both local anesthetics and narcotics. It has been observed that obese patients are more likely to have greater cephalad spread of sympathetic block than normal weight patients and may be more susceptible to the respiratory depressant effects of neuraxially administered opioids.[28,29] Obese patients will also experience greater respiratory embarrassment from a high regional block than will normal weight patients.[30]

The overall impact of epidural analgesia in regard to measurable patient outcomes remains controversial. The increasing use of laparoscopic techniques to replace procedures that once required open laparotomy in obese patients has simplified postoperative care, particularly in regard to pain management. In obese patients who require open laparotomy, vital capacity is known to decrease significantly in the postoperative period. Given that low-thoracic epidural analgesia has been shown to reduce this decline in vital capacity, it may be considered as a strategy to mitigate this effect.[31]

The continuing trend toward ambulatory surgery ensures that many obese patients will present for outpatient procedures. Many of these procedures, particularly orthopedic, dermatologic, and plastic, can be performed under local anesthesia, or peripheral nerve block with or without sedation. Many of these patients may benefit from a peripheral nerve block to reduce postoperative pain. The development of continuous catheter techniques for postoperative pain relief offers the potential to significantly reduce discomfort well beyond the analgesic window provided by a single injection of local anesthetic, and should allow for substantial reduction in the doses of opioid necessary in the postoperative period. The enthusiasm for regional analgesia in anesthesia should nevertheless be tempered by a recent report of more than 9000 peripheral nerve blocks that documented high patient satisfaction with peripheral nerve block in obese patients while also finding a higher rate of block failure rate and a higher complication rate (including pneumothorax, preseizure

excitation, seizure, subdural block, and epidural spread of local anesthetic). Based on these findings, the authors suggest that obese patients should not be excluded from consideration for peripheral nerve blocks in the ambulatory setting.[32]

PERIOPERATIVE MONITORING FOR OBESE PATIENTS

There is little evidence to suggest that the presence of obesity per se increases the intensity of monitoring required for the delivery of an anesthetic. Anesthesia for gastroplasty can be safely provided with or without invasive monitoring.[33] The presence of comorbidities, which will be more common among obese patients presenting for surgery may, however, lead to more frequent use of invasive monitoring. Selected obese patients (such as those with obesity-hypoventilation syndrome and hence more likely to have pulmonary hypertension and cor pulmonale), may benefit from cardiovascular monitoring with a pulmonary artery catheter or transesophageal echocardiography. Technical difficulty with peripheral venous access may necessitate central line placement. Given the technical challenges associated with landmark identification in these patients, strong consideration should be given to the use of ultrasound guidance when placing these devices. It may also be necessary to insert an arterial line to obtain reliable blood pressure readings in some morbidly obese individuals, as body habitus may interfere with the performance of blood pressure cuffs.

LAPAROSCOPY IN OBESE PATIENTS

There is accumulating evidence to suggest that bariatric surgery offers continued reduction in comorbidities and may offer the possibility of long-term weight reduction to obese patients.[7] The widespread introduction of laparoscopic gastric bypass has significantly augmented the experience with laparoscopy in morbidly obese individuals. Laparoscopy requires intra-abdominal insufflation of a gas, usually carbon dioxide, to provide a pneumoperitoneum that allows visualization of, and access to, intra-abdominal structures. The creation of a pneumoperitoneum increases intra-abdominal pressure (IAP), which has cardiovascular consequences that vary with the level of intra-abdominal pressure. Systemic vascular resistance increases with the creation of pneumoperitoneum, and low levels of IAP (>10 mm Hg) increase venous return, with a resultant increase in arterial blood pressure and cardiac output. Higher levels of IAP can obstruct the vena cava, leading to decreased venous return and hence decreased cardiac output.[34]

Increased intra-abdominal pressure can reduce urine output, but experience with laparoscopic kidney donation documents that a management strategy designed to avoid hypovolemia and preserve renal perfusion pressure results in excellent renal function in both the donated and remaining kidneys.[35] In the absence of hemorrhage and with intra-abdominal pressure limited to 12 to 15 mm Hg, it does not appear to be necessary to administer excess fluid to ensure preservation of renal function.

Respiratory mechanics are impaired by both severe obesity and by the creation of pneumoperitoneum. Functional residual capacity is reduced in obesity, and atelectasis can be a significant clinical problem in the perioperative period.[36] Decreased pulmonary compliance has been documented in obese patients undergoing laparoscopy, and pneumoperitoneum worsens compliance at the same time as it leads to increased requirements for CO_2 elimination, which will require increases in ventilation. Supine anesthetized morbidly obese patients had 29% lower pulmonary compliance than normal weight patients in one study, and unfortunately neither a doubling of tidal volume nor a doubling of respiratory frequency reduced the A-a gradient.[37] Endotracheal tube position must be carefully monitored in obese patients undergoing laparoscopy, as head-down position and abdominal insufflation can cause migration of the endotracheal tube into the right mainstem bronchus.[38] Despite these problems, laparoscopy is usually well tolerated as long as the pneumoperitoneum pressure is maintained at less than 15 mm Hg, and many studies show reductions in overall morbidity when a laparoscopic technique is used.[39]

MINIMIZING HYPOXEMIA DURING ANESTHESIA

It has been recognized for many years that obese individuals are more likely to become hypoxemic during anesthesia and surgery than normal weight patients.[40] Obese patients desaturate more quickly when apnea is caused by general anesthesia, which makes careful preoxygenation extremely important.[41] Morbid obesity is associated with reductions in expiratory reserve volume, forced vital capacity, forced expiratory volume in 1 second (FEV1), functional residual capacity (FRC), and maximum voluntary ventilation.[42] Marked derangements in lung and chest wall mechanics have been well documented in mechanically ventilated and paralyzed morbidly obese patients, including reduced respiratory system compliance, increased

respiratory system resistance, severely reduced FRC, and impaired arterial oxygenation.[43] BMI is an important determinant of lung volumes, respiratory mechanics, and oxygenation, with increasing BMI leading to exponential decreases in FRC, total lung compliance, and oxygenation index (PaO2/PAO2), whereas chest wall compliance is only minimally affected.[44] Hypoxemia during mechanical ventilation in obese patients is at least in part mediated through unopposed increases in intra-abdominal pressure that reduce lung volumes, resulting in ventilation/perfusion mismatch.[45]

The numerous contributors to respiratory dysfunction described in the preceding paragraph make it important to take advantage of techniques that can reduce the degree of intraoperative hypoxemia that occurs in obese patients. Induction of anesthesia in obese patients requires an additional degree of caution. If careful preoperative evaluation raises any question about the adequacy of the mask airway, an awake intubation technique should be considered. Proper positioning for direct laryngoscopy will maximize the likelihood of success on the first attempt, and will likely require significant elevation of the upper body and head.[46] Positioning obese patients in a "ramped position" (with blankets used to elevate both the upper body and head of the patient) has been shown to result in improved laryngeal exposure with direct laryngoscopy, which might predict fewer failed intubations.[47] The difficulty of repositioning a morbidly obese patient during a failed intubation should not be underestimated. If direct laryngoscopy is unsuccessful, laryngeal mask airways are frequently effective at establishing ventilation, and should be immediately available.[48]

The prevention or reduction of atelectasis from the induction and maintenance of general anesthesia will improve arterial oxygenation. Preoxygenation with 100% oxygen and 10 cm positive end expiratory pressure (PEEP) for 5 minutes before the induction of general anesthesia, followed by 10 cm PEEP during mask ventilation and after intubation reduces immediate postintubation atelectasis as assessed by CT scan, and improves immediate postintubation arterial oxygenation on FiO2 100% (PaO2 of 457 ± 130 mm Hg versus 315 ± 100 in the control group).[49] Whether or not this reduction is maintained, and for how long it, is not known. The application of 10 cm of PEEP during the maintenance phase of general anesthesia has been shown to provide a sustained improvement in arterial oxygenation in morbidly obese patients through alveolar recruitment.[50] Although these maneuvers are quite safe in the vast majority of patients, further clinical studies with PEEP in obese patients would be helpful, particularly concerning the application of PEEP during induction.

ANESTHETIC MANAGEMENT OF PATIENTS WITH SLEEP APNEA

Sleep apnea is a general term for several conditions that involve sleep-disordered breathing. The most common type of sleep apnea is obstructive sleep apnea (OSA), which involves obstruction of the airway during sleep. The perioperative period is hazardous for patients with OSA because of, as might be expected, an increased risk of airway obstruction. As airway management is discussed elsewhere in this monograph, this section will say only that both mask ventilation and endotracheal intubation are more likely to be difficult in patients with OSA. The anesthetic care of patients with OSA is challenging because anesthetic drugs profoundly influence control of the already dysfunctional respiratory system, because airway management is more likely to be difficult, and because many patients with OSA have significant comorbidities.[51,52] In addition, many patients with OSA have not been formally diagnosed, and it is impossible to tailor an anesthetic plan for the benefit of a patient with OSA unless the diagnosis has been made (less common) or considered (becoming more common). In modern surgical and anesthetic practice, there is often minimal time allowed for in-depth preoperative evaluation. Outpatient surgical practice continues to expand, and there has been significant controversy regarding the suitability of the outpatient arena for patients with sleep apnea. For a patient with sleep apnea who requires a surgical procedure, one of the first questions that must be addressed is whether or not it is reasonable to expect the procedure to be done on an ambulatory basis. In an effort to provide some guidance to practitioners, the American Society of Anesthesiologists (ASA) published "Practice Guidelines for the Perioperative Management of Patients with Obstructive Sleep Apnea" in 2006.[53] This publication provides useful tools for identifying and screening patients who may not have a formal diagnosis of OSA. Physical characteristics, signs of obstruction during sleep, and the presence or absence of daytime somnolence form the basis of this screening (**Box 1**). Once sleep study results are reviewed, or consideration of obtaining a sleep study occurs, the practitioner can use this tool to estimate perioperative risk. This risk estimation considers the severity of sleep apnea, the invasiveness of the surgery, and the projected need for postoperative opioids. Patients at high risk

---

Box 1
Preoperative screening tool for obstructive sleep apnea

A. Clinical signs and symptoms suggesting the possibility of OSA

  1. Predisposing physical characteristics

      a. BMI 35 kg/m² (95th percentile for age and gender)[a]
      b. Neck circumference 17 in (men) or 16 in (women)
      c. Craniofacial abnormalities affecting the airway
      d. Anatomic nasal obstruction
      e. Tonsils nearly touching or touching in the midline

  2. History of apparent airway obstruction during sleep (two or more of the following are present; if patient lives alone or sleep is not observed by another person, then only one of the following needs to be present)

      a. Snoring (loud enough to be heard through closed door)
      b. Frequent snoring
      c. Observed pauses in breathing during sleep
      d. Awakens from sleep with choking sensation
      e. Frequent arousals from sleep
      f. Intermittent vocalization during sleep[a]
      g. Parental report of restless sleep, difficulty breathing, or struggling respiratory efforts during sleep[a]

  3. Somnolence (one or more of the following is present)

      a. Frequent somnolence or fatigue despite adequate "sleep"
      b. Falls asleep easily in a nonstimulating environment (eg, watching TV, reading, riding in or driving a car) despite adequate "sleep"
      c. Parent or teacher comments that child appears sleepy during the day, is easily distracted, is overly aggressive, or has difficulty concentrating[a]
      d. Child often difficult to arouse at usual awakening time[a]

[a] Signifies pediatric patients.

From Gross JB, Bachenberg KL, Benumof JL, et al. Practice guidelines for the perioperative management of patients with obstructive sleep apnea: a report by the American Society of Anesthesiologists Task Force on Perioperative Management of patients with obstructive sleep apnea. Anesthesiology 2006;104:1081–93; [quiz 1117–1088]; with permission.

should be steered away from the ambulatory surgical arena (**Table 1**).

The OSA scoring system presented in **Table 1** is a guide intended to reduce perioperative morbidity and mortality. Consistent preoperative use of continuous positive airway pressure (CPAP) reduces the score by 1, and an elevated resting carbon dioxide tension raises the score by 1. A score of 4 is thought to convey increased risk, and scores of 5 or 6 may indicate significantly increased perioperative risk. Please note that the scoring system attempts to integrate the severity of the disease (which may be hard to accurately do without a sleep study), the invasiveness of the surgery and the anesthetic that will be required

(which can be predicted fairly well), and the requirement for postoperative opioids (which must be honestly addressed).

Regardless of the type of anesthetic used, management of the airway should be conservative, with measures taken to minimize hypoxemia incident to airway obstruction and/or apnea. It is mandatory that patients be monitored and observed if sedation is administered in the preoperative period, and sedative drugs should be administered in a titrated fashion. In the operating suite, if spontaneous ventilation is to be abolished, strict attention to adequate preoxygenation is essential, and laryngeal mask airways and other emergency airway devices should be immediately available.

Table 1
Scoring system for estimating perioperative risk for patients with sleep apnea

	Points
A. Severity of sleep apnea based on sleep study (or clinical indicators if sleep study not available). Point score _____ (0–3)[a,b]	
Severity of OSA (see **Box 1**)	
None	0
Mild	1
Moderate	2
Severe	3
B. Invasiveness of surgery and anesthesia. Point score _____ (0–3)	
Type of surgery and anesthesia	
Superficial surgery under local or peripheral nerve block anesthesia without sedation	0
Superficial surgery with moderate sedation or general anesthesia	1
Peripheral surgery with spinal or epidural anesthesia (with no more than moderate sedation)	1
Peripheral surgery with general anesthesia	2
Airway surgery with moderate sedation	2
Major surgery, general anesthesia	3
Airway surgery, general anesthesia	3
C. Requirement for postoperative opioids. Point score _____ (0–3)	
Opioid requirement	
None	0
Low-dose oral opioids	1
High-dose oral opioids, parenteral or neuraxial opioids	3
D. Estimation of perioperative risk. Overall sore = the score for A plus the greater of the score for either B or C. Point score _____ (0–6)[c]	

[a] Signifies that one point may be subtracted if a patient has been on CPAP (continuous positive airway pressure) or noninvasive positive pressure ventilation (NIPPV) before surgery and will be using his or her appliance consistently during the postoperative period.
[b] Signifies that one point should be added if a patient with mild or moderate OSA also has a resting arterial carbon dioxide tension greater than 50 mmHG.
[c] Signifies that patients with a score of 4 may be at increased perioperative risk from OSA; patients with a score of 5 or 6 may be at significantly increased perioperative risk.
From Gross JB, Bachenberg KL, Benumof JL, et al. Practice guidelines for the perioperative management of patients with obstructive sleep apnea: a report by the American Society of Anesthesiologists Task Force on Perioperative Management of patients with obstructive sleep apnea. Anesthesiology 2006;104:1081–93; [quiz 1117–1088]; with permission.

Imaging studies have demonstrated that pharyngeal cross-sectional area is larger in the lateral position than in the supine position. This may attenuate the effects of sedation on airway obstruction in procedures performed under regional anesthesia in the lateral position,[54] although potentially complicating emergency airway management if intubation becomes necessary.

Many questions central to the anesthetic management of patients with OSA have not been addressed by definitive clinical trials. A recent review of the implications of OSA for anesthesiologists has collected the numerous case reports documenting adverse perioperative outcomes that are almost uniformly associated with the use of perioperative opioids. The authors note that OSA is frequently undiagnosed, that the incidence of OSA in the surgical population is higher than in the general population, and that the many comorbidities associated with OSA may make it difficult to separate the impact of OSA itself from the impact of the associated conditions.[55] For nonairway surgery in patients with OSA, little information exists on which to base decisions regarding the appropriate postoperative setting and the degree of special, if any, postoperative monitoring required by these patients. The literature does not provide evidence-based guidance regarding whether patients with OSA can safely have outpatient surgery or whether all patients with OSA require in-hospital monitoring after their surgery. However, anesthesiologists, nurse anesthetists, and recovery nurses are very attuned to the detection and rapid management of airway obstruction. Life-threatening airway obstruction typically happens to patients with OSA when they transition to a less intensively monitored environment (eg, home after ambulatory surgery or an unmonitored hospital floor bed after inpatient surgery). Although it seems rational and prudent to use CPAP or bilevel positive airway pressure (BiPAP) for patients who used these devices at home before surgery, it is not clear whether or not their application in the recovery room can reliably mitigate the occurrence of postoperative respiratory complications.

THE EFFECT OF ANESTHETIC DRUGS ON VENTILATORY RESPONSES IN PATIENTS WITH OBSTRUCTIVE SLEEP APNEA

There is evidence that many anesthetic agents cause exaggerated responses in patients with sleep apnea. Drugs such as pentothal, propofol, opioids, benzodiazepines, and nitrous oxide may reduce the tone of the pharyngeal musculature that acts to maintain airway patency.[56,57] The response to carbon dioxide in children with OSA and tonsillar hypertrophy is diminished during halothane anesthesia.[58] Intubated, spontaneously breathing children with sleep apnea who are anesthetized with a volatile anesthetic have depressed ventilation when compared with normal children, and up to a 50% incidence of apnea after 0.5 μg/kg of fentanyl is administered.[59] Although the studies cited previously regarding ventilatory response to carbon dioxide and apnea after modest doses of fentanyl were performed in children, prudence dictates that these data be considered when formulating anesthetic plans for adult patients with OSA. Patients with more severe sleep apnea as judged by lower oxygen saturation nadirs during polysomnography and higher preoperative apnea-hypopnea index (AHI) are more likely to have respiratory complications after surgery.[60,61] It is reasonable to infer from these, and many other studies, that sleep apnea may be worsened postoperatively, and that the worse the sleep apnea is, the more prone to postoperative respiratory disturbance and airway obstruction the patient will be.

ANESTHETIC TECHNIQUE

Unfortunately, there is no definitive evidence supporting one anesthetic technique over another for patients with OSA. The available information suggests the type of surgery (minor versus major, airway versus nonairway, noninvasive versus invasive surgery) performed is what makes a difference in regard to outcome. Anesthetic techniques that use shorter acting agents that allow for a more rapid restoration of consciousness and a more rapid return to baseline respiratory function after emergence from general anesthesia should be desirable for patients with OSA. Regional anesthesia offers the possibility of minimally affecting respiratory drive, and can reduce the impact of anesthetic agents on subsequent sleep patterns as well as maintaining arousal responses during apneic episodes. Sedation used during regional anesthesia must be carefully monitored, as sedatives are known to worsen hypoventilation in patients with sleep apnea.[62]

INTENSITY OF INTRAOPERATIVE AND POSTOPERATIVE MONITORING

There is no evidence to suggest that patients with OSA need more aggressive or invasive intraoperative monitoring than other patients do. The type of surgery planned and the other comorbidities the patient brings to the operating room should rather dictate the intensity of monitoring. The placement of an arterial line may be necessary if noninvasive blood pressure monitoring is inaccurate or impossible. The measurement of arterial blood gases may also assist in optimizing intraoperative ventilation. Metabolic alkalosis can result in mild hypoventilation, a condition that is undesirable in these patients. Thus, maintenance of the patient's baseline bicarbonate is optimal. Transesophageal echocardiography is often used as a monitor of ventricular function and filling for noncardiac surgery, but cannot be used when the surgical site involves the airway or esophagus, and may have limited utility with certain upper abdominal procedures.

Maintenance of general anesthesia can be managed with either volatile anesthetic or intravenous agents, and the availability of newer, shorter-acting drugs may minimize the duration of postoperative ventilatory depression. Ultra–short-acting opioids such as remifentanil can be used to increase the depth of general anesthesia and reduce the necessity for postintubation neuromuscular blockade in some cases. Extubation should be done only when the patient is fully awake and able to follow commands. The return of protective airway reflexes should be ensured. In addition, there should be an assessment of the patient's strength, with special attention given to the careful antagonism of neuromuscular blockade.

The provision of adequate postoperative analgesia is an integral part of the anesthetic plan, and it should be accomplished, to the extent possible, in a multimodal fashion. Sedation and narcotic-based analgesia may exacerbate symptoms of sleep apnea; however, there are no adequately powered studies to guide analgesic therapy of these patients. There are case reports documenting adverse respiratory events occurring with opioid-based analgesia via both the parenteral or epidural route including patient-controlled analgesia.[63,64] The use of nonsteroidal anti-inflammatory drugs, local anesthetics for incision infiltration, and epidural analgesia and peripheral nerve blocks where appropriate can minimize, or perhaps even eliminate the need for postoperative opioids. Regional analgesic techniques may be helpful in postoperative management of these patients, although whether or not these techniques reduce the incidence of sleep-disordered breathing postoperatively is unknown.

The ASA Practice Guidelines make several consensus-based recommendations regarding the postoperative care of patients with OSA. When patients use CPAP preoperatively, it should be reinstituted as soon as possible after surgery. It is recommended that the supine position be avoided in favor of the prone, sitting, or lateral positions during recovery. Supplemental oxygen should be administered to patients with OSA until they return to their resting arterial oxygen tension (PaO_2) while breathing room air. Patients with OSA should be observed for 3 hours longer than a patient who does not have OSA before discharge to an unmonitored area. If a significant episode of airway obstruction or apnea occurs during the postoperative period, the consultants recommend that postoperative monitoring continue for 7 hours.[53] Although these recommendations are based on expert consensus and not clinical trials, until proper trials are performed, a conservative and cautious approach to the postoperative monitoring of patients with OSA seems eminently reasonable.

REFERENCES

1. World Health Organization. Obesity and overweight fact sheet. Available at: http://web.who.int/mediacentre/factsheets/fs311/en/index.html. Accessed January 25, 2009.
2. Hedley AA, Ogden CL, Carroll MD, et al. Prevalence of overweight and obesity among US children, adolescents, and adults, 1999–2002. J Am Med Assoc 2004;291:2847–50.
3. Birkmeyer NJ, Charlesworth DC, Hernandez F, et al. Obesity and risk of adverse outcomes associated with coronary artery bypass surgery. Northern New England Cardiovascular Disease Study Group. Circulation 1998;97:1689–94.
4. Ahmad S, Nagle A, McCarthy RJ, et al. Postoperative hypoxemia in morbidly obese patients with and without obstructive sleep apnea undergoing laparoscopic bariatric surgery. Anesth Analg 2008;107:138–43.
5. Dindo D, Muller MK, Weber M, et al. Obesity in general elective surgery. Lancet 2003;361:2032–5.
6. Collier B, Goreja MA, Duke BE 3rd. Postoperative rhabdomyolysis with bariatric surgery. Obes Surg 2003;13:941–3.
7. Sjostrom L, Lindroos AK, Peltonen M, et al. Lifestyle, diabetes, and cardiovascular risk factors 10 years after bariatric surgery. N Engl J Med 2004;351:2683–93.
8. Cheymol G. Effects of obesity on pharmacokinetics implications for drug therapy. Clin Pharmacokinet 2000;39:215–31.
9. Rowland M, Tn T. Distribution. In: Clinical pharmacokinetics: concepts and applications. 3rd edition. Baltimore (MD): Williams and Wilkins; 1995. p. 137–55.
10. Reisin E, Tuck ML. Obesity-associated hypertension: hypothesized link between etiology and selection of therapy. Blood Press Monit 1999;4(Suppl 1):S23–6.

11. Messerli FH, Christie B, DeCarvalho JG, et al. Obesity and essential hypertension. Hemodynamics, intravascular volume, sodium excretion, and plasma renin activity. Arch Intern Med 1981; 141:81–5.

12. Servin F, Farinotti R, Haberer JP, et al. Propofol infusion for maintenance of anesthesia in morbidly obese patients receiving nitrous oxide. A clinical and pharmacokinetic study. Anesthesiology 1993; 78:657–65.

13. Egan TD, Huizinga B, Gupta SK, et al. Remifentanil pharmacokinetics in obese versus lean patients. Anesthesiology 1998;89:562–73.

14. Slepchenko G, Simon N, Goubaux B, et al. Performance of target-controlled sufentanil infusion in obese patients. Anesthesiology 2003;98:65–73.

15. Shibutani K, Inchiosa MA Jr, Sawada K, et al. Accuracy of pharmacokinetic models for predicting plasma fentanyl concentrations in lean and obese surgical patients: derivation of dosing weight ("pharmacokinetic mass"). Anesthesiology 2004;101:603–13.

16. Schwartz AE, Matteo RS, Ornstein E, et al. Pharmacokinetics and pharmacodynamics of vecuronium in the obese surgical patient. Anesth Analg 1992;74:515–8.

17. Leykin Y, Pellis T, Lucca M, et al. The pharmacodynamic effects of rocuronium when dosed according to real body weight or ideal body weight in morbidly obese patients. Anesth Analg 2004;99:1086–9 [table of contents].

18. Leykin Y, Pellis T, Lucca M, et al. The effects of cisatracurium on morbidly obese women. Anesth Analg 2004;99:1090–4 [table of contents].

19. Torri G, Casati A, Albertin A, et al. Randomized comparison of isoflurane and sevoflurane for laparoscopic gastric banding in morbidly obese patients. J Clin Anesth 2001;13:565–70.

20. Sollazzi L, Perilli V, Modesti C, et al. Volatile anesthesia in bariatric surgery. Obes Surg 2001;11:623–6.

21. Strum EM, Szenohradszki J, Kaufman WA, et al. Emergence and recovery characteristics of desflurane versus sevoflurane in morbidly obese adult surgical patients: a prospective, randomized study. Anesth Analg 2004;99:1848–53 [table of contents].

22. Juvin P, Vadam C, Malek L, et al. Postoperative recovery after desflurane, propofol, or isoflurane anesthesia among morbidly obese patients: a prospective, randomized study. Anesth Analg 2000;91:714–9.

23. Bostanjian D, Anthone GJ, Hamoui N, et al. Rhabdomyolysis of gluteal muscles leading to renal failure: a potentially fatal complication of surgery in the morbidly obese. Obes Surg 2003;13:302–5.

24. Mathews PV, Perry JJ, Murray PC. Compartment syndrome of the well leg as a result of the hemilithotomy position: a report of two cases and review of literature. J Orthop Trauma 2001;15:580–3.

25. Hood DD, Dewan DM. Anesthetic and obstetric outcome in morbidly obese parturients. Anesthesiology 1993;79:1210–8.

26. Shnaider R, Ezri T, Szmuk P, et al. Combined spinal-epidural anesthesia for Cesarean section in a patient with peripartum dilated cardiomyopathy. Can J Anaesth 2001;48:681–3.

27. Coker LL. Continuous spinal anesthesia for cesarean section for a morbidly obese parturient patient: a case report. AANA J 2002;70:189–92.

28. Hodgkinson R, Husain FJ. Obesity and the cephalad spread of analgesia following epidural administration of bupivacaine for Cesarean section. Anesth Analg 1980;59:89–92.

29. Hodgkinson R, Husain FJ. Obesity, gravity, and spread of epidural anesthesia. Anesth Analg 1981; 60:421–4.

30. von Ungern-Sternberg BS, Regli A, Bucher E, et al. Impact of spinal anaesthesia and obesity on maternal respiratory function during elective Caesarean section. Anaesthesia 2004;59:743–9.

31. von Ungern-Sternberg BS, Regli A, Reber A, et al. Effect of obesity and thoracic epidural analgesia on perioperative spirometry. Br J Anaesth 2005;94:121–7.

32. Nielsen KC, Guller U, Steele SM, et al. Influence of obesity on surgical regional anesthesia in the ambulatory setting: an analysis of 9,038 blocks. Anesthesiology 2005;102:181–7.

33. Capella JF, Capella RF. Is routine invasive monitoring indicated in surgery for the morbidly obese? Obes Surg 1996;6:50–3.

34. Ogunnaike BO, Jones SB, Jones DB, et al. Anesthetic considerations for bariatric surgery. Anesth Analg 2002;95:1793–805.

35. Biancofiore G, Amorose G, Lugli D, et al. Perioperative anesthetic management for laparoscopic kidney donation. Transplant Proc 2004;36:464–6.

36. Eichenberger A, Proietti S, Wicky S, et al. Morbid obesity and postoperative pulmonary atelectasis: an underestimated problem. Anesth Analg 2002; 95:1788–92.

37. Sprung J, Whalley DG, Falcone T, et al. The effects of tidal volume and respiratory rate on oxygenation and respiratory mechanics during laparoscopy in morbidly obese patients. Anesth Analg 2003;97:268–74.

38. Ezri T, Hazin V, Warters D, et al. The endotracheal tube moves more often in obese patients undergoing laparoscopy compared with open abdominal surgery. Anesth Analg 2003;96:278–82.

39. Lamvu G, Zolnoun D, Boggess J, et al. Obesity: physiologic changes and challenges during laparoscopy. Am J Obstet Gynecol 2004;191:669–74.

40. Vaughan RW, Wise L. Intraoperative arterial oxygenation in obese patients. Ann Surg 1976;184:35–42.

41. Jense HG, Dubin SA, Silverstein PI, et al. Effect of obesity on safe duration of apnea in anesthetized humans. Anesth Analg 1991;72:89–93.

42. Biring MS, Lewis MI, Liu JT, et al. Pulmonary physiologic changes of morbid obesity. Am J Med Sci 1999;318:293–7.

43. Pelosi P, Croci M, Ravagnan I, et al. Total respiratory system, lung, and chest wall mechanics in sedated-paralyzed postoperative morbidly obese patients. Chest 1996;109:144–51.

44. Pelosi P, Croci M, Ravagnan I, et al. The effects of body mass on lung volumes, respiratory mechanics, and gas exchange during general anesthesia. Anesth Analg 1998;87:654–60.

45. Pelosi P, Croci M, Ravagnan I, et al. Respiratory system mechanics in sedated, paralyzed, morbidly obese patients. J Appl Physiol 1997;82:811–8.

46. Brodsky JB, Lemmens HJ, Brock-Utne JG, et al. Anesthetic considerations for bariatric surgery: proper positioning is important for laryngoscopy. Anesth Analg 2003;96:1841–2 [author reply: 1842].

47. Collins JS, Lemmens HJ, Brodsky JB, et al. Laryngoscopy and morbid obesity: a comparison of the "sniff" and "ramped" positions. Obes Surg 2004;14:1171–5.

48. Frappier J, Guenoun T, Journois D, et al. Airway management using the intubating laryngeal mask airway for the morbidly obese patient. Anesth Analg 2003;96:1510–5 [table of contents].

49. Coussa M, Proietti S, Schnyder P, et al. Prevention of atelectasis formation during the induction of general anesthesia in morbidly obese patients. Anesth Analg 2004;98:1491–5 [table of contents].

50. Pelosi P, Ravagnan I, Giurati G, et al. Positive end-expiratory pressure improves respiratory function in obese but not in normal subjects during anesthesia and paralysis. Anesthesiology 1999;91:1221–31.

51. Hillman DR, Loadsman JA, Platt PR, et al. Obstructive sleep apnoea and anaesthesia. Sleep Med Rev 2004;8:459–71.

52. Loadsman JA, Hillman DR. Anaesthesia and sleep apnoea. Br J Anaesth 2001;86:254–66.

53. Gross JB, Bachenberg KL, Benumof JL, et al. Practice guidelines for the perioperative management of patients with obstructive sleep apnea: a report by the American Society of Anesthesiologists Task Force on Perioperative Management of patients with obstructive sleep apnea. Anesthesiology 2006;104:1081–93 [quiz 1117–1088].

54. Isono S, Tanaka A, Nishino T. Lateral position decreases collapsibility of the passive pharynx in patients with obstructive sleep apnea. Anesthesiology 2002;97:780–5.

55. Chung SA, Yuan H, Chung F. A systemic review of obstructive sleep apnea and its implications for anesthesiologists. Anesth Analg 2008;107:1543–63.

56. Dhonneur G, Combes X, Leroux B, et al. Postoperative obstructive apnea. Anesth Analg 1999;89:762–7.

57. Benumof JL. Obstructive sleep apnea in the adult obese patient: implications for airway management. J Clin Anesth 2001;13:144–56.

58. Strauss SG, Lynn AM, Bratton SL, et al. Ventilatory response to CO2 in children with obstructive sleep apnea from adenotonsillar hypertrophy. Anesth Analg 1999;89:328–32.

59. Waters KA, McBrien F, Stewart P, et al. Effects of OSA, inhalational anesthesia, and fentanyl on the airway and ventilation of children. J Appl Physiol 2002;92:1987–94.

60. Kim JA, Lee JJ, Jung HH. Predictive factors of immediate postoperative complications after uvulopalatopharyngoplasty. Laryngoscope 2005;115:1837–40.

61. Pang KP. Identifying patients who need close monitoring during and after upper airway surgery for obstructive sleep apnoea. J Laryngol Otol 2006;120:655–60.

62. Dolly FR, Block AJ. Effect of flurazepam on sleep-disordered breathing and nocturnal oxygen desaturation in asymptomatic subjects. Am J Med 1982;73:239–43.

63. Stone JG, Cozine KA, Wald A. Nocturnal oxygenation during patient-controlled analgesia. Anesth Analg 1999;89:104–10.

64. VanDercar DH, Martinez AP, De Lisser EA. Sleep apnea syndromes: a potential contraindication for patient-controlled analgesia. Anesthesiology 1991;74:623–4.

Obesity in the Intensive Care Unit

Shyoko Honiden, MS, MD, John R. McArdle, MD*

KEYWORDS

- Obesity • Intensive care unit • Drug dosing
- Mechanical ventilation • Critical illness

Nearly a third of United States adults older than 20 years are obese (defined as a body mass index [BMI] greater than 30) according to the National Health and Nutrition Evaluation Survey (NHANES) data from 2001 to 2004.[1] More recent data published by the US Centers for Disease Control and Prevention show only one state with a prevalence of obesity less than 20% (http://www.cdc.gov/nccdphp/dnpa/obesity/trend/maps/). In 2007, 30 states reported a prevalence of obesity of at least 25%, and 3 states reported a prevalence of more than 30%. The concept of an "obesity pandemic" is a real one; 66% of the United States population is currently overweight (BMI greater than 25), and the figure is expected to rise to 75% by 2015.[2] It has been estimated that the total health care costs attributable to obesity may double every decade, and may amount to more than $900 billion by 2030, accounting for 16% to 18% of the total United States health care costs.[3] Prevalence data for obesity among critically ill patients depend on the cohort examined but may be as high as 25% in medical/surgical intensive care units (ICUs).[4]

This article systematically reviews the physiologic changes attributable to obesity that may be relevant in critical illness, outlines the common disease processes encountered, highlights the practical challenges to care of the critically ill obese patient, and briefly touches on the effect of obesity on ICU outcome. Sleep-disordered breathing and the obesity-hypoventilation syndrome are common complications of obesity that are discussed in detail elsewhere in this issue and will not be addressed in depth here.

CARDIOVASCULAR PHYSIOLOGY IN OBESITY

Increases in body mass associated with obesity cause significant changes in cardiac performance and structure that can have pathophysiologic consequences even in patients who do not have coexistent hypertension. Early studies of the effect of obesity on hemodynamics focused on the morbidly obese. Alexander and colleagues demonstrated that morbidly obese patients had increased blood volume and cardiac output, which were in proportion to the degree of obesity.[5] Cardiac output was in the normal range when indexed for body mass, and the increases in output were likewise in proportion to increases in circulating blood volume. The increases in cardiac output were the result of increased stroke volume alone, with heart rates found to be in the normal range.[5] In normotensive obese patients, systemic vascular resistance decreased in conjunction with the increases in cardiac output.

The hemodynamic response to exercise also differs in obese and lean persons. In extremely obese patients, the increase in cardiac output associated with exercise may result in elevations in mean pulmonary artery pressure, mean pulmonary capillary wedge pressure, and left ventricular end-diastolic pressure.[6–8] These hemodynamic responses to exercise suggest that obesity itself may lead to diastolic dysfunction, which has also been suggested by echocardiographic studies demonstrating prolongation in mitral deceleration half time and lower left ventricular peak filling rates in normotensive obese patients compared with lean patients.[9–11] Diastolic dysfunction associated

Department of Medicine, Section of Pulmonary and Critical Care Medicine, Yale University School of Medicine, 333 Cedar Street, PO Box 208057, New Haven, CT 06520-8057, USA
* Corresponding author.
E-mail address: john.mcardle@yale.edu (J.R. McArdle).

Clin Chest Med 30 (2009) 581–599
doi:10.1016/j.ccm.2009.05.007
0272-5231/09/$ – see front matter © 2009 Published by Elsevier Inc.

chestmed.theclinics.com

with obesity could certainly lead to a higher propensity toward the development of pulmonary edema during high cardiac output states or conditions of fluid loading in critical illness.

The elevations in cardiac output and circulating blood volume can lead to left ventricular dilation. Echocardiographic studies comparing ventricular dimensions and wall thickness have consistently revealed increased left ventricular chamber size in obese subjects.[12,13] The increases in chamber size, even in the absence of hypertension, are associated with increases in wall tension, with a compensatory development of eccentric left ventricular hypertrophy. The increase in left ventricular mass associated with obesity is correlated with BMI and with waist/hip ratio. The left ventricular hypertrophy decreases wall stress in the face of left ventricular dilation. If the degree of hypertrophy does not keep pace with the degree of chamber dilation, systolic dysfunction or so-called "obesity cardiomyopathy" may ensue. Clinically meaningful systolic dysfunction most commonly occurs in patients with a BMI greater than 40 and in patients with a longer duration of obesity.[14,15] Obesity cardiomyopathy occurs in roughly 10% of this population[14] (see the article by Dela Cruz and Matthay in this issue).

Obesity is also associated with an increased risk for systemic hypertension.[15] Systemic hypertension leads to pressure overload of the left ventricle, which predisposes to concentric, as opposed to the eccentric, left ventricular hypertrophy that occurs with conditions of volume overload alone. Obese patients with systemic hypertension develop greater increases in left ventricular wall thickness and end-diastolic pressure than normal-weight hypertensive patients.[16] The mixed pressure and volume overload leads to increased wall stress of the left ventricle. Diastolic dysfunction is common in obese patients, and coexistent hypertension increases the risk for overt systolic dysfunction.[15]

PULMONARY PHYSIOLOGY IN OBESITY

Obesity can alter respiratory physiology substantially, leading to abnormalities in compliance, resistance, ventilation and perfusion relationships, the workload of the respiratory muscles, upper airway caliber and tone, and ventilatory control.[17] Both pulmonary and chest wall compliance may be reduced in obese patients. Pulmonary compliance is reduced by up to 25% in simple obesity and by as much as 40% in patients with the obesity-hypoventilation syndrome.[18,19] The primary mechanism of reduced lung compliance is increased blood volume in the pulmonary circulation, although small

airway closure related to reductions in functional residual capacity is also a factor.[20] The primary mechanism of reduced chest wall compliance is the increased mechanical load of adipose tissues in the abdomen and chest wall. The compliance is further reduced by recumbent posture, which leads to increased mechanical loading of the diaphragm.[20] The supine posture may be associated with significant reductions in lung volumes, leading to alterations in oxygenation and upper airway dimensions.[21] Such changes may have added importance in patients with respiratory failure.

Obese patients also have elevated airway resistance as a result of their having a smaller cross-sectional area of the upper airway than normal weight persons. Other causes of increased upper airway resistance include increased parapharyngeal soft tissue, impaired pharyngeal dilator activity owing to altered pharyngeal shape, and decreased pharyngeal volume owing to lower tractional forces by the trachea in the setting of diminished lung volumes.[21] In a study of 103 obese nonsmokers and 190 nonobese nonsmokers, Rubinstein and colleagues found that the obese subjects had significantly higher airway resistance, lower forced expiratory volume in 1 second (FEV_1), and lower expiratory flow rates at mid and low lung volumes than the nonobese subjects.[22]

In obese patients, the oxygen consumption by the muscles of respiration is increased substantially compared with nonobese persons. The oxygen cost of breathing increases 4-fold in simple obesity and as much as 10-fold in patients with the obesity-hypoventilation syndrome.[20] Kress and colleagues[23] compared the oxygen consumption of subjects during spontaneous breathing with that in obese patients who had mechanical ventilation and neuromuscular blockade in gastric bypass surgery. Total oxygen consumption was reduced by 16% after intubation and paralysis in the obese patients compared with 1% in nonobese control subjects undergoing surgery. Obese persons typically have normal maximal inspiratory and expiratory pressures (with the exception of patients with obesity-hypoventilation syndrome who may have inspiratory muscle weakness), but respiratory muscle endurance, as measured by maximum voluntary ventilation is reduced by 20% in simple obesity and by 45% in the obesity-hypoventilation syndrome.[24,25] This increase in respiratory muscle work and decreased respiratory muscle endurance may predispose obese patients to respiratory failure during situations that further tax the respiratory system.

Obesity is also associated with gas exchange abnormalities related to alterations in ventilation and perfusion (V/Q) matching. In normal weight subjects, the lung bases receive the bulk of both ventilation and perfusion. In obese patients, the lung bases continue to be perfused preferentially related to gravitational effects, but ventilation to the lung bases may be impaired because of the closure of small airways and the tendency toward atelectasis as a result of low lung volumes.[17] Overt hypoxemia may occur in the severely obese and is likely to be most evident with supine posture.

IMMUNOLOGIC CHANGES IN OBESITY

Adipocytes, the cells that primarily compose adipose tissue, were once thought to function solely as storage depots for excess energy balance, but these cells are now known to produce signaling molecules, called adipokines, that can significantly alter inflammatory cell and immune function. White adipose tissue (WAT) contains leukocytes, macrophages, and pre-adipocytes (fibroblastlike adipocyte precursors) in addition to the adipocytes.[26] Macrophages constitute approximately 10% of the cells in WAT from lean subjects, but the percentage of macrophages is substantially higher in obese persons.[27]

Pre-adipocytes produce macrophage colony-stimulating factor (M-CSF) and peroxisome proliferation activated receptor gamma (PPARγ), both of which promote macrophage activation.[28] Increased production of interleukin (IL)-6 and tumor necrosis factor alpha (TNF-α) in these macrophages likely contributes to obesity-related inflammation. Altered immune cell function, such as increased monocyte and granulocyte oxidative burst, have been found in obese subjects.[29]

One such adipokine is leptin, which acts to decrease food intake and increase energy consumption by promoting production of anorexigenic factors (**Fig. 1**).[26] T lymphocytes express high levels of leptin receptors, and leptin exerts specific effects on T-helper lymphocytes. These effects include increasing production of IL-2 and interferon-gamma (IFNγ) while decreasing IL-4 production, thus promoting a TH1 immune response.[26] Adiponectin, an anti-inflammatory adipokine that reduces macrophage activity and proinflammatory cytokine production, is produced in decreased amounts in obese patients.

Adipocytes also appear to stimulate innate immune responses. Expression of toll-like receptor-2, which is associated with obesity, can lead to innate immune responses on stimulation with bacterial products, such as peptidoglycan.[28] The net effect of these alterations in immune function is a chronic proinflammatory state that may promote insulin resistance, atherogenesis, and perhaps other sequelae of obesity.

Adipocytes also appear to affect endothelial cells and to have prothrombotic effects. Plasminogen activator inhibitor-1 (PAI-1) inhibits activation of plasminogen, thus promoting thrombosis and reducing normal fibrin clearance.[30] PAI-1 levels are increased in such thrombotic conditions as myocardial infarction and deep venous thrombosis (DVT). Leptin-deficient mice, which become obese, have markedly higher levels of PAI-1 activity than lean mice, and high levels of PAI-1 gene expression in adipose tissue. TNF-α, insulin,

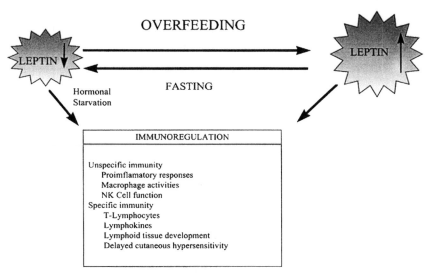

Fig. 1. Leptin involvement in immunoregulation. (*Adapted from* Marti A, Marcos A, Martinez JA. Obesity and immune function relationships. Obes Rev 2001;2:131–40; with permission.)

and transforming growth factor beta, which are all elevated in obesity, have been shown to increase PAI-1 levels in an animal model (**Fig. 2**).[30] Therefore, the proinflammatory, prothrombotic state that exists in obese patients might significantly affect their response to systemic infection and sepsis, although this is an area in need of ongoing investigation. (Also, see article by McCallister, Adkins, and O'Brien in this issue.)

COMMON DISORDERS IN CRITICALLY ILL OBESE PATIENTS
Thromboembolic Disease

The incidence of thromboembolic disease varies greatly among various types of hospitalized patients, from 10% to 20% in general medical patients to 40% in patients with major trauma and as high as 80% in critical care patients.[31] Alterations in PAI-1 and fibrinolytic activity in obese patients may contribute to their increased risk for venous thromboembolism (VTE).[30] Pulmonary embolism (PE) is the leading cause of death in patients who undergo bariatric surgery, with the risk being higher in patients with the obesity-hypoventilation syndrome or sleep apnea.[32–34]

Goldhaber and colleagues[35] found an increased risk for VTE among the obese members of the Nurses' Health Study.[35] The relative risk for PE in these initially healthy women was 1.7 in those with a BMI greater than 25 and 3.2 for those with a BMI greater than 29. The Study of Men Born in 1913 found a significant increase in the risk of VTE in men with a waist circumference of 100 cm or larger compared with those with waist circumference smaller than 100 cm, with a relative risk of 3.92 for VTE in the obese subjects.[36] Stein and colleagues found an increased risk for VTE in obese men and women compared with nonobese patients[37] (see the article by Stein in this issue).

Morbidly obese patients are frequently excluded from clinical trials of thromboprophylaxis because of altered pharmacokinetics in such patients and the difficulty of accurately diagnosing DVT or PE in the obese.[38] Therapy with enoxaparin, 40 mg subcutaneously every 12 hours, was associated with lower rates of postoperative DVT than was a dose of 30 mg every 12 hours in a nonrandomized prospective study of patients undergoing bariatric surgery.[39] A multicenter retrospective study of enoxaparin therapy after bariatric surgery found that regimens including 30 mg of enoxaparin begun preoperatively or 40 mg every 12 to 24 hours initiated postoperatively resulted in very low rates of VTE.[40] Therapy with nadroparin or tinzaparin has also been associated with low rates of VTE in obese patients.[41,42] Subcutaneous unfractionated heparin, which has not been well studied in the obese, is commonly used for VTE prophylaxis, with suggested doses of 5000 IU every 8 hours.

Abdominal obesity affects alveolar patency in the lower lung zones, which may predispose obese patients to atelectasis and arterial hypoxemia, particularly when immobile and in the supine position.[17] PE may be a concern in these situations, but diagnosis of PE is a challenge in patients with morbid obesity. Compression ultrasonography with venous imaging is not as sensitive in

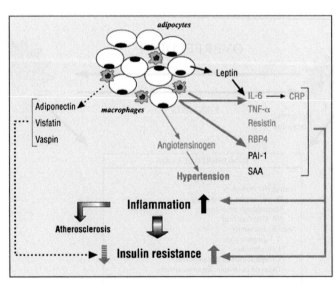

Fig. 2. Adipose tissue, adipokines, and its downstream pathways. (*From* Antuna-Puente B, Feve B, Fellahi S, et al. Adipokines: The missing link between insulin resistance and obesity. Diabetes Metab 2008;34:3; with permission.)

patients with severe obesity and/or significant leg edema.[43] Morbid obesity may limit CT angiography because of weight limits of the scanning table or mismatches between the patient's dimensions and the diameter of the CT scanner. Ventilation-perfusion scanning or perfusion scanning alone is a potential alternative, but neither modality can give a definitive diagnosis.[43] Therefore, patients at risk for PE and a persistent suspicion for the disorder may be unnecessarily exposed to full-dose anticoagulation and its attendant risks.

Aspiration

Obesity, especially central adiposity, is a significant risk factor for gastroesophageal reflux disease (GERD).[44,45] Proposed mechanisms include increased intra-abdominal pressure, decreased lower esophageal sphincter pressure, increased frequency of hiatal hernia, and perhaps alterations in esophageal motility and gastric emptying in the obese.[46] The use of narcotic analgesics and other drugs that alter intestinal motility may increase the risk of reflux and complications of aspiration in obese patients. Obesity is a recognized risk factor for aspiration in the perioperative period.[47] Histamine H_2 antagonists and proton pump inhibitors, which increase gastric pH and decrease the volume of gastric secretions,[48,49] might minimize the deleterious effects of gastric acid aspiration on the lung, but the loss of the antimicrobial effects of gastric acid has been suggested as a potential risk factor for pneumonia. Elevation of the patient's head may decrease intra-abdominal pressure and reduce the risk for aspiration after intubation.[50] The use of special endotracheal tubes that allow for continuous suctioning of subglottic secretions may also decrease the risk for aspiration and ventilator-associated pneumonia, although the use of these devices has not been studied in obese patients.[51]

Abdominal Compartment Syndrome

Intra-abdominal pressure (IAP) may be elevated because of ascites, hemorrhage, or visceral organ edema in patients with multiple traumas, pancreatitis, massive hemorrhage, and vigorous fluid resuscitation.[38] As intra-abdominal hypertension (IAH) develops, it can lead to the abdominal compartment syndrome with multiorgan dysfunction, including decreased urine output, low cardiac output owing to impaired venous return and perhaps increased afterload, decreased respiratory system compliance, intracranial pressure elevation, hypotension, and metabolic acidosis. Abdominal decompression is the mainstay of therapy for IAH, often necessitating decompressive laparotomy.

Obese patients have higher IAP than nonobese control subjects. Lambert and colleagues compared preoperative IAP in 45 morbidly obese patients (mean BMI 55) before open gastric bypass surgery with nonobese controls undergoing abdominal surgery. The nonobese patients had a mean IAP of 0 cm H_2O, the morbidly obese patients had a mean IAP of 12 cm H_2O. Patients with GERD, incontinence, diabetes mellitus, hypertension, and venous insufficiency had higher IAP than obese patients without these comorbidities.[52]

The incidence of clinically significant abdominal compartment syndrome in critically ill obese patients is unknown. Their increased resting IAP suggests that they would have an increased susceptibility to dangerous elevations in IAP with critical illness. The abdominal compartment syndrome should be suspected in the setting of increased IAP with attendant poor urine output, respiratory acidosis, or metabolic acidosis. In these settings, abdominal decompression should be considered, with treatment of ileus, large volume paracentesis, or laparotomy.[53]

COMPLICATIONS OF GASTRIC BYPASS SURGERY

The type and frequency of complications from weight-reduction surgery vary depending on whether the surgery is performed laparoscopically or as an open procedure.[54] A recent review of approximately 3500 patients who underwent laparoscopic gastric bypass surgery found that laparoscopic procedures were associated with fewer iatrogenic splenectomies, wound infections, incisional hernias, and overall mortality compared with open surgical procedures. However, with laparoscopic procedures there appears to be an increase in both early and late bowel obstruction, gastrointestinal hemorrhage, and stomal stenosis. Pneumonia, PE, and anastomotic leak occur with equal frequency in both procedures, with PE and anastomotic leak accounting for a significant proportion of postoperative death. PE accounted for half of the deaths for both open and laparoscopic procedures.

Persistent tachycardia and respiratory failure are independent predictors of postoperative anastomotic leak.[55] Other findings may include left shoulder pain, increasing abdominal pain, and left pleural effusion. Although contrast-enhanced upper gastrointestinal imaging is useful in assessing the integrity of the anastomotic site, a normal study does not exclude the diagnosis. Unrecognized, the disorder can lead to rapid deterioration and death. In patients who are persistently tachycardic or hypoxemic and in whom PE and other disorders have been excluded, urgent exploratory laparotomy is often necessary.[56,57]

PROLONGED RESPIRATORY FAILURE AND DIFFICULTIES WITH VENTILATOR WEANING

Physiologic changes associated with obesity can affect weaning from mechanical ventilation. Increased blood volume, systolic or diastolic dysfunction, increased chest wall loading, decreased respiratory muscle endurance, elevated IAP, upper airway narrowing, and potential alterations in central ventilatory drive that have been discussed here may impair the ability to breathe spontaneously. Diminished level of arousal may play a greater role in obese patients, who already may have significant narrowing of the upper airway and low lung volumes. The use of an endotracheal tube may blunt the reflexes of the upper airway, and the use of sedation may diminish tone in pharyngeal dilator muscles.[21] All of these features may result in upper airway obstruction after extubation.

Several large observational studies have shown that ventilator days and mortality rates are increased in obese trauma victims,[58,59] compared with lean patients, but these findings are not seen uniformly in obese, nontrauma, critically ill patients.[60] Although some studies have noted increased ventilator days in obese medical ICU patients, others have failed to find an association between obesity and ventilator days.[61–63] El Solh and colleagues[64] compared extubation outcomes in 62 consecutive patients with BMI of 35 or more who were treated immediately after extubation with noninvasive ventilation (NIV) with outcomes of similarly obese historical controls treated with conventional methods. The authors found that the use of NIV was associated with a statistically significant 16% reduction in postextubation respiratory failure. Rescue NIV given after the development of respiratory failure in the historical controls enabled a minority of these patients to avoid reintubation, with a resultant trend toward decreased need for reintubation (10% for the NIV group versus 21% from the historical control group), which did not reach statistical significance. (Also, see article by El Solh in this issue.)

Mechanical loading of the diaphragm by abdominal adipose tissue, viscera, and/or ascites can increase the work of breathing, thereby reducing the likelihood of successful extubation of obese patients with tenuous respiratory status. Positioning may also play a role in the optimization of respiratory mechanics in obese patients. Burns

and colleagues[65] showed the effect of reverse Trendelenburg posture on spontaneous breathing parameters in 19 patients with abdominal distension related to obesity, ascites, or intestinal distension. They found that positioning patients in this posture at an angle of 45 degrees was associated with increased tidal volumes and decreased respiratory rate compared with upright posture, and tidal volume was superior to that seen with head elevation of 45 degrees without Trendelenburg position. These findings suggest that reverse Trendelenburg positioning at a 45-degree angle be considered as default positioning for obese patients being weaned from mechanical ventilation in the absence of contraindications. The use of reverse Trendelenburg position is further supported by observations in the operating room during anesthesia induction. In a study in which morbidly obese patients were randomly assigned to one of three positions for induction of anesthesia, patients placed in the reverse Trendelenburg position had the fastest recovery to an oxygen saturation of 97% after reaching a nadir oxygenation that was similar to that of the other two groups.[66] Furthermore, the safe apnea period, defined as the apnea time during which the capillary oxygen saturation remains above 92% after induction of general anesthesia, was the longest for the reverse Trendelenburg position (**Fig. 3**).

CHALLENGES IN THE CARE OF CRITICALLY ILL OBESE PATIENTS
Airway Management

Morbidly obese patients often have anatomic changes that make intubation difficult, such as a short and thick neck, redundant soft tissue in the oropharynx, and limited mouth opening, and the availability of two experienced intubators is

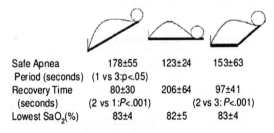

Safe Apnea Period (seconds)	178±55 (1 vs 3:p<.05)	123±24	153±63
Recovery Time (seconds)	80±30 (2 vs 1:P<.001)	206±64	97±41 (2 vs 3: P<.001)
Lowest SaO$_2$(%)	83±4	82±5	83±4

Data are Mean±Standard Deviation.

Fig. 3. Desaturation and recovery times after anesthesia induction in three positions: reverse Trendelenburg (30°) versus Supine versus 30° Back-Up Fowler. (*Adapted from* Boyce JR, Ness T, Castroman P, et al. A preliminary study of the optimal anesthesia positioning for the morbidly obese patient. Obes Surg 2003;13(1):4–9; with permission.)

preferable. Indeed, several studies have established an association between increasing BMI and difficulties with intubation.[67] Proper positioning, with the head elevated above the shoulders in the "sniffing position," is important.[68] Because of the upper airway anatomy and reduction in functional residual capacity when the patient is supine, ideal preoxygenation before intubation may not be possible, and the patient may rapidly desaturate and become unstable. Bilevel positive airway pressure (BiPAP) has been used to oxygenate patients before rapid sequence intubation when conventional methods of preoxygenation have failed to bring the saturation above 90%.[69] Laryngeal mask airways (LMA) can provide temporary airways in this setting, and there has been some success and relatively low complications with the use of intubating LMAs.[70] Ultimately, when other advanced airway techniques fail, skilled operators may need to intubate under fiber-optic guidance or with the aid of newer devices (for example, LMA CTrach, Airtraq, Glidescope) that allow for video-assisted intubation without the need to align the oral and pharyngeal axes.[71] If such methods are not successful, an emergent tracheostomy should be considered.

A review of nearly 25,000 patients in the postanesthesia care unit found that obese patients have twice the rate of critical respiratory events (such as upper airway obstruction, hypoventilation, unforeseen hypoxemia) requiring emergent management after extubation than nonobese patients.[72] One group reported on the use of a Cook airway exchange catheter as a bridge to extubation, when lingering concerns remained in a patient who was felt to have a borderline readiness (and whose original intubation was difficult). The catheter was successfully left in place for 35 minutes after extubation to serve as an intratracheal guide in case reintubation were necessary and as a means of insufflating oxygen intratracheally if needed emergently.[73] With administration of laryngotracheal lidocaine for airway anesthesia at the time of extubation, the patient tolerated this procedure without any excessive coughing or discomfort.

Central Venous Access

Because of the distortion of normal anatomic landmarks in obese patients, establishing central venous access can be time-consuming and challenging. In a randomized, crossover study in obese or anticoagulated patients, real-time ultrasound guidance improved success rates at cannulation and led to fewer complications.[74] Longer needles (for example, spinal needles) may be required in obese patients because standard needles may be too short to clear excessive soft tissue. Careful dressing changes and site maintenance are paramount because central venous catheters tend to be left in place longer in obese patients[63] (presumably because of technical difficulties and lack of alternative sites). Vigilance for infection and catheter-related phlebitis and thrombosis is important as well because intertriginous folds predispose these patients to local skin infections.

Surgical Airways

Longer tubes with sharper angles may be required for tracheostomy in obese patients because of their increased soft tissue, but such tubes carry a higher risk of becoming dislodged or occluded. Some investigators have preferentially used adjustable length tubes, but adverse events related to tracheal ulceration have been described, in part related to tube straightening after placement.[75,76] Higher complication rates have also been reported with tube placement itself (whether via a surgical[77] or percutaneous route), although the magnitude of excess risk in experienced hands is not clear.[78]

Hemodynamic Monitoring

Noninvasive blood pressure monitoring by cuff sphygmomanometer has unpredictable accuracy because of difficulties with cuff size selection. Inaccuracies may persist, even when an appropriately sized cuff is available.[79]

Invasive hemodynamic monitoring techniques are sometimes used in obese patients in whom other methods are impractical or inaccurate. Hemodynamic parameters are often adjusted according to body surface area. Beutler and colleagues highlight the potential variations in calculated indexed values depending on weight chosen (actual, adjusted, or ideal), which could lead to different conclusions regarding a patient's status, and, ultimately, treatment.[80] Ideal body weight is not optimal because oxygen demand and cardiac output are higher in obese patients than in nonobese patients. However, the increases in hemodynamic parameters are unlikely to rise continuously at extremes of weight, and using adjusted weights seems most reasonable. As a compromise, a 40% adjustment for weight above ideal body weight is commonly used as in drug dosing, but no study has rigorously validated this adjustment. Some investigators have shown that changes in hemodynamic parameters are predictable, relatively small, and most pronounced only at the extremes of BMI, and that standard indexing (using actual weight) for body surface area adequately attenuates this effect.[81]

Nursing Care

All staff caring for the obese ICU patient should be aware of the potential effect of personal prejudices toward the obese, who may have insecurities about body image.[82] In one survey of patients undergoing gastric bypass, 55% felt they had been treated disrespectfully by health care providers because of their weight.[83]

Skin integrity can be particularly problematic in obese patients. Admission Braden scores (**Table 1**) may inaccurately predict the need for skin care in obese patients.[84] Multiple skinfolds can lead to the buildup of moisture, posing a threat to skin integrity. Limited mobility, difficulty in nurse-assisted turning, decreased vascularity within adipose tissue, and excessive weight all contribute to pressure ulcer risk.[38] Pressure ulcers that begin in skin folds may go undetected during their early stages unless all such regions are examined carefully during routine turning. Turning the patient, particularly those at the upper extremes of BMI, can present a risk for injury to the patient and staff but can be minimized with proper training, staffing, and equipment.[85] The physical demands of turning can lead to suboptimal visualization of dependent skin regions. Patients with a BMI greater than 40 generally require at least four staff members to assist with repositioning.[84] Executing turns with clear roles for each participant (for example, one person at the patient's head to secure support devices and to communicate with the patient and several persons on each side of the patient to assist with turning, cleaning, and skin inspection) can ensure that the details of care are not neglected in the physical stress of the task.[86]

Mobilization and rehabilitation in obese patients may require increased personnel and equipment. Over-bed trapeze lifts and specialty beds that can shift to a chair egress mode to shift the burden of supporting weight to the patient may help to facilitate the gradual return of strength and mobility. The patient's knees should be carefully supported at the onset of standing to avoid buckling. Physical therapy staff experienced in the treatment of obese patients are pivotal to help the patient and staff so that transfers and weight bearing can occur safely.[86]

Imaging and Tests

Variable lead positioning owing to indistinct landmarks and excessive soft tissue can lead to low voltages and make accurate interpretation of electrocardiograms (ECG) difficult. Specifically, application of ECG-based criteria for the assessment of left ventricular hypertrophy and chamber enlargements is limited.[87] Similarly, image acquisition using an echocardiogram is poor.

Inadequate soft tissue penetration makes interpretation of portable radiographs difficult. Confluence of shadows from overlying soft tissue can mimic abnormalities, such as pleural thickening. Distinguishing the nature of parenchymal opacities (infiltrate versus edema, for example) can be difficult. Computed tomography (CT) is limited by load limits of the scanning tables as well as the diameter of the aperture. Some veterinary hospitals have specialized CT equipment to accommodate large animals and may be willing to perform scans in morbidly obese patients who cannot fit into conventional human scanners.

Nutritional Support

Obesity and malnutrition can coexist, particularly in the setting of critical illness, and appropriate nutritional support of obese patients is essential. Accelerated protein breakdown can lead to a rapid reduction in lean body mass. Hypocaloric, high-protein feeding theoretically prevents overfeeding (and its consequences, such as hyperglycemia) and allows for net protein anabolism and secondary fat weight loss.[88–91] Although small studies have suggested improved morbidity end points with this approach, including shorter ICU stay and ventilator days, it remains controversial.[4,91]

Estimation of the metabolic need of the critically ill obese patient is difficult. Direct calculations using indirect calorimetry may be helpful. There is much debate as to whether ideal body weight or actual weight should be used when using metabolic formulas, such as the Harris-Benedict equation. Some investigators have advocated the use of an obesity-adjusted weight with a 25% correction for excess weight above ideal body weight as follows: adjusted body weight = (actual weight − IBW) 0.25 + IBW, where IBW = ideal body weight.

This approach has not been validated for standard practice.[92]

DRUG DOSING

The physiologic changes in obesity markedly affect distribution, binding, and elimination of medications commonly prescribed in the ICU. Although systemic absorption of oral drugs is not significantly altered in obese patients, the increase in fat body mass and relative decrease in percentage contribution of lean mass and water can cause dramatic changes in the volume of

Table 1
Braden scale for predicting pressure sore risk

Patient's Name _____   Evaluator's Name _____   Date of Assessment _____

Category	1	2	3	4				
Sensory perception: ability to respond meaningfully to pressure-related discomfort	1. Completely limited. Unresponsive (does not moan, flinch, or grasp) to painful stimuli, owing to diminished level of consciousness or sedation OR limited ability to feel pain over most of body.	2. Very limited. Responds only to painful stimuli. Cannot communicate discomfort except by moaning or restlessness OR has a sensory impairment that limits the ability to feel pain or discomfort over half of body.	3. Slightly limited. Responds to verbal commands, but cannot always communicate discomfort or the need to be turned. OR has some sensory impairment that limits ability to feel pain or discomfort in 1 or 2 extremities.	4. No impairment. Responds to verbal commands. Has no sensory deficit that would limit ability to feel or voice pain or discomfort				
Moisture: degree to which skin is exposed to moisture	1. Constantly moist. Skin is kept moist almost constantly by perspiration, urine, etc. Dampness is detected every time patients is moved or turned.	2. Very moist. Skin is often, but not always moist. Linen must be changed at least once a shift.	3. Occasionally moist. Skin is occasionally moist, requiring an extra linen change approximately once a day.	4. Rarely moist. Skin is usually dry, linen requires changing only at routine intervals.				
Activity: degree to which skin is exposed to moisture	1. Bedfast. Confined to bed.	2. Chairfast. Ability to walk severely limited or nonexistent. Cannot bear own weight and/or must be assisted into chair or wheelchair.	3. Walks occasionally. Walks occasionally during day, but for very short distances, with or without assistance. Spends majority of each shift in bed or chair.	4. Walks frequently. Walks outside room at least twice a day and inside room at least once every 2 hours during walking hours.				
Mobility: ability to change and control body position	1. Completely immobile. Does not make even slight changes in body or extremity position without assistance.	2. Very limited. Makes occasional slight changes in body or extremity position but unable to make frequent or significant changes independently.	3. Slightly limited. Makes frequent though slight changes in body or extremity position independently.	4. No limitation. Makes major and frequent changes in position without assistance.				
Nutrition: usual food intake pattern	1. Very poor. Never eats a complete meal. Rarely eats more than 1/2 of any food offered. Eats 2 servings or less of protein (meat or dairy products) per day. Takes fluids poorly. Does not take a liquid dietary supplement OR is NPO and/or maintained on clear liquids or IVs for more than 5 days.	2. Probably inadequate. Rarely eats a complete meal and generally eats only about 1/2 of any food offered. Protein intake includes only 3 servings of meat or dairy products per day. Occasionally will take a dietary supplement OR receives less than optimum amount of liquid diet or tube feeding.	3. Adequate. East over half of most meals. Eats a total of 4 servings of protein (meat, dairy products) per day. Occasionally will refuse a meal, but will usually take a supplement when offered OR is on a tube feeding or TPN regimen that probably meets most of nutritional needs.	4. Excellent. Eats most of every meal. Never refuses a meal. Usually eats a total of 4 or more servings of meat and dairy products. Occasionally eats between meals. Does not require supplementation.				
Friction & shear	1. Problem. Requires moderate to maximum assistance in moving. Complete lifting without sliding against sheets is impossible. Frequently slides down in bed or chair, requiring frequent repositioning with maximum assistance. Spasticity contractures or agitation leads to almost constant friction.	2. Potential problem. Moves feebly or requires minimum assistance during a move. Skin probably slides to some extent against sheets, chair, restraints or other devices. Maintains relatively good position in chair or bed most of the time but occasionally slides down.	3. No apparent problem. Moves in bed and in chair independently and has sufficient muscle strength to lift up completely during move. Maintains good position in bed or chair.	—				

Total Score _____

Copyright © Barbara Braden and Nancy Bergstrom, 1988. Reprinted with permission. All Rights Reserved.

NPO, nothing by mouth; TPN, total parenteral nutrition.
Courtesy of Barbara Braden and Nancy Bergstrom; with permission

distribution. Other important changes include increases in total blood volume and cardiac output, alterations in plasma protein binding, and obesity-induced changes in liver and kidney function that may affect drug elimination.[93]

Appropriate drug dosing in obese patients for drugs commonly prescribed in the ICU is poorly understood given the lack of sufficient evidence in this population, in part because of the exclusion of the morbidly obese from many clinical trials (actual weight ≥200% ideal body weight or BMI >40).

For many lipophilic medications, such as aminoglycosides, with a large volume of distribution, the use of adjusted body weight is recommended. The distribution is presumed to be approximately 20% to 50% of the weight above ideal body weight. A typical calculation using 40% of excess weight is as follows: adjusted body weight = (Actual body weight − IBW) 0.4 + IBW However in the ICU, measurement of weight itself can be affected by temporary changes in body water from third spacing, which may or may not influence the distribution of medications. Pharmacokinetic effects of medications under these conditions are not well studied, particularly among obese patients. Elimination of medications is also often altered by concurrent renal or hepatic dysfunction in critical illness. Summary recommendations for medications commonly prescribed in the ICU are in **Table 2**.

Analgesia and Sedatives

Opioids
Opioids are generally lipophilic. However, because of significant individual variation in opioid requirements,[94] dosing based purely on predicted distribution in adipose tissue is difficult.[95] Some investigators have assumed that increased endogenous opioid concentrations in obese patients may be reflected into lower postoperative requirements for narcotics adjusted for weight,[96] but this assumption has not been replicated. Shibutani and colleagues[97] have attempted to formulate a nonlinearly adjusted model for fentanyl dosing. Others have studied the pharmacokinetics of remifentanil among 12 obese and 12 matched lean patients undergoing elective surgery and have concluded that dosing regimens are best based on ideal body weight in this setting.[98]

No single calculation or adjustment adequately accounts for variations in clinical response and dynamic changes in distribution and elimination encountered in the ICU. Initial dosing therefore should be guided by severity of pain and respiratory status (spontaneous, NIV, mechanical ventilation). The best approach when initiating opioid

therapy is to provide a series of small intravenous doses of rapid-acting agents given frequently (every 15 minutes) until the pain is controlled. Frequent pain assessment and appropriate dose titration are important.

Benzodiazepines
Benzodiazepines are highly lipophilic, a property that enables the drug to be widely distributed within fat tissue and that affects the terminal elimination half-life owing to alterations in volumes of distribution. The volume of distribution for both long-acting (diazepam) and short-acting (midazolam) benzodiazepines is significantly greater in obese patients than in normal weight controls, even after correction for total body weight.[99,100] For example, after a single 5-mg intravenous bolus dose of midazolam, the mean elimination half-life in obese patients was 5.94 hours compared with 2.27 hours in the nonobese.

Because of the excess distribution of the drug into fat, a relatively large loading dose may be necessary before a maintenance regimen is initiated. However, a series of smaller loading doses is preferable, titrated to clinical effect. Because of the prolonged half-life of benzodiazepines, maintenance doses are calculated using ideal body weight.

Propofol
Only one study has compared the pharmacokinetics of propofol in morbidly obese and normal weight patients.[101] In this small study, both volume of distribution and clearance increased with higher total body weight—taken together, these increases essentially canceled each other out, leading to similar elimination half-lives in obese and normal weight patients. Therefore, propofol dosing should theoretically be based on actual body weight, as in lean subjects. However, the risk for precipitous drops in blood pressure limits administration of very large intravenous doses of propofol. A more rational approach would be to start with a conservative dose using ideal body weight or an adjusted weight, and then rapidly titrating to clinical response.

Anticoagulants

Heparin
Weight-based heparin nomograms have been formulated to facilitate attainment of therapeutic targets. The efficacy of standard nomograms, however, in morbidly obese patients is not known. Although Spruill and colleagues[102] reported no significant difference between obese and lean patients when using standard actual body weight–based nomograms, their study was

Table 2
Recommended drug dosing for critically ill obese patients

Drugs for Dosing Using IBW or "Usual Dosing"	Drugs for Dosing Using Actual BW	Drugs for Dosing Using Adjusted BW	Too Little Data to Recommend
Opioids (with titration as needed according to pain scale)	LMWH[a] (with probable ceiling dose that may differ for different drugs)	Propofol	Beta-lactams
Benzodiazepine (with titration as needed according to sedation scale)	Thrombolytics (with maximal allowable ceiling dose)	Unfractionated heparin (probably, with PTT monitoring)	Amiodarone
Propofol Propofol is also listed in column three	Vancomycin – higher end of accepted range or actual BW with therapeutic drug monitoring	Aminoglycosides, with therapeutic drug monitoring for prolonged dosing	Vasopressors
Fluoroquinolones (very obese patients with severe infections may benefit from higher end of usual dosing range)	Activated protein C (drotrecogin alpha) (limited data)	Corticosteroids (for short courses of high-dose therapy for emergent situations; eg, acute spinal cord injury)	Inotropes
Digoxin	—	Lidocaine, verapamil (may need adjusted BW dosing for LOADING doses only)	—
Procainamide	—	—	—
Beta-blockers	—	—	—
Lidocaine, verapamil (usual dosing for maintenance doses)	—	—	—
H$_2$-blockers	—	—	—
Corticosteroids	—	—	—
Neuromuscular blockers	—	—	—

Abbreviations: BW, body weight; IBW, ideal body weight; LMWH, low-molecular-weight heparin.

[a] Per American College of Chest Physicians guidelines, for therapeutic dosing for LMWHs. Limited data available for weight up to 144 kg for enoxaparin, 190 kg for dalteparin, and 165 kg for tinzaparin. Concerns remain regarding subcutaneous absorption in obese patients.

retrospective, small, and did not include patients weighing more than 109 kg.

Heparin binds to endothelial cells and is then internalized and eliminated via the kidneys.[103] As with lean patients, the volume of distribution of heparin in obese patients mimics plasma volume. Because heparin does not distribute to adipose tissue and because adipose tissue is less vascularized than lean tissue, use of actual body weight may lead to overdosing and attaining a higher than desired activated partial thromboplastin time (aPTT).[104] Anticoagulant effects are nonlinear at (and above) therapeutic doses, and, therefore, a significantly higher aPTT than desired may place the patient at an increased risk for bleeding.[105] However, simply using ideal body weight may lead to underdosing, because extra vasculatures present in obese patients are excluded from consideration.

Several studies have evaluated the role of using actual body weight, modified dosing, and ideal body weight for heparin therapy in obese patients. Some advocate lowering the initial infusion rate from 18 units/kg/h to 15 units/kg/h when using actual body weight, with a ceiling bolus dose and initial infusion rate.[106] Others have used modified dosing weights: one such example described by Schwiesow and colleagues led to a therapeutic aPTT within 10 hours in a 54-year-old woman with a BMI of 75 using the following calculation: dosing weight = IBW + 0.26 (Actual body weight − IBW).[107] There is much controversy, however, about heparin dosing in obese patients, and until further definitive evidence emerges, the recently published American College of Chest Physicians (ACCP) evidence-based clinical practice guidelines on antithrombotic therapy have made no clear recommendations on how to manage the use of unfractionated heparin in the morbidly obese.[108]

There are no systematic studies of the use of low molecular weight heparin (LMWH) in morbidly obese patients, and information on dosing and efficacy is largely extrapolated from case series and other retrospective data. For prophylactic dalteparin given after bariatric surgery, standard dosing regimens may not achieve optimal anti–factor Xa levels in morbidly obese patients.[109] Therefore, some investigators support the use of higher doses of enoxaparin (40–60 mg, rather than the usual 30 mg, every 12 hours) in fixed-dose prophylaxis settings.[39,110,111] The most recent ACCP guidelines recommend weight-based dosing when using LMWH at therapeutic doses in obese patients.[108] In a pooled subgroup analysis of patients with a BMI greater than 30 in the ESSENCE[112] and TIMI11B[113] trials, there was no apparent risk of major bleeding when therapeutic doses were administered according to total body weight.[114] Although there is conflicting evidence about the strength of association between anti–factor Xa levels and patient outcome, anti–factor Xa levels seem to increase appropriately up to a total body weight of 144 kg for enoxaparin.[115] Similar determinations have been made for dalteparin for weights up to 190 kg[116,117] (despite the manufacturer's suggested dose limit for patients weighing more than 90 kg), and tinzaparin up to 165 kg.[42] Although subcutaneous dosing options are an alternative among very obese patients with difficult venous access, it is important to note that the reliability of absorption during critical illness is unclear, irrespective of body weight.[118,119]

Thrombolytic agents

In major trials that investigated the use of thrombolytic agents in acute myocardial infarction and stroke, the drugs were typically dosed in a weight-based manner with a maximum dose threshold.[120,121] There are no recommendations for dose adjustments in obese patients, and there are no data on whether the maximum allowable dose provides the same efficacy as that expected in a lean patient.

Antibiotics

Commonly used antibacterial agents (for example, aminoglycosides, fluoroquinolones, and vancomycin) are moderately lipophilic, and, therefore, dosing becomes relevant in the treatment of critically ill overweight patients.

Aminoglycosides

There is more pharmacokinetic information available on aminoglycosides than other antibiotics. Initial doses are usually calculated based on creatinine clearance, usually derived by use of the Cockroft-Gault equation, which takes into account the patient's serum creatinine concentration, age, total body weight, and sex. Such calculations tend to result in overdosing when based on total body weight, whereas calculations based on ideal body weight lead to underdosing. Use of a 40% correction factor that accounts for the larger volume of distribution in obese patients has the most support in the literature: adjusted weight = IBW + 0.4 (Actual body weight − IBW).[122] An arbitrarily established upper dose limit has been advocated for once-daily dosing in morbidly obese patients. Meanwhile, dosing intervals should be based on the estimated renal function. Many of the available pharmacokinetic studies, however, were based on observations after a single dose and were performed before the era of once-daily dosing regimens. Careful drug monitoring is essential if treatment is planned for more than 3 days.

Beta-lactams (cephalosporins and penicillins)

Beta-lactams are the largest and most commonly prescribed class of antibiotic, but very little is known about their optimal use in obese patients. Reliable data on penicillins are particularly lacking. Clearance and distribution appear to increase with excess weight for cephalosporins.[123–125] At least one study recommends the use of a higher surgical prophylactic dose of cefazolin (2 g rather than 1 g) for extremely obese patients and has documented decreased infection rates,[126] although a more recent small retrospective review failed to show any difference in outcome.[127]

Fluoroquinolones

A pharmacokinetic study with ciprofloxacin demonstrated a larger volume of distribution and higher clearance among moderately obese patients, and recommended adding 45% of the excess weight to the ideal body weight to calculate appropriate dosage.[128] This dosing recommendation was used in a 226-kg patient and achieved appropriate therapeutic concentrations.[129] In contrast, other investigators have shown no significant difference in volume of distribution and clearance with ciprofloxacin but a significantly lower tissue penetration (as measured in interstitial fluid) and advocated the use of actual body weight, particularly for wound and soft tissue infections.[130] Therefore, it may be reasonable to treat very obese patients with severe infections at the higher end of the recommended treatment ranges until further data become available.

Vancomycin

The volume of distribution and clearance of vancomycin are both increased in morbidly obese patients. Vancomycin dosing should, therefore, be based on actual body weight, and more frequent dosing may be required in patients with normal renal function because of the drug's shorter half-life as a result of enhanced clearance.[131,132] Therapeutic drug monitoring is advisable for all obese patients, probably regardless of renal function.

Cardiac Medications

Amiodarone

Amiodarone is lipophilic with a very large volume of distribution, and, therefore, adequate loading and tissue saturation may take several weeks. Obese patients would, therefore, likely require higher than usual doses. However, the anti-arrhythmic action of amiodarone does not necessarily track pharmacokinetic data.[133] In addition, there is significant interpatient variability in pharmacokinetic data even among lean patients, and no studies have systematically evaluated drug dosing in obese patients. Therefore, no recommendation can be made regarding dose adjustments for the obese population.

Other cardiac medications

Limited data in moderately obese patients support the use of ideal body weight when calculating loading and maintenance regimens for digoxin,[134] procainamide,[135] and propranolol. Propranolol is the exception to the general rule that lipophilic drugs have an increased volume of distribution in obese patients. Despite being lipophilic, propranolol and other lipophilic β-blockers, such as labetalol and nebivolol, do not appear to have substantial distribution into adipose tissue.[136]

Limited pharmacokinetic data suggest actual body weight can be used for loading regimens for lidocaine and verapamil, but because of the relative paucity of data, a more conservative approach using adjusted body weight seems reasonable. Usual, non–weight-based dosing and adjustments can be made for maintenance doses.[137]

Gastrointestinal Agents

Histamine H₂ antagonists

Gastrointestinal prophylaxis with histamine H_2 antagonists is standard of care in mechanically ventilated patients. Most dosing regimens are fixed, with no consideration for weight in particular, except in special situations, such as in patients with the Zollinger-Ellison syndrome. H_2 blockers are not distributed into excess body fat, and there is no evidence of altered drug clearance or half-life in obese patients.[138,139] Ideal body weight should, therefore, be used when calculating weight-based dosing for these agents.

Corticosteroids

Most corticosteroid treatment regimens are fixed and not based on weight. When weight-based dosing is used, such as in emergent therapy for acute spinal cord injury, data are limited, and patients weighing more than 109 kg were excluded from enrollment in studies.[140] One pharmacokinetic study suggested that the volume of distribution and drug clearance were decreased when adjusted for weight.[141] In general, corticosteroid dosing should be based on ideal body weight, particularly when concerns for toxicity are heightened (for example, in patients who will require prolonged administration). When rapid clinical efficacy is of utmost importance and therapy is given for a short period of time, as in acute spinal cord injury, use of adjusted body weight is probably reasonable to avoid complications from underdosing.

Neuromuscular blockers

Neuromuscular blockers are polar and hydrophilic compounds. Although a few studies suggested that obese patients require dosing based on actual body weight,[142,143] most studies recommend dosing based on ideal body weight.[144–146] Initial maintenance infusions are therefore best based on ideal body weight, with close monitoring via peripheral nerve stimulation and adjustments as clinically appropriate.

One exception may be succinylcholine, a depolarizing muscle relaxant whose duration of action is determined by pseudocholinesterase activity in the blood and the volume of extracellular fluid space. Obesity has been associated with both increased psuedocholinesterase activity and volume of extracellular fluid space.[147]

Vasoactive agents

No studies have evaluated pharmacokinetic and pharmacodynamic parameters among obese patients with regard to commonly used vasopressor and inotropic agents. However, because of the large inter- and intrapatient variation in drug concentrations in lean and healthy patients, systematic predictable changes are unlikely to occur owing to obesity. For example, when nine healthy male volunteers were infused with dopamine at 3 μg/kg/min for 90 minutes, steady-state drug concentrations varied widely, ranging from 1880 to 18,300 ng/L. The variation was even more dramatic at higher drug doses.[148] Similarly, steady-state dobutamine concentrations had poor correlation with infusion rates among 16 surgical critical care patients.[149] In this study, steady-state concentrations appeared to have little correlation with such factors as age, weight, estimated creatinine clearance, and net cumulative fluid balance. Dose titration should, therefore, be based on clinical response and adjusted according to objective goals, such as mean arterial pressure.

Recombinant human activated protein C (drotrecogin alpha)

Although obese patients were excluded from the original PROWESS trial, which examined the benefit of recombinant activated protein C in severe sepsis,[150] a follow-up phase IV study reported similar pharmacokinetics when morbidly obese patients were dosed according to actual body weight (without limitation in total dosage).[151]

ICU OUTCOMES

Although one might assume that obesity is associated with poor ICU outcomes, current evidence fails to establish this association consistently; several studies have shown obesity to be protective during critical illness, whereas others have shown a negative or equivocal effect.[58,59,61,62,152–155] A recent meta-analysis of 14 studies and more than 15,000 obese patients (BMI >30) in medical and surgical ICUs showed no significant difference in ICU mortality rate for obese patients compared with normal weight patients. However, ICU length of stay and days requiring mechanical ventilation were increased. In this study, a subgroup analysis of moderately obese patients (BMI >30 but <40) found an increase in ICU survival rate among these obese patients compared with normal weight patients (relative risk 0.86; confidence interval 0.81–0.91; $P < .001$).[156] (Also, see article by O'Brien in this issue.)

SUMMARY

Obesity poses unique challenges for the ICU team. Important changes in cardiovascular, pulmonary, and immunologic physiology predispose such patients to respiratory failure, thromboembolic disease, abdominal compartment syndrome, and aspiration. Special attention is required when performing routine ICU procedures, such as intubation and insertion of central venous catheters, and limitations in testing capabilities may lead the astute ICU clinician to rely solely on clinical suspicion when making therapeutic decisions. Daily management can be further hampered by uncertainties regarding drug metabolism and pharmacokinetics, nutritional needs, and challenges in bedside nursing care. Dedicated research is much needed in obese patients to allow for formulation of evidence-based guidelines that would further enhance delivery of ICU care for this challenging population.

REFERENCES

1. Ogden CL, Carroll MD, Curtin LR, et al. Prevalence of overweight and obesity in the United States, 1999–2004. JAMA 2006;295:1549.
2. Wang Y, Beydoun MA. The obesity epidemic in the United States—gender, age, socioeconomic, racial/ethnic, and geographic characteristics: a systematic review and meta-regression analysis. Epidemiol Rev 2007;29:6.

3. Wang Y, Beydoun MA, Liang L, et al. Will all Americans become overweight or obese? Estimating the progression and cost of the US obesity epidemic. Obesity (Silver Spring) 2008;16:2323.

4. Joffe A, Wood K. Obesity in critical care. Curr Opin Anaesthesiol 2007;20:113.

5. Alexander JK, Dennis EW, Smith WG, et al. Blood volume, cardiac output, and distribution of systemic blood flow in extreme obesity. Cardiovasc Res Cent Bull 1962;1:39.

6. Alpert MA, Singh A, Terry BE, et al. Effect of exercise on left ventricular systolic function and reserve in morbid obesity. Am J Cardiol 1989;63:1478.

7. de Divitiis O, Fazio S, Petitto M, et al. Obesity and cardiac function. Circulation 1981;64:477.

8. Alexander JK. Obesity and cardiac performance. Am J Cardiol 1964;14:860.

9. Nakajima T, Fujioka S, Tokunaga K, et al. Noninvasive study of left ventricular performance in obese patients: influence of duration of obesity. Circulation 1985;71:481.

10. Karason K, Wallentin I, Larsson B, et al. Effects of obesity and weight loss on left ventricular mass and relative wall thickness: survey and intervention study. BMJ 1997;315:912.

11. Ku CS, Lin SL, Wang DJ, et al. Left ventricular filling in young normotensive obese adults. Am J Cardiol 1994;73:613.

12. Alpert MA, Lambert CR, Terry BE, et al. Effect of weight loss on left ventricular diastolic filling in morbid obesity. Am J Cardiol 1995;76:1198.

13. Zema MJ, Caccavano M. Feasibility of detailed M-mode echocardiographic examination in markedly obese adults: prospective study of 50 patients. J Clin Ultrasound 1982;10:31.

14. Alpert MA. Obesity cardiomyopathy: pathophysiology and evolution of the clinical syndrome. Am J Med Sci 2001;321:225.

15. Alpert MA, Hashimi MW. Obesity and the heart. Am J Med Sci 1993;306:117.

16. Messerli FH, Sundgaard-Riise K, Reisin E, et al. Disparate cardiovascular effects of obesity and arterial hypertension. Am J Med 1983;74:808.

17. Parameswaran K, Todd DC, Soth M. Altered respiratory physiology in obesity. Can Respir J 2006;13:203.

18. Sharp JT, Henry JP, Sweany SK, et al. The total work of breathing in normal and obese men. J Clin Invest 1964;43:728.

19. Pelosi P, Croci M, Ravagnan I, et al. Total respiratory system, lung, and chest wall mechanics in sedated-paralyzed postoperative morbidly obese patients. Chest 1996;109:144.

20. Koenig SM. Pulmonary complications of obesity. Am J Med Sci 2001;321:249.

21. Malhotra A, Hillman D. Obesity and the lung: 3. Obesity, respiration and intensive care. Thorax 2008;63:925.

22. Rubinstein I, Zamel N, DuBarry L, et al. Airflow limitation in morbidly obese, nonsmoking men. Ann Intern Med 1990;112:828.

23. Kress JP, Pohlman AS, Alverdy J, et al. The impact of morbid obesity on oxygen cost of breathing (VO(2RESP)) at rest. Am J Respir Crit Care Med 1999;160:883.

24. Fritts HW Jr, Filler J, Fishman AP, et al. The efficiency of ventilation during voluntary hyperpnea: studies in normal subjects and in dyspneic patients with either chronic pulmonary emphysema or obesity. J Clin Invest 1959;38:1339.

25. Kaufman BJ, Ferguson MH, Cherniack RM. Hypoventilation in obesity. J Clin Invest 1959;38:500.

26. Marti A, Marcos A, Martinez JA. Obesity and immune function relationships. Obes Rev 2001;2:131.

27. Dixit VD. Adipose-immune interactions during obesity and caloric restriction: reciprocal mechanisms regulating immunity and health span. J Leukoc Biol 2008;84:882.

28. Karagiannides I, Pothoulakis C. Obesity, innate immunity and gut inflammation. Curr Opin Gastroenterol 2007;23:661.

29. Lamas O, Marti A, Martinez JA. Obesity and immunocompetence. Eur J Clin Nutr 2002;56(Suppl 3): S42.

30. Loskutoff DJ, Samad F. The adipocyte and hemostatic balance in obesity: studies of PAI-1. Arterioscler Thromb Vasc Biol 1998;18:1.

31. Geerts WH, Pineo GF, Heit JA, et al. Prevention of venous thromboembolism: the Seventh ACCP Conference on antithrombotic and thrombolytic therapy. Chest 2004;126:338S.

32. Carmody BJ, Sugerman HJ, Kellum JM, et al. Pulmonary embolism complicating bariatric surgery: detailed analysis of a single institution's 24-year experience. J Am Coll Surg 2006;203:831.

33. Hamad GG, Bergqvist D. Venous thromboembolism in bariatric surgery patients: an update of risk and prevention. Surg Obes Relat Dis 2007;3:97.

34. Davis G, Patel JA, Gagne DJ. Pulmonary considerations in obesity and the bariatric surgical patient. Med Clin North Am 2007;91:433.

35. Goldhaber SZ, Grodstein F, Stampfer MJ, et al. A prospective study of risk factors for pulmonary embolism in women. JAMA 1997;277:642.

36. Hansson PO, Eriksson H, Welin L, et al. Smoking and abdominal obesity: risk factors for venous thromboembolism among middle-aged men: "the study of men born in 1913." Arch Intern Med 1886;159:1999.

37. Stein PD, Beemath A, Olson RE. Obesity as a risk factor in venous thromboembolism. Am J Med 2005;118:978.

38. El-Solh AA. Clinical approach to the critically ill, morbidly obese patient. Am J Respir Crit Care Med 2004;169:557.

39. Scholten DJ, Hoedema RM, Scholten SE. A comparison of two different prophylactic dose regimens of low molecular weight heparin in bariatric surgery. Obes Surg 2002;12:19.

40. Hamad GG, Choban PS. Enoxaparin for thromboprophylaxis in morbidly obese patients undergoing bariatric surgery: findings of the prophylaxis against VTE outcomes in bariatric surgery patients receiving enoxaparin (PROBE) study. Obes Surg 2005;15:1368.

41. Kalfarentzos F, Stavropoulou F, Yarmenitis S, et al. Prophylaxis of venous thromboembolism using two different doses of low-molecular-weight heparin (nadroparin) in bariatric surgery: a prospective randomized trial. Obes Surg 2001;11:670.

42. Hainer JW, Barrett JS, Assaid CA, et al. Dosing in heavy-weight/obese patients with the LMWH, tinzaparin: a pharmacodynamic study. Thromb Haemost 2002;87:817.

43. Tapson VF, Carroll BA, Davidson BL, et al. The diagnostic approach to acute venous thromboembolism. Clinical practice guideline. American Thoracic Society. Am J Respir Crit Care Med 1999;160:1043.

44. Nilsson M, Johnsen R, Ye W, et al. Obesity and estrogen as risk factors for gastroesophageal reflux symptoms. JAMA 2003;290:66.

45. Corley DA, Kubo A, Zhao W. Abdominal obesity, ethnicity and gastro-oesophageal reflux symptoms. Gut 2007;56:756.

46. Friedenberg FK, Xanthopoulos M, Foster GD, et al. The association between gastroesophageal reflux disease and obesity. Am J Gastroenterol 2008;103:2111.

47. Kalinowski CP, Kirsch JR. Strategies for prophylaxis and treatment for aspiration. Best Pract Res Clin Anaesthesiol 2004;18:719.

48. Andrews AD, Brock-Utne JG, Downing JW. Protection against pulmonary acid aspiration with ranitidine. A new histamine H2-receptor antagonist. Anaesthesia 1982;37:22.

49. Nishina K, Mikawa K, Maekawa N, et al. A comparison of lansoprazole, omeprazole, and ranitidine for reducing preoperative gastric secretion in adult patients undergoing elective surgery. Anesth Analg 1996;82:832.

50. Drakulovic MB, Torres A, Bauer TT, et al. Supine body position as a risk factor for nosocomial pneumonia in mechanically ventilated patients: a randomised trial. Lancet 1851;354:1999.

51. Valles J, Artigas A, Rello J, et al. Continuous aspiration of subglottic secretions in preventing ventilator-associated pneumonia. Ann Intern Med 1995;122:179.

52. Lambert DM, Marceau S, Forse RA. Intra-abdominal pressure in the morbidly obese. Obes Surg 2005;15:1225.

53. Malbrain ML, De laet IE. Intra-abdominal hypertension: evolving concepts. Clin Chest Med 2009;30:45.

54. Podnos YD, Jimenez JC, Wilson SE, et al. Complications after laparoscopic gastric bypass: a review of 3464 cases. Arch Surg 2003;138:957.

55. Hamilton EC, Sims TL, Hamilton TT, et al. Clinical predictors of leak after laparoscopic Roux-en-Y gastric bypass for morbid obesity. Surg Endosc 2003;17:679.

56. Levi D, Goodman ER, Patel M, et al. Critical care of the obese and bariatric surgical patient. Crit Care Clin 2003;19:11.

57. Pieracci FM, Barie PS, Pomp A. Critical care of the bariatric patient. Crit Care Med 2006;34:1796.

58. Brown CV, Neville AL, Rhee P, et al. The impact of obesity on the outcomes of 1,153 critically injured blunt trauma patients. J Trauma 2005;59:1048.

59. Bochicchio GV, Joshi M, Bochicchio K, et al. Impact of obesity in the critically ill trauma patient: a prospective study. J Am Coll Surg 2006;203:533.

60. Oliveros H, Villamor E. Obesity and mortality in critically ill adults: a systematic review and meta-analysis. Obesity (Silver Spring) 2008;16:515.

61. Ray DE, Matchett SC, Baker K, et al. The effect of body mass index on patient outcomes in a medical ICU. Chest 2005;127:2125.

62. Goulenok C, Monchi M, Chiche JD, et al. Influence of overweight on ICU mortality: a prospective study. Chest 2004;125:1441.

63. El-Solh A, Sikka P, Bozkanat E, et al. Morbid obesity in the medical ICU. Chest 2001;120:1989.

64. El-Solh AA, Aquilina A, Pineda L, et al. Noninvasive ventilation for prevention of post-extubation respiratory failure in obese patients. Eur Respir J 2006;28:588.

65. Burns SM, Egloff MB, Ryan B, et al. Effect of body position on spontaneous respiratory rate and tidal volume in patients with obesity, abdominal distension and ascites. Am J Crit Care 1994;3:102.

66. Boyce JR, Ness T, Castroman P, et al. A preliminary study of the optimal anesthesia positioning for the morbidly obese patient. Obes Surg 2003;13:4.

67. Grant P, Newcombe M. Emergency management of the morbidly obese. Emerg Med Australas 2004;16:309.

68. Rao SL, Kunselman AR, Schuler HG, et al. Laryngoscopy and tracheal intubation in the head-elevated position in obese patients: a randomized, controlled, equivalence trial. Anesth Analg 2008;107:1912.

69. El-Khatib MF, Kanazi G, Baraka AS. Noninvasive bilevel positive airway pressure for preoxygenation of the critically ill morbidly obese patient. Can J Anaesth 2007;54:744.

70. Frappier J, Guenoun T, Journois D, et al. Airway management using the intubating laryngeal mask

airway for the morbidly obese patient. Anesth Analg 2003;96:1510.

71. Dhonneur G, Abdi W, Ndoko SK, et al. Video-assisted versus conventional tracheal intubation in morbidly obese patients. Obes Surg 2008.

72. Rose DK, Cohen MM, Wigglesworth DF, et al. Critical respiratory events in the postanesthesia care unit. Patient, surgical, and anesthetic factors. Anesthesiology 1994;81:410.

73. Moyers G, McDougle L. Use of the Cook airway exchange catheter in "bridging" the potentially difficult extubation: a case report. AANA J 2002;70:275.

74. Gilbert TB, Seneff MG, Becker RB. Facilitation of internal jugular venous cannulation using an audio-guided Doppler ultrasound vascular access device: results from a prospective, dual-center, randomized, crossover clinical study. Crit Care Med 1995;23:60.

75. Papadimos TJ, Flores AS, Schmidt MS, et al. Bivona hyperflex tracheostomy tube occlusion causing spurious tachypnoea and tracheal ulceration. Eur J Anaesthesiol 2007;24:472.

76. Tibballs J, Robertson C, Wall R. Tracheal ulceration and obstruction associated with flexible Bivona tracheostomy tubes. Anaesth Intensive Care 2006;34:495.

77. El Solh AA, Jaafar W. A comparative study of the complications of surgical tracheostomy in morbidly obese critically ill patients. Crit Care 2007;11:R3.

78. Byhahn C, Lischke V, Meininger D, et al. Peri-operative complications during percutaneous tracheostomy in obese patients. Anaesthesia 2005;60:12.

79. Maxwell MH, Waks AU, Schroth PC, et al. Error in blood-pressure measurement due to incorrect cuff size in obese patients. Lancet 1982;2:33.

80. Beutler S, Schmidt U, Michard F. Hemodynamic monitoring in obese patients: a big issue. Crit Care Med 1981;32:2004.

81. Stelfox HT, Ahmed SB, Ribeiro RA, et al. Hemodynamic monitoring in obese patients: the impact of body mass index on cardiac output and stroke volume. Crit Care Med 2006;34:1243.

82. Charlebois D, Wilmoth D. Critical care of patients with obesity. Crit Care Nurse 2004;24:19.

83. Rand CS, Macgregor AM. Morbidly obese patients' perceptions of social discrimination before and after surgery for obesity. South Med J 1990;83:1390.

84. Winkelman C, Maloney B. Obese ICU patients: resource utilization and outcomes. Clin Nurs Res 2005;14:303.

85. Hurst S, Blanco K, Boyle D, et al. Bariatric implications of critical care nursing. Dimens Crit Care Nurs 2004;23:76.

86. Nasraway SA Jr, Hudson-Jinks TM, Kelleher RM. Multidisciplinary care of the obese patient with chronic critical illness after surgery. Crit Care Clin 2002;18:643.

87. Nath A, Alpert MA, Terry BE, et al. Sensitivity and specificity of electrocardiographic criteria for left and right ventricular hypertrophy in morbid obesity. Am J Cardiol 1988;62:126.

88. Malone AM. Permissive underfeeding: its appropriateness in patients with obesity, patients on parenteral nutrition, and non-obese patients receiving enteral nutrition. Curr Gastroenterol Rep 2007;9: 317.

89. Miller JP, Choban PS. Feeding the critically ill obese patient: the role of hypocaloric nutrition support. Respir Care Clin N Am 2006;12:593.

90. Dickerson RN. Hypocaloric feeding of obese patients in the intensive care unit. Curr Opin Clin Nutr Metab Care 2005;8:189.

91. Dickerson RN, Boschert KJ, Kudsk KA, et al. Hypocaloric enteral tube feeding in critically ill obese patients. Nutrition 2002;18:241.

92. Cutts ME, Dowdy RP, Ellersieck MR, et al. Predicting energy needs in ventilator-dependent critically ill patients: effect of adjusting weight for edema or adiposity. Am J Clin Nutr 1997;66:1250.

93. Casati A, Putzu M. Anesthesia in the obese patient: pharmacokinetic considerations. J Clin Anesth 2005;17:134.

94. Bennett R, Batenhorst R, Graves DA, et al. Variation in postoperative analgesic requirements in the morbidly obese following gastric bypass surgery. Pharmacotherapy 1982;2:50.

95. Cheymol G. Effects of obesity on pharmacokinetics implications for drug therapy. Clin Pharmacokinet 2000;39:215.

96. Rand CS, Kuldau JM, Yost RL. Obesity and postoperative pain. J Psychosom Res 1985;29:43.

97. Shibutani K, Inchiosa MA Jr, Sawada K, et al. Pharmacokinetic mass of fentanyl for postoperative analgesia in lean and obese patients. Br J Anaesth 2005;95:377.

98. Egan TD, Huizinga B, Gupta SK, et al. Remifentanil pharmacokinetics in obese versus lean patients. Anesthesiology 1998;89:562.

99. Abernethy DR, Greenblatt DJ, Divoll M, et al. Prolonged accumulation of diazepam in obesity. J Clin Pharmacol 1983;23:369.

100. Greenblatt DJ, Abernethy DR, Locniskar A, et al. Effect of age, gender, and obesity on midazolam kinetics. Anesthesiology 1984;61:27.

101. Servin F, Farinotti R, Haberer JP, et al. Propofol infusion for maintenance of anesthesia in morbidly obese patients receiving nitrous oxide. A clinical and pharmacokinetic study. Anesthesiology 1993; 78:657.

102. Spruill WJ, Wade WE, Huckaby WG, et al. Achievement of anticoagulation by using a weight-based heparin dosing protocol for obese and nonobese patients. Am J Health Syst Pharm 2001;58:2143.

103. Kandrotas RJ. Heparin pharmacokinetics and pharmacodynamics. Clin Pharmacokinet 1992;22:359.

104. Ellison MJ, Sawyer WT, Mills TC. Calculation of heparin dosage in a morbidly obese woman. Clin Pharm 1989;8:65.

105. Hirsh J, Warkentin TE, Shaughnessy SG, et al. Heparin and low-molecular-weight heparin: mechanisms of action, pharmacokinetics, dosing, monitoring, efficacy, and safety. Chest 2001;119:64S.

106. Yee WP, Norton LL. Optimal weight base for a weight-based heparin dosing protocol. Am J Health Syst Pharm 1998;55:159.

107. Schwiesow SJ, Wessell AM, Steyer TE. Use of a modified dosing weight for heparin therapy in a morbidly obese patient. Ann Pharmacother 2005;39:753.

108. Hirsh J, Guyatt G, Albers GW, et al. Executive summary: American College of Chest Physicians evidence-based clinical practice guidelines (8th edition). Chest 2008;133:71S.

109. Simoneau MD, Vachon A, Picard F. Effect of prophylactic dalteparin on anti-factor Xa levels in morbidly obese patients after bariatric surgery. Obes Surg 2008.

110. Rowan BO, Kuhl DA, Lee MD, et al. Anti-Xa levels in bariatric surgery patients receiving prophylactic enoxaparin. Obes Surg 2008;18:162.

111. Simone EP, Madan AK, Tichansky DS, et al. Comparison of two low-molecular-weight heparin dosing regimens for patients undergoing laparoscopic bariatric surgery. Surg Endosc 2008;22:2392.

112. Cohen M, Demers C, Gurfinkel EP, et al. A comparison of low-molecular-weight heparin with unfractionated heparin for unstable coronary artery disease. Efficacy and Safety of Subcutaneous Enoxaparin in Non-Q-Wave Coronary Events Study Group. N Engl J Med 1997;337:447.

113. Antman EM, McCabe CH, Gurfinkel EP, et al. Enoxaparin prevents death and cardiac ischemic events in unstable angina/non-Q-wave myocardial infarction. Results of the thrombolysis in myocardial infarction (TIMI) 11B trial. Circulation 1999;100:1593.

114. Spinler SA, Inverso SM, Cohen M, et al. Safety and efficacy of unfractionated heparin versus enoxaparin in patients who are obese and patients with severe renal impairment: analysis from the ESSENCE and TIMI 11B studies. Am Heart J 2003;146:33.

115. Sanderink GJ, Le Liboux A, Jariwala N, et al. The pharmacokinetics and pharmacodynamics of enoxaparin in obese volunteers. Clin Pharmacol Ther 2002;72:308.

116. Smith J, Canton EM. Weight-based administration of dalteparin in obese patients. Am J Health Syst Pharm 2003;60:683.

117. Wilson SJ, Wilbur K, Burton E, et al. Effect of patient weight on the anticoagulant response to adjusted therapeutic dosage of low-molecular-weight heparin for the treatment of venous thromboembolism. Haemostasis 2001;31:42.

118. Priglinger U, Delle Karth G, Geppert A, et al. Prophylactic anticoagulation with enoxaparin: Is the subcutaneous route appropriate in the critically ill? Crit Care Med 2003;31:1405.

119. Rutherford EJ, Schooler WG, Sredzienski E, et al. Optimal dose of enoxaparin in critically ill trauma and surgical patients. J Trauma 2005;58:1167.

120. Topol EJ. Reperfusion therapy for acute myocardial infarction with fibrinolytic therapy or combination reduced fibrinolytic therapy and platelet glycoprotein IIb/IIIa inhibition: the GUSTO V randomised trial. Lancet 1905;357:2001.

121. Tissue plasminogen activator for acute ischemic stroke. The National Institute of Neurological Disorders and Stroke rt-PA Stroke Study Group. N Engl J Med 1995;333:1581.

122. Pai MP, Bearden DT. Antimicrobial dosing considerations in obese adult patients. Pharmacotherapy 2007;27:1081.

123. Chiba K, Tsuchiya M, Kato J, et al. Cefotiam disposition in markedly obese athlete patients, Japanese sumo wrestlers. Antimicrobial Agents Chemother 1989;33:1188.

124. Mann HJ, Buchwald H. Cefamandole distribution in serum, adipose tissue, and wound drainage in morbidly obese patients. Drug Intell Clin Pharm 1986;20:869.

125. Yost RL, Derendorf H. Disposition of cefotaxime and its desacetyl metabolite in morbidly obese male and female subjects. Ther Drug Monit 1986;8:189.

126. Forse RA, Karam B, MacLean LD, et al. Antibiotic prophylaxis for surgery in morbidly obese patients. Surgery 1989;106:750.

127. Mehta U, Malone M, Alger S. Cefazolin use in clinically severe obese patients undergoing gastric restrictive surgery. Ann Pharmacother 1995;29:935.

128. Allard S, Kinzig M, Boivin G, et al. Intravenous ciprofloxacin disposition in obesity. Clin Pharmacol Ther 1993;54:368.

129. Caldwell JB, Nilsen AK. Intravenous ciprofloxacin dosing in a morbidly obese patient. Ann Pharmacother 1994;28:806.

130. Hollenstein UM, Brunner M, Schmid R, et al. Soft tissue concentrations of ciprofloxacin in obese and lean subjects following weight-adjusted dosing. Int J Obes Relat Metab Disord 2001;25:354.

131. Bauer LA, Black DJ, Lill JS. Vancomycin dosing in morbidly obese patients. Eur J Clin Pharmacol 1998;54:621.

132. Erstad BL. Dosing of medications in morbidly obese patients in the intensive care unit setting. Intensive Care Med 2004;30:18.

133. Roden DM. Pharmacokinetics of amiodarone: implications for drug therapy. Am J Cardiol 1993;72:45F.

134. Abernethy DR, Greenblatt DJ, Smith TW. Digoxin disposition in obesity: clinical pharmacokinetic investigation. Am Heart J 1981;102:740.

135. Christoff PB, Conti DR, Naylor C, et al. Procainamide disposition in obesity. Drug Intell Clin Pharm 1983;17:516.

136. Cheymol G, Poirier JM, Carrupt PA, et al. Pharmacokinetics of beta-adrenoceptor blockers in obese and normal volunteers. Br J Clin Pharmacol 1997; 43:563.

137. Abernethy DR, Greenblatt DJ. Lidocaine disposition in obesity. Am J Cardiol 1984;53:1183.

138. Abernethy DR, Greenblatt DJ, Matlis R, et al. Cimetidine disposition in obesity. Am J Gastroenterol 1984;79:91.

139. Davis RL, Quenzer RW, Bozigian HP, et al. Pharmacokinetics of ranitidine in morbidly obese women. DICP 1990;24:1040.

140. Bracken MB, Shepard MJ, Holford TR, et al. Administration of methylprednisolone for 24 or 48 hours or tirilazad mesylate for 48 hours in the treatment of acute spinal cord injury. Results of the Third National Acute Spinal Cord Injury Randomized Controlled Trial. National Acute Spinal Cord Injury Study. JAMA 1997;277:1597.

141. Nichols AI, D'Ambrosio R, Pyszczynski NA, et al. Pharmacokinetics and pharmacodynamics of prednisolone in obese rats. J Pharmacol Exp Ther 1989;250:963.

142. Tsueda K, Warren JE, McCafferty LA, et al. Pancuronium bromide requirement during anesthesia for the morbidly obese. Anesthesiology 1978;48:438.

143. Varin F, Ducharme J, Theoret Y, et al. Influence of extreme obesity on the body disposition and neuromuscular blocking effect of atracurium. Clin Pharmacol Ther 1990;48:18.

144. Leykin Y, Pellis T, Lucca M, et al. The pharmacodynamic effects of rocuronium when dosed according to real body weight or ideal body weight in morbidly obese patients. Anesth Analg 2004;99:1086.

145. Puhringer FK, Keller C, Kleinsasser A, et al. Pharmacokinetics of rocuronium bromide in obese female patients. Eur J Anaesthesiol 1999;16:507.

146. Schwartz AE, Matteo RS, Ornstein E, et al. Pharmacokinetics and pharmacodynamics of vecuronium in the obese surgical patient. Anesth Analg 1992; 74:515.

147. Bentley JB, Borel JD, Vaughan RW, et al. Weight, pseudocholinesterase activity, and succinylcholine requirement. Anesthesiology 1982;57:48.

148. MacGregor DA, Smith TE, Prielipp RC, et al. Pharmacokinetics of dopamine in healthy male subjects. Anesthesiology 2000;92:338.

149. Klem C, Dasta JF, Reilley TE, et al. Variability in dobutamine pharmacokinetics in unstable critically ill surgical patients. Crit Care Med 1994; 22:1926.

150. Bernard GR, Vincent JL, Laterre PF, et al. Efficacy and safety of recombinant human activated protein C for severe sepsis. N Engl J Med 2001; 344:699.

151. Levy H, Small D, Heiselman DE, et al. Obesity does not alter the pharmacokinetics of drotrecogin alfa (activated) in severe sepsis. Ann Pharmacother 2005;39:262.

152. Diaz JJ Jr, Norris PR, Collier BR, et al. Morbid obesity is not a risk factor for mortality in critically ill trauma patients. J Trauma 2009;66:226.

153. Frat JP, Gissot V, Ragot S, et al. Impact of obesity in mechanically ventilated patients: a prospective study. Intensive Care Med 2008;34:1991.

154. Peake SL, Moran JL, Ghelani DR, et al. The effect of obesity on 12-month survival following admission to intensive care: a prospective study. Crit Care Med 2006;34:2929.

155. O'Brien JM Jr, Welsh CH, Fish RH, et al. Excess body weight is not independently associated with outcome in mechanically ventilated patients with acute lung injury. Ann Intern Med 2004;140:338.

156. Akinnusi ME, Pineda LA, El Solh AA. Effect of obesity on intensive care morbidity and mortality: a meta-analysis. Crit Care Med 2008; 36:151.

Obesity and Respiratory Diseases in Childhood

Elizabeth K. Fiorino, MD, Lee J. Brooks, MD*

KEYWORDS

- Obesity • Children • Pulmonary mechanics • Asthma
- Sleep apnea • Obesity-hypoventilation syndrome

Obesity is a major public health problem in children. According to the latest National Health and Nutrition Examination Survey (NHANES) data from 2003 to 2004, 17.1% of children in the United States are overweight, with an age- and sex-specific body mass index, (BMI, kg/m^2) greater than the 95th percentile. This represents a vast increase when compared with the 1960s, when fewer than 5% of children aged 6 to 19 were overweight (**Fig. 1**).[1,2] Associated comorbidities in the adult, such as metabolic syndrome, an increased risk for obstructive sleep apnea (OSA), and increased cardiovascular complications are well known. In children, however, the risks of obesity are less clearly defined. Moreover, the impact of obesity on the growing individual, in particular the growing lung, may be unique and particularly detrimental. Nevertheless, a recent textbook of pediatric pulmonary medicine devoted less than one page in toto to discussions of obesity.[3]

The economic burden of childhood obesity also cannot be discounted. For children aged 6 to 17 years, obesity-related health costs more than tripled from $35 million during the period 1979 to 1981 to $127 million from 1997 to 1999. A significant proportion of hospitalizations listed asthma as the primary discharge diagnosis; over this time period, the diagnosis of sleep apnea increased by five.[4]

Obesity's impact on respiratory disease in children can be categorized as follows: impact on pulmonary mechanics, its possible link with and impact on asthma, and the risk factor it poses for sleep-disordered breathing. Concerns that also deserve special mention are the interaction of obesity and physical fitness and perioperative risks in obese children.

PULMONARY MECHANICS

The leptin-deficient (ob/ob) mouse is massively obese, largely because of increased food intake. It demonstrates higher airway resistance and smaller lung volumes than lean mice. Shore and colleagues[5] hypothesized that this may be because of altered lung growth owing to deficiency of leptin, restrictive effects of increased fat mass on the growing lung, or a combination of the two.

In adult humans, functional residual capacity (FRC) and expiratory reserve volume (ERV) decrease with increasing BMI. These changes are seen particularly with BMI greater than 30 kg/m^2 and are most pronounced in the supine position.[6] Vital capacity, ERV, and maximal voluntary ventilation (MVV) were decreased in a sample of morbidly obese young adults, and these values improved with weight loss.[7] These changes may be attributable to increased loading of the chest wall and abdomen. Mechanical chest wall loading, performed in healthy adults to simulate the effects of obesity, resulted in a decrease in lung volumes and peak work rate during exercise, suggesting that obesity mechanically limits an individual's exercise capacity.[8] Conversely, diffusing capacity (DLCO) increases with obesity in adults.[6,7]

In children, growth, development, and changes with puberty complicate the study of lung function

---

Division of Pulmonary Medicine and Sleep Center, The Children's Hospital of Philadelphia, University of Pennsylvania School of Medicine, 34th Street and Civic Center Boulevard, 5 Wood, Philadelphia, PA 19104, USA
* Corresponding author.
E-mail address: brooksl@email.chop.edu (L.J. Brooks).

Clin Chest Med 30 (2009) 601–608
doi:10.1016/j.ccm.2009.05.010
0272-5231/09/$ – see front matter © 2009 Published by Elsevier Inc.

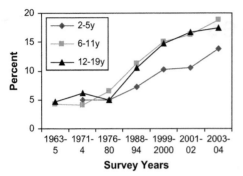

Fig. 1. The prevalence of overweight in children has increased over the past 40 years, nearly quadrupling in pre-teens and adolescents. (*From* CDC National Center for Health Statistics Report, "Prevalence of overweight among children and adolescents: United States, 2003–2004." Available at: http://www.cdc.gov/nchs/products/pubs/pubd/hestats/overweight/overwght_child_03.htm. Accessed June 24, 2009).

over time; growth of the lungs, airways, and body do not occur symmetrically.[9] Marcus and colleagues[10] demonstrated essentially normal spirometry in a group of 22 obese children, but there was no control group. In a population cohort of 2464 schoolchildren in Australia, ranging in age from 9 to 15 years, FVC and forced expiratory volume in 1 second (FEV1) decreased with increasing percentage of total body fat. The actual difference in mean FVC between children in the lower and upper tertiles of total body fat was 90 mL, approximately 4%; however, those children with "gross obesity," with a mean body weight 212% of ideal, demonstrated a more significant reduction in FVC and FEV1 (to 78% and 73% predicted, respectively).[11] A smaller group of 64 obese children underwent dual-energy x-ray absorptiomety (DEXA) scans and a full complement of pulmonary function testing, including spirometry, lung volumes, and DLCO. A low FRC was the most common abnormality observed, seen in 46% of children, and FRC was inversely proportional to the percent total body fat as measured by DEXA.[12] In contrast to adults, 33% of subjects had moderately reduced DLCO, even when corrected for lung volume. Three children demonstrated a mild obstructive pattern on spirometry; these children all had BMI in excess of 34 kg/m^2.

ASTHMA

The relationship between asthma and obesity is controversial. Although the prevalence of both conditions has increased in children over the past several decades,[13] the significance of the association is unclear.

In an examination of the data from NHANES III, von Mutius and colleagues[13] described a significant association between BMI and asthma prevalence, but not atopy. Other studies, however, have found no clear increase in asthma in the obese, or in obesity in those with asthma. Brenner and colleagues[14] studied a group of 256 adolescents with asthma and 482 nonasthmatic controls and found no significant relationship between asthma and obesity. In another study, children with asthma had higher nitric oxide (ENO) and leukotriene B4 in exhaled breath condensate than controls; obese children did not have increased levels of these inflammatory markers when compared with children of normal weight.[15] Mansell and colleagues[16] found no significant difference in the dose of methacholine required to induce bronchoconstriction in obese and non-obese adolescents with asthma. In addition, obesity alone was not associated with broncho-constriction in response to methacholine.

Flaherman and Rutherford[17] completed a meta-analysis of 12 studies examining the relationship between weight and asthma. Results of their analysis suggest that a high weight at birth and in childhood confer an increased risk of asthma. Another examination of a large dataset of school children in Great Britain, however, failed to demonstrate such an association.[18] Several epidemiologic studies have demonstrated an association between obesity and atopy,[19] especially in pubertal females;[20–22] others have shown no such association.[23]

Obese children may have more severe asthma than normal weight children. Children with asthma and obesity who are admitted to the intensive care unit during an exacerbation require more medication, supplemental oxygen for a greater period of time, and longer duration of care in the intensive care unit.[24] Pianosi and Davis[25] found that obese children reported more medication use. In a cohort of 1322 inner-city children with asthma, subjects who were also obese required more medication, reported more wheezing, and sought care in an emergency department setting more often than children with asthma who were of normal weight.[26]

There are several considerations in the interpretation of studies of asthma and obesity. Was asthma defined by parental report, physician diagnosis, or pulmonary function tests? Obese children may describe dyspnea with exercise; this may represent asthma, deconditioning, or both. The complaint of dyspnea on exertion may prompt an increase in medication, which may or may not signify more severe asthma. Similarly, definitions of obesity have varied from study to study.

Sleep-disordered breathing (SDB) may complicate any association between obesity and asthma. Sulit and colleagues[27] performed polysomnography (PSG) in a cohort of 788 children who wheezed or had asthma. Children who wheezed and had asthma were more likely to be obese; however, when the analysis was adjusted for SDB, the association between obesity and wheezing weakened, although those who were obese were still more likely to have asthma.

Pathophysiology

Several factors may contribute to the potential relationship between asthma and obesity. These include psychological factors, mechanical factors, gastroesophageal reflux (GER), and hormonal factors.

Asthma may create a psychological barrier to exercise, rendering children more sedentary, and thus at more risk for obesity.[28] This is supported by data suggesting that children who have asthma and are obese have a poor self-perceived quality of life.[29]

A model has been proposed that may explain the effects of obesity on mechanical airway narrowing, and provide a link between asthma and obesity. If the normal "dynamic equilibrium" between actin and myosin is disrupted, and at a cellular level, the muscle motor unit remains in a single position and not in its normal state of movement, intrinsic bronchodilatory mechanisms may be lost. One innate bronchodilating mechanism is tidal breathing. Lung inflation transmits strain to airway smooth muscle, leading to disruption of the actin-myosin cross-bridge; essentially, in a normal individual breathing over a normal range of tidal volumes, airway smooth muscle cross bridges are disrupted resulting in decreased contractile force by the airway smooth muscle.[30] The obese individual, who may have a lower lung capacity and breathe at lower, more fixed tidal volumes, likely does not exhibit this protective mechanism to the same degree; airway smooth muscle cross-bridges are disrupted to a lesser degree, leading to potentially greater baseline contractile force. As such, the usual "dynamic

equilibrium," and balance between the lungs and chest wall, and airway smooth muscle is lost, leading to airway narrowing, without airway hyperreactivity per se.[31]

Obesity is associated with an increased incidence of GER in adults.[32] Asthmatic and overweight children report increased reflux symptoms when compared with controls.[33,34] Overweight children are also more likely to have abnormal esophageal pH probe results.[34] GER may result in increased airway reactivity through neural mechanisms, and/or increase airway inflammation because of microaspiration.

An intriguing possibility is that adipokines may increase airway inflammation and reactivity. Previously conceptualized as a metabolically dormant repository for energy, adipocytes release a variety of hormonal products with roles in glucose and lipid homeostasis. They are also potential mediators in asthma and allergy. Included among the adipokines are leptin, adiponectin, and resistin (**Table 1**).

Leptin, the product of the Ob gene, is involved in body weight and appetite homeostasis, decreasing appetite and increasing energy expenditure; its levels increase with body fat mass, perhaps secondary to a mechanism akin to insulin resistance. Glucocorticoid administration stimulates leptin production in rats and humans.

Although leptin's principal site of action is in the hypothalamus, receptors exist in the lung as well, but their role there is less clear. In vitro, leptin seems to play a role in lung growth and surfactant homeostasis.[35,36] Children with asthma have higher leptin levels than do nonasthmatic children.[37] Obese children have higher levels of leptin than controls, and, in obese children with asthma, leptin levels are increased twofold over normal weight, nonasthmatic controls.[38] Leptin levels correlate positively with BMI, airway reactivity, and total IgE.[38]

In contrast to leptin, adiponectin may have anti-inflammatory properties. Airway smooth muscle cells contain adiponectin receptors.[39] In obese mice, adiponectin infusion decreased allergic and airway hyperresponsiveness to an allergen challenge.[40] In addition, the act of allergen

| Table 1 |
| Several adipokines and their effects or associations |

Adipokine	Effect or association with obesity and inflammation
Leptin	Increased in the obese; may be proinflammatory; may be associated with asthma
Adiponectin	Decreased in the obese; anti-inflammatory; decreased levels associated with asthma
Resistin	Correlation with methacholine PC20

challenge itself diminished serum adiponectin levels. Some studies have demonstrated a positive correlation between low cord blood adiponectin and development of wheeze at the age of two.[41] Typically, adiponectin levels are low in obese individuals and increase with weight loss. In children, as in adults, adiponectin demonstrates an inverse correlation with BMI.[42,43]

Resistin's mechanism of action is not clear. In a study of children with asthma, lower levels of resistin were found in those whose asthma was atopic in nature, and there was an inverse correlation with eosinophil count, IgE, and airway reactivity measured by methacholine challenge. Higher resistin levels were shown to have negative predictive value for the presence of asthma. In this study, higher levels of leptin were associated with lower FEV1 and forced expiratory flow (FEF)25%–75%, although there was no specific relationship between leptin and asthma symptoms.[44]

Clinical Evaluation

Children and their parents may feel the child's dyspnea is because he or she is "out of shape." Conversely, obese children may be treated for asthma simply based on respiratory symptoms with exercise. Obese children with asthma reported more activity limitation than did asthmatic children of healthy weight, but did not display worse spirometry than those of normal weight.[25] Pulmonary function testing, including lung volumes, spirometry before and after administration of a bronchodilator, and, if appropriate, exercise challenge, can help distinguish asthma from deconditioning.

Treatment and Outcome

Weight loss is associated with a more favorable adipokine profile, and, at least in adults, an improvement in asthma symptoms. Several studies have demonstrated short-term efficacy of residential weight loss centers in children. However, long-term duration of these changes is unknown. Gastric banding is a controversial treatment for morbid obesity in adolescents. One study demonstrated success 1 year following surgery in maintaining lower weight, as well as a resolution of several comorbidities, including asthma.[45]

OBSTRUCTIVE SLEEP APNEA

In 1977, the case of a child with "obesity, cyanosis, and somnolence" was reported. This child had airway obstruction, apneas, and disturbed sleep, but a normal ventilatory response to carbon dioxide. The child's symptoms improved with weight loss.[46] In the same year, Stool and colleagues described three children with obesity, adenotonsillar hypertrophy, and abnormal gas exchange whose respiratory symptoms resolved following adenotonsillectomy. They termed this the "chubby puffer" syndrome, now recognized as obstructive sleep apnea.[47] Obesity is a well-documented risk factor for the development of OSA in adults. In contrast, children with OSA are very often of normal weight and some may even fail to thrive.[48] However, obesity has been increasingly recognized as a risk factor for the development of obstructive sleep apnea syndrome (OSAS) in the pediatric population.[10,49,50]

Approximately one third of obese children have abnormal polysomnograms.[10] In another study of 33 children who were referred for the evaluation of suspected OSA, obesity was the major predictor of the respiratory disturbance index (number of apneas and hypopneas per hour of sleep) and the lowest oxyhemoglobin saturation (**Fig. 2**).[51] In a large epidemiologic study of 399 children and adolescents aged 2 to 18 years, obesity (defined by a BMI >28) was the strongest predictor of sleep disordered breathing, with an odds ratio of 4.59.[52]

Pathophysiology of Obstructive Sleep Apnea Syndrome Attributable to Obesity

There are several hypotheses to explain the relationship between obesity and obstructive sleep apnea,[53] including excess adiposity in the upper airway, subnormal ventilatory drive in response

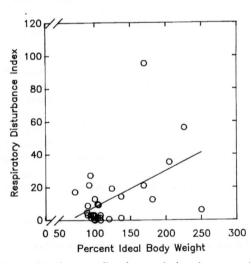

Fig. 2. Respiratory disturbance index increases in proportion with increasing body weight in children (r = 0.49, P < .01). (*From* Brooks LJ, Stephens BM, Bacevice AM. Adenoid size is related to severity but not the number of episodes of obstructive apnea in children. J Pediatr 1998;132(4):682–6; with permission.)

to elevated carbon dioxide levels, and change in pulmonary mechanics.

Obesity results in the deposition of adipose tissue within the muscles and soft tissues surrounding the upper airway.[54] This, along with external compression from the neck and jowls results in narrowing of the upper airway.[55] In children, several studies have evaluated the location of most prominent upper airway narrowing. Isono and colleagues[56] demonstrated via endoscopy the minimum airway diameter to be at the adenoid and soft palate. Several studies using MRI to evaluate airway structure and dimensions also demonstrate the narrowest portion to be at the point at which the adenoids and soft palate overlap.[57,58] Obese children with OSA also demonstrate adenotonsillar hypertrophy. Increased deposits of fat in airway muscles and supporting tissues may alter their airway dynamics. Obesity may also result in increased pharyngeal floppiness if adipose tissue contributes to a relative uncoupling of the pharyngeal mucosa from the effects of the upper airway dilator muscles.

Obesity Hypoventilation Syndrome

The increased chest wall and abdominal mass in obese patients results in reduced lung volumes and restricted movement of the diaphragm,[10] especially when recumbent. This can contribute to hypoventilation, compounded by the reduced respiratory drive that occurs during sleep.

Rosen[59] studied 326 children referred for evaluation of obstructive sleep apnea specifically for obesity hypoventilation syndrome (OHS), that is, recurrent episodes of upper airway obstruction resulting in hypoxemia, hypercapnia, and poor sleep quality. African American ethnicity and adenotonsillar hypertrophy increased the likelihood of OHS; in this study, gender and obesity did not confer an increased risk, unlike in adults. However, the authors note that the incidence of obesity in this population was 28%, nearly double that in the childhood population at large at the time.

Children with severe OHS may have severe OSA, hypoxia, hypercapnia both awake and asleep, hypersomnolence, and cor pulmonale.[60] Hypercapnic ventilatory responses may be severely reduced, and may take several weeks to normalize after treatment for OSA. The fact that it does normalize, however, suggests that the respiratory control dysfunction probably represents habituation of brainstem centers rather than a primary defect in neurologic control of breathing.[60]

Clinical Sequelae

Obesity may increase the child's risk for consequences of OSA, including daytime sleepiness and hypertension. In a study of 50 habitually snoring children, the likelihood of excessive daytime sleepiness (EDS) as quantitated by Epworth sleepiness score and multiple sleep latency testing was much greater for obese than nonobese children.[61] Obesity alone, without frank OSA, was also associated with EDS. When the analysis controlled for obstructive AHI and hypoxemia, elevated respiratory arousal index was associated most clearly with decreased sleep latency. EDS is associated with increased inflammatory markers,[62] and the authors speculate that a constant state of low-grade inflammation may lead to EDS in obese children.

Hypertension has been linked to obesity and OSA in children. OSA and BMI z-scores are independently associated with both systolic and diastolic blood pressure z-scores in sleeping children.[63] In a study of 96 children who underwent polysomnography and ambulatory blood pressure monitoring, both elevated AHI and elevated BMI correlated with elevated diastolic blood pressure during sleep.[64] Reade and colleagues[65] retrospectively studied a group of 90 children who had undergone polysomnography; 56 of these were obese, 40 had OSA, and 42 had hypertension. Obesity and hypertension were both more common in the patients with OSA. In addition, those patients who were obese and had high blood pressure were more likely to have OSA than obese patients without evidence of sleep-disordered breathing. In another study, 306 school-aged children underwent polysomnography and subsequent ambulatory blood pressure monitoring. Children with moderate to severe OSA were more than three times more likely to have hypertension than those children without OSA. Obesity, however, did not increase the likelihood of hypertension.[66]

Treatment and Outcome

Children with OSA, including those who are obese, usually improve after adenotonsillectomy.[67,68] Some studies suggest that obese children are more likely to have persistent OSA following adenotonsillectomy.[69] O'Brien and colleagues[70] evaluated 69 children with OSA, 29 of whom were obese. Postoperative polysomnograms demonstrated persistent abnormalities in the obese children. Seventy-seven percent of normal weight children demonstrated improvement in their symptoms, compared with only 45% of those who were obese. Other studies have found no predictive link between body weight and elevated AHI following surgical treatment.[67,71] Suen and colleagues[67] found that baseline respiratory disturbance index (RDI), plus hypoapneas per hour of sleep was the only factor that predicted a postoperative RDI of less than 5. In obese children, follow-up polysomnography after adenotonsillectomy may be necessary to determine whether to initiate other treatments such as noninvasive ventilatory support with positive airway pressure in conjunction with weight loss. Diagnosis and treatment of comorbid disorders, such as asthma, allergic rhinitis, and gastroesophageal reflux, are also crucial.

PERIOPERATIVE MORBIDITY

Perioperative morbidity is increased in obese children.[72,73] Obesity can alter the metabolism of some anesthetic medications by increasing the volume of distribution in adipose tissue, which increases the elimination half-life of commonly used medications such as benzodiazepines. Obese children with OSA admitted for adenotonsillectomy are more likely to have a longer and more complicated postoperative course than their normal weight peers. Not only do obese children have more comorbid conditions, such as asthma and type 2 diabetes, than their normal weight counterparts, but obese children are also at increased risk for perioperative respiratory complications. In two large studies investigating anesthesia outcome in both obese and normal weight children,[72,73] subjects with obesity had more complications regarding airway obstruction, including difficult intubation, significant desaturation, and critical respiratory events. A history of obstructive sleep apnea and younger age increased the risk of these potentially critical respiratory events.

SUMMARY

Childhood obesity continues to increase, bringing along with it a risk for increased respiratory complications. The risk of health compromise, however, is not limited to childhood. Several of these problems may influence health outcome in adulthood. Children who are obese are more likely to be obese adults.[74] Obesity and/or OSA may influence development of the metabolic syndrome in childhood.[75,76] OSA in childhood and adolescence may lead to a state of chronic inflammation, perhaps influencing the development of cardiac and vascular disease into adulthood. In addition, as lung growth tracks over time, so does the decline in pulmonary function in adulthood. If obese children have even a small decrement in pulmonary function, this may lead to increased morbidity in middle and even young adulthood.

REFERENCES

1. Strauss RS, Pollack HA. Epidemic increase in childhood overweight. JAMA 2001;286(22):2845–8.
2. Ogden CL, Carroll MD, Curtin LR, et al. Prevalence of overweight and obesity in the United States, 1999–2004. JAMA 2006;295(13):1549–55.
3. Chernick V, Boat TF, Wilmott RW, et al. Kendig's disorders of the respiratory tract in children. Philadelphia: Elsevier; 2006.
4. Wang G, Dietz WH. Economic burden of obesity in youths aged 6 to 17 years: 1979–1999. Pediatrics 2002;109:e81.
5. Shore SA. Obesity and asthma: lessons from animal models. J Appl Physiol 2007;102:516–28.
6. Jones RL, Nzekwu MU. The effects of body mass index on lung volumes. Chest 2006;130(3):827–33.
7. Ray CS, Sue DY, Bray G, et al. Effects of obesity on respiratory function. Am Rev Respir Dis 1983;128:501–6.
8. Wang L, Cerny FJ. Ventilatory response to exercise in simulated obesity by chest loading. Med Sci Sports Exerc 2004;35:780–6.
9. Wang X, Dockery D, Wypij D, et al. Pulmonary function between 6 and 18 years of age. Pediatr Pulmonol 1993;15:75–88.
10. Marcus C, Curtis S, Koerner C, et al. Evaluation of pulmonary function and polysomnography in obese children and adolescents. Pediatr Pulmonol 1996;21:176–83.
11. Lazarus RL, Colditz G, Berkey CS, et al. Effects of body fat on ventilatory function in children and adolescents: cross-sectional findings from a random population sample of school children. Pediatr Pulmonol 1997;24(3):187–94.
12. Li AM, Chan D, Wong E, et al. The effects of obesity on pulmonary function. Arch Dis Child 2003;88:361–3.
13. von Mutius E, Schwartz J, Neas LM, et al. Relation of body mass index to asthma and atopy in children: the National Health and Nutrition Examination Study III. Thorax 2001;56:835–8.
14. Brenner JS, Kelly CS, Wenger AD, et al. Asthma and obesity in adolescents: is there an association? J Asthma 2001;38(6):509–15.
15. Leung TF, Li CY, Lam CW, et al. The relation between obesity and asthmatic airway inflammation. Pediatr Allergy Immunol 2004;15(4):344–50.
16. Mansell AL, Walders N, Wamboldt MZ, et al. Effect of body mass index on response to methacholine bronchial provocation in healthy and asthmatic adolescents. Pediatr Pulmonol 2006;41:434–40.

17. Flaherman V, Rutherford GW. A meta-analysis of the effect of high weight on asthma. Arch Dis Child 2006;91:334–9.

18. Chinn S, Rona RJ. Can the increase in body mass index explain the rising trend in asthma in children? Thorax 2001;56:845–50.

19. Visness CM, London SJ, Daniels JL, et al. Association of obesity with IgE levels and allergy symptoms in children and adolescents: results from the National Health and Nutrition Examination Survey 2005–2006. J Allergy Clin Immunol 2009;123(5):1163–9.

20. Huang SL, Shiao G, Chou P. Association between body mass index and allergy in teenage girls in Taiwan. Clin Exp Allergy 1999;29(3):323–9.

21. Schachter LM, Peat JK, Salome CM. Asthma and atopy in overweight children. Thorax 2003;58(12):1031–5.

22. Hancox RJ, Milne BJ, Pouton R, et al. Sex differences in the relation between body mass index and asthma and atopy in a birth cohort. Am J Respir Crit Care Med 2005;171(5):440–5.

23. VanGysel D, Govaere E, Verhamme K, et al. Body mass index in Belgian schoolchildren and its relationship with sensitization and allergic symptoms. Pediatr Allergy Immunol 2008 [Epub ahead of print]. DOI:10.1111/j.1399-3038.2008.00774.x.

24. Carroll CL, Bhandari A, Zucker AR, et al. Childhood obesity increases duration of therapy during severe asthma exacerbations. Pediatr Crit Care Med 2006;7:527–31.

25. Pianosi PT, Davis HS. Determinants of physical fitness in children with asthma. Pediatrics 2004;113(3 Pt 1):e225–9.

26. Belamarich F, Luder E, Kattan M, et al. Do obese inner-city children with asthma have more symptoms than nonobese children with asthma? Pediatrics 2000;106:1436–41.

27. Sulit LG, Storfer-Iser A, Rosen CL, et al. Associations of obesity, sleep-disordered breathing, and wheezing in children. Am J Respir Crit Care Med 2005;171:659–64.

28. Glazebrook C, McPherson AC, Macdonald IA, et al. Asthma as a barrier to children's physical activity: implications for body mass index and mental health. Pediatrics 2006;118:2443–9.

29. van Gent R, van der Ent CK, Rovers MM, et al. Excessive body weight is associated with additional loss of quality of life in children with asthma. J Allergy Clin Immunol 2007;119(3):591–6.

30. Fredberg JF, Inouye DS, Mijailovich SM, et al. Perturbed equilibrium of myosin binding in airway smooth muscle and its implications in bronchospasm. Am J Respir Crit Care Med 1999;159:959–67.

31. Fredberg JJ. Bronchospasm and its biophysical basis in airway smooth muscle. Available at: Respir Res 2004; http://respiratory-research.com/content/5/1/2.

32. Friedenberg FK, Xanthopoulos M, Foster GD, et al. The association between gastroesophageal reflux disease and obesity. Am J Gastroenterol 2008;103:2111–22.

33. Størdal K, Johannesdottir GB, Bentsen BS, et al. Asthma and overweight are associated with symptoms of gastro-oesophageal reflux. Acta Paediatr 2006;95(10):1197–201.

34. Pashankar DS, Corbin Z, Shah SK, et al. Increased prevalence of gastroesophageal reflux symptoms in obese children evaluated in an academic medical center. J Clin Gastroenterol 2008 Dec 18 [Epub ahead of print].

35. Bergen HT, Cherlet TC, Manuel P, et al. Identification of leptin receptors in lung and isolated fetal type II cells. Am J Respir Cell Mol Biol 2002;27:71–7.

36. Torday JS, Sun H, Wang L, et al. Leptin mediates the parathyroid hormone-related protein paracrine stimulation of fetal lung maturation. Am J Physiol Lung Cell Mol Physiol 2002;282:L405–10.

37. Guler N, Kirerleri E, Ones U, et al. Leptin: does it have any role in childhood asthma? J Allergy Clin Immunol 2004;114:254–9.

38. Mai XM, Bottcher MF, Leijon I. Leptin and asthma in overweight children at 12 years of age. Pediatr Allergy Immunol 2004;15(6):523–30.

39. Shin JH, Kim JH, Lee WY, et al. The expression of adiponectin receptors and the effects of adiponectin and leptin on airway smooth muscle cells. Yonsei Med J 2008;49(5):804–10.

40. Shore SA, Terry RD, Flynt L, et al. Adiponectin attenuates allergen-induced airway inflammation and hyperresponsiveness in mice. J Allergy Clin Immunol 2006;118:389–95.

41. Rothenbacher D, Weyermann M, Fantuzzi G, et al. Adipokines in cord blood and risk of wheezing disorders within the first two years of life. Clin Exp Allergy 2007;37(8):1143–9.

42. Nagel G, Koenig W, Rapp K, et al. Associations of adipokines with asthma, rhinoconjunctivitis, and eczema in German schoolchildren. Pediatr Allergy Immunol 2009;20:81–8.

43. Nemet D, Wang P, Funahashi T, et al. Adipocytokines, body composition, and fitness in children. Pediatr Res 2003;53(1):148–52.

44. Kim KW, Shin YH, Lee KE, et al. Relationship between adipokines and manifestations of childhood asthma. Pediatr Allergy Immunol 2008;19:535–40.

45. Yitzhak A, Mizrahi S, Avinoach E. Laparoscopic gastric banding in adolescents. Obes Surg 2006;16(10):1318–22.

46. Simpser MD, Strieder DJ, Wohl ME, et al. Sleep apnea in a child with the pickwickian syndrome. Pediatrics 1977;60(3):290–3.

47. Stool SE, Eavey RD, Stein SL, et al. The "chubby puffer" syndrome. Upper airway obstruction and obesity, with intermittent somnolence and cardiorespiratory embarrassment. Clin Pediatr 1977;16(1):43–50.

48. Brouillette RT, Fernbach SK, Hunt CE. Obstructive sleep apnea in infants and children. J Pediatr 1982;100(1):31–40.

49. Mallory GB Jr, Fiser DH, Jackson R. Sleep-associated breathing disorders in morbidly obese children and adolescents. J Pediatr 1989;115(6):892–7.

50. Silvestri JM, Weese-Mayer DE, Bass MT, et al. Polysomnography in obese children with a history of sleep associated breathing disorders. Pediatr Pulmonol 1993;16(2):124–9.

51. Brooks LJ, Stephens BM, Bacevice AM. Adenoid size is related to severity but not the number of episodes of obstructive apnea in children. J Pediatr 1998;132(4):682–6.

52. Redline S, Tishler PV, Schluchter S, et al. Risk factors for sleep-disordered breathing in children. Associations with obesity, race, and respiratory problems. Am J Respir Crit Care Med 1999;159(5 Pt 1): 1527–32.

53. Bandla P, Brooks LJ, Trimarchi T, et al. Obstructive sleep apnea in children. Anesthesiology Clin N Am 2005;23:535–49.

54. Horner RL, Mohiaddin RH, Lowell DG, et al. Sites and sizes of fat deposits around the pharynx in obese patients with obstructive sleep apnoea and weight matched controls. Eur Respir J 1989;2(7): 613–22.

55. Suratt PM, Dee P, Atkinson RL, et al. Fluoroscopic and computed tomographic features of the pharyngeal airway in obstructive sleep apnea. Am Rev Respir Dis 1983;127(4):487–92.

56. Isono S, Shimada A, Utsugi M, et al. Comparison of static mechanical properties of the passive pharynx between normal children and children with sleep-disordered breathing. Am J Respir Crit Care Med 1998;157(4 Pt 1):1204–12.

57. Arens R, Marcus CL. Pathophysiology of upper airway obstruction: a developmental perspective. Sleep 2004;27(5):997–1018.

58. Fregosi RF, Quan SF, Kaemingk KL, et al. Sleep-disordered breathing, pharyngeal size, and soft tissue anatomy in children. J Appl Physiol 2003;95: 2030–8.

59. Rosen CL. Clinical features of obstructive sleep apnea hypoventilation syndrome in otherwise healthy children. Pediatr Pulmonol 1999;27(6):403–9.

60. Keens TG, Ward SLD. Syndromes affecting respiratory control during sleep. In: Loughlin GM, Carroll JL, Marcus CL, editors. Sleep and breathing in children: a developmental approach. New York: Maracel Dekker; 2000. p. 525–53.

61. Gozal D, Kheirandish-Gozal L. Obesity and excessive daytime sleepiness in prepubertal children with obstructive sleep apnea. Pediatrics 2009; 123(1):13–8.

62. Vgontzas AN, Papanicolau DA, Bixler EO, et al. Elevation of plasma cytokines in disorders of excessive daytime sleepiness: role of sleep disturbance and obesity. J Clin Endocrinol Metab 1997;82(5):1313–6.

63. Brooks LJ, Chng SY, Marcus CL, et al. Blood pressure, sleep, and sleep disordered breathing in children [abstract]. Am J Respir Crit Care Med 2008; 177:A705.

64. Leung LC, Ng DK, Lau MW, et al. Twenty-four hour ambulatory BP in snoring children with obstructive sleep apnea syndrome. Chest 2006;130(4): 1009–17.

65. Reade EP, Whaley C, Lin JJ, et al. Hypopnea in pediatric patients with obesity hypertension. Pediatr Nephrol 2004;19(9):1014–20.

66. Li AM, Au CT, Sung RY, et al. Ambulatory blood pressure in children with obstructive sleep apnoea: a community based study. Thorax 2008;63(9):803–9.

67. Suen JS, Arnold JE, Brooks LJ. Adenotonsillectomy for treatment of obstructive sleep apnea in children. Arch Otolaryngol Head Neck Surg 1995;121(5):525–30.

68. Kudoh F, Sanai A. Effect of tonsillectomy and adenoidectomy on obese children with sleep-associated breathing disorders. Acta Otolaryngol Suppl 1996;523:216–8.

69. Morton S, Rosen C, Larkin E, et al. Predictors of sleep-disordered breathing in children with a history of tonsillectomy and adenoidectomy. Sleep 2001; 24(7):823–9.

70. O'Brien LM, Sitha S, Baur LA, et al. Obesity increases the risk for persisting obstructive sleep apnea after treatment in children. Int J Pediatr Otorhinolaryngol 2006;70:1555–60.

71. Apostolidou MT, Alexopoulos EI, Chaidas K, et al. Obesity and persisting sleep apnea after adenotonsillectomy in Greek children. Chest 2008;134: 1149–55.

72. Nafiu OO, Reynolds PI, Bamgbade OA, et al. Childhood body mass index and perioperative complications. Paediatr Anaesth 2007;17(5):426–30.

73. Tait AR, Voepel-Lewis T, Burke C, et al. Incidence and risk factors for perioperative adverse respiratory events in children who are obese. Anesthesiology 2008;108(3):375–80.

74. Singh AS, Mulder C, Twisk JW, et al. Tracking of childhood overweight into adulthood: a systematic review of the literature. Obes Rev 2008;9(5):474–88.

75. Redline S, Storfer-Isser A, Rosen CL, et al. Association between metabolic syndrome and sleep disordered breathing in adolescents. Am J Respir Crit Care Med 2007;176(4):401–8.

76. Verhulst SL, Schrauwen N, Haentjens D, et al. Sleep-disordered breathing and the metabolic syndrome in overweight and obese children and adolescents. J Pediatr 2007;150(6):612–6.

Obesity and Aging

John Harrington, MD, MPH*, Teofilo Lee-Chiong, MD

KEYWORDS

- Aging • Elderly • Obesity • Respiratory disorders
- Pulmonary function

The percentage of the United States population aged 65 years and older is growing rapidly and is predicted to increase to 18% by 2025.[1] The prevalence of obesity also has increased dramatically over past 25 years in all age groups in the United States.[2]

Epidemiologic estimates suggest that the prevalence of obesity among elderly persons in the United States will likely increase by 5.4% to 20.9 million by the year 2010.[3] The National Health and Nutrition Examination Survey (NHANES) found that 31% of persons aged 60 years or older were overweight in 2003 to 2004.[4] Data from the 2003 Behavioral Risk Factor Surveillance System (BRFSS) survey further demonstrated that 20.3% of persons aged 65 years and older were classified as obese, defined as a body mass index (BMI) of 30 or greater, with those aged 65 to 74 years having the highest prevalence at 40.8%, followed by 16.6% and 9.9% for those aged 75 to 84 years and 85 and older, respectively.[5]

The incidence of obesity among the aged is not limited to community-dwelling persons. In United States nursing homes, the proportion of newly admitted residents who were classified as obese increased from less than 15% to more than 25% from 1992 to 2002. In addition, those residents indentified as obese had increased rates of comorbidities.[6]

OBESITY AND AGING CONSEQUENCES

The associated health consequences of obesity in this population are not always consistent, and may be related to how obesity is measured and defined in older persons compared with younger persons, and whether other factors (eg, smoking status and survival effect) contribute to the reported findings.[7]

A large prospective study assessed the potential association of midlife BMI and health outcomes in later life. The results of this analysis suggest that obesity in midlife portend significantly higher rates of hospitalization and mortality in those participants who survived beyond 65 years of age compared with normal weight subjects with comparable cardiovascular profiles at baseline.[8]

Elevated BMI is also associated with various health conditions in older persons. In a cross-sectional cohort analysis of 73,003 adults aged 50 to 76 years, 90% of the adverse conditions examined were associated with obesity in women and 71% in men.[9] Results from the Women's Health Initiative (WHI) indicate that age and obesity are important risk factors for self-reported osteo-arthritis among postmenopausal women aged 50 to 79 years.[10] Health complaints, such as chronic pain, are also increased among the obese elderly. Another study found that in a sample of older adults, mean age of 80 years, obese subjects were twice as likely to complain of recurrent pain of at least moderate severity compared with individuals of normal weight, and that those who were severely obese were four times as likely to report chronic pain; these findings remained consistent even after adjusting for factors such as age, sex, education, and health conditions, including diabetes mellitus, hypertension, depression, and anxiety.[11]

Obesity is also related with frailty among older persons. In a study of participants aged 70 to 79 years in the Women's Health and Aging Studies, obesity was significantly associated with frailty syndrome even after controlling for covariates.[10,12] Functional limitations appear to be associated with obesity in elderly persons. However, the rate of functional disability may be increased

Department of Internal Medicine, Division of Sleep Medicine, National Jewish Health, 1400 Jackson Street, Denver, CO 80206, USA
* Corresponding author.
E-mail address: harringtonj@njc.org (J. Harrington).

Clin Chest Med 30 (2009) 609–614
doi:10.1016/j.ccm.2009.05.011
0272-5231/09/$ – see front matter © 2009 Elsevier Inc. All rights reserved.

for older obese women compared with men.[13–15] As part of the NHANES, investigators found that in women older than 60 years, indicators of overall and abdominal obesity (ie, BMI and waist circumference) were independently related to increased prevalence of functional impairment.[16] However, gender has not been a consistent prognosticator of disability in obesity. In a large 5-year prospective cohort study, obese community-dwelling adults of both genders aged 65 years and older were noted to have increased relative risks of decrements in both physical performance and in activities of daily living (ADL).[17]

Despite these associations, other studies have not demonstrated consistent negative effects related to obesity in aging. In regard to mortality risk, a retrospective cohort analysis of a large community-dwelling population as part of the Longitudinal Study of Aging (LSOA) noted lower mortality rates for obese persons in this cohort compared with thin or normal weight, even after controlling for several confounders.[18] The potential association between obesity and excess mortality among nursing home residents may be more complicated. In one study, although an increase in mortality was noted during the early admission period for newly admitted morbidly obese residents compared with normal weight subjects, excess mortality was not increased in this population after the initial period.[19] The longitudinal Cardiovascular Health Study also demonstrated that higher BMI was a negative predictor of mortality, represented by a decrease in mortality of 12% for each standard deviation increase in BMI in this elderly sample.[20] Other investigators[21] reported similar findings in their study after a median follow-up period of nearly 15 years. Elderly subjects with lower BMIs had consistently higher mortality compared with those with high BMI.

The risk of perioperative complications associated with weight in older persons undergoing cardiovascular surgery was evaluated in a retrospective review. Elderly subjects aged 75 to 94 years of age were divided into tertiles based on BMI measurements (<23, 23–26, and >26). Multivariate analysis demonstrated that cardiovascular complications and stroke were highest for the first tertile compared with the second and third tertiles. Increased weight was not associated with increased complications, except for sternal wound infections.[22] In a more recent population retrospective trial, researchers attempted to determine whether obesity was associated with cardiac complications following urgent hip fracture repair in persons aged 65 years and older. In this study, underweight patients were noted to have higher rates of myocardial infarction and arrhythmia

compared with normal weight patients. Overweight and obese patients in this sample, however, had no increased risk of cardiac complications.[23]

The potential association between BMI and hospital use in elderly subjects (aged 65 to 100 years) was analyzed as part of a large retrospective cohort study using the Medicare Current Beneficiary Survey (1992–1994). The results of this investigation found that although hospitalization risk was modestly increased in those in the two highest BMI categories for those aged 65 to 75, BMI was not related to hospitalization for those 75 years of age and older.[24]

AGING AND RESPIRATORY ANATOMY AND PHYSIOLOGY

Aging is a not uniform process, and there is considerable variability in its effect on organ systems among different individuals as well as in a specific individual over time. In addition, it is important to distinguish the changes in respiratory anatomy and physiology among older adults that might be related to the aging process itself from those that are attributable to the cumulative effects of environmental exposure to noxious gases and particles.[25]

Significant changes in pulmonary function occur with aging (**Box 1**).[26] A number of factors are responsible for the decline in lung function, including reductions in the strength of the

---

Box 1
Changes in pulmonary function with aging

1. Decreased expiratory flow rates (forced expiratory volume in 1 s [FEV1] and forced vital capacity [FVC])
2. Increase in residual volume (RV), functional residual capacity (FRC)
3. Decline in strength of respiratory muscles, including diaphragm (maximal inspiratory pressure [Pimax] and maximal expiratory pressure [PEmax])
4. Reduction in diffusing capacity for carbon monoxide (DLCO)
5. Decline in maximum oxygen consumption (VO2max)
6. Decrease in arterial partial pressure of oxygen (PaO2)
7. Higher alveolar arterial oxygen gradient
8. Reduction in ventilatory responses to hypoxia or hypercapnia
9. Blunting in perception of airflow resistance
10. Increase in pulmonary compliance
11. Reduced pulmonary elastic recoil
12. Decrease in chest wall compliance

respiratory muscles (diaphragm and intercostals), decreased lung elasticity, changes in chest wall compliance, and decline in maximal oxygen consumption (VO2max).[27]

Maximal aerobic capacity, as determined by VO2max, declines with aging. In one meta-analysis, VO2max was inversely related to both age and aerobic exercise status, with VO2max being lowest in sedentary women, higher in active women, and highest in endurance-trained women. However, the rate of decline in VO2max with increasing age was greatest in endurance-trained women (−6.2 mL/kg/min/decade) compared with sedentary women (−3.5 mL/kg/min/decade) and active women (−4.4 mL/kg/min/decade, all $P < .001$). The greater rate of decline in VO2max among endurance-trained aging women is not related to the rate of decline in maximal heart rate with aging; rather, it may be influenced by higher baseline values during young adulthood, or may reflect greater reductions in exercise over time.[28] In contrast, other studies have suggested that the rate of decline in VO2max with aging is greater among sedentary than endurance-trained men.[29,30]

The rate of decline in VO2max is not linear but rather accelerates with advancing age. In the Baltimore Longitudinal Study of Aging, VO2max was determined serially in 810 community-dwelling adults (375 women and 435 men) aged 21 to 87 years, who were free of heart disease, over a median follow-up period of about 8 years. In both genders, VO2max declined progressively in each of the 6 age-decades, with the rate of decline in VO2max accelerating from 3% to 6% per decade in the 20s and 30s to about 20% per decade in the 70s and older. Starting from the fourth decade, the rate of decline in VO2max was greater in men compared with women.[31]

VO2max decreases as do performance test scores in frail obese older adults.[32] A 10-year longitudinal study of 62 healthy, ambulatory, and community-dwelling older adults (34 men with a mean age of 73.5 ± 6.4 years, and 28 women with a mean age of 72.1 ± 5.3 years) demonstrated a decline in VO2max (14% in men and 7% in women). Men had a faster rate of decline in VO2max (−0.43 mL/kg/min/year) compared with women (−0.19/mL/kg/min/year) ($P < .05$). The rate of decline in VO2max was similar in men who were considered young-old (65–72 years at follow-up) compared with the old-old (73–90 years at follow-up). In contrast, whereas a significant decline in VO2max was noted in young-old women, there was no loss in VO2max among old-old women. The fall in VO2max was primarily because of a reduction in maximal heart rate rather

than any changes in maximum oxygen (O2) pulse, and was not related to physical activity scores. Mean body and fat-free mass remained unchanged over this 10-year period.[33]

OBESITY AND PULMONARY FUNCTION IN OLDER ADULTS

Obesity can lead to abnormalities in pulmonary function, the most important of which is a restrictive ventilatory impairment, with reductions in forced expiratory volume in 1 second (FEV1), forced vital capacity (FVC), total lung capacity (TLC), functional residual capacity (FRC), and expiratory reserve volume (ERV).[34] This is generally believed to be a result of the added mechanical load in the chest wall and diaphragm that, in turn, reduces thoracic compliance and impedes diaphragmatic descent. Work of breathing is often increased. Respiratory muscle strength can be reduced. The changes in pulmonary function parameters are generally mild but may become considerable in persons with massive obesity and significant central fat deposition.[35]

Airflow limitation, such as a reduced FEV1/FVC ratio is usually absent. Nonetheless, obesity may give rise to peripheral airways disease and air trapping may develop in obese individuals. Finally, obesity can occasionally increase diffusion capacity for carbon monoxide (DLCO) and decrease exercise capacity (ie, VO2max).[36,37]

An inverse relationship between abdominal obesity and respiratory function has been described. A study examined this relationship in 9674 men and 11,876 women (aged 45–79 years) in the European Prospective Investigation into Cancer and Nutrition–Norfolk (EPIC-Norfolk) cohort. Both FEV1 and FVC were inversely and linearly related to waist-hip ratio, a measure of abdominal obesity, in both men and women, even after adjusting for age, cigarette smoking, and BMI. Values for FEV1 and FVC were about 17% lower among subjects in the top quintile of waist-hip ratio compared with those in the bottom quintile in both genders. Lung function was lowest in men belonging to the top waist-hip ratio quartile and bottom BMI quartile, and in women in the top waist-hip ratio and BMI quartiles.[38]

Body composition and the pattern of distribution of body fat are more important than overall weight in determining the changes in pulmonary function in older adults. These include the amount of abdominal fat, fat-free mass, and waist-hip ratio. In the British Regional Heart Study, which involved 2744 adult men aged 60 to 79 years who were free of cardiovascular disease, diabetes and cancer, height-standardized FEV1 diminished in both lean (BMI < 22.5) and obese (BMI > 30) men, whereas FVC decreased with increasing BMI ($P <$ .01). Waist circumference, waist-hip ratio, and fat mass were inversely related to FEV1 and FVC in obese as well as nonobese men. Conversely, fat-free mass correlated positively with FEV1 ($P = .03$). The combination of a higher BMI and fat-free mass decreased the odds of a low FEV1/FVC ratio.[39] Thus, central obesity negatively affects pulmonary function, whereas fat-free mass enhances the latter. In another study, pulmonary function parameters were measured in 507 subjects over the course of 30 years. The FEV1/FVC ratio was positively correlated, whereas FVC was negatively correlated, with BMI; the latter was more pronounced in middle-aged groups than in subjects aged 70 to 79 years.[40] Similar findings were observed in 97 men, aged 67 to 78 years, in whom a significant negative correlation was noted between FEV1 and FVC on one hand and indices of fat distribution, such as sagittal abdominal diameter. Conversely, FVC and fat-free mass were directly correlated.[41]

The simultaneous loss of fat-free mass and increase in abdominal fat, referred to as sarcopenic obesity, contribute to worsening lung function among older adults. A longitudinal 7-year clinical study was conducted involving 47 elderly women (aged 71.6 ± 2.3 years) and 30 elderly men (aged 71.6 ± 2.3 years). Baseline BMI values were 24.96 ± 3.28 and 27.04 ± 3.35 kg/m^2 for women and men, respectively. At the 7-year follow-up, there were reductions in FEV1 (height-adjusted), FVC, and fat-free mass. The decline in FEV1 and FVC were inversely related to sagittal abdominal diameter, a surrogate of visceral fat, whereas the decrease in FVC was directly correlated to a reduction in fat-free mass. The greatest decline in FEV1 and FVC was observed in persons with increased sagittal abdominal diameter and decreased fat-free mass.[42]

OBESITY AND RESPIRATORY DISORDERS IN OLDER ADULTS

Excess weight, especially central obesity, increases the risk and severity of several respiratory disorders, including asthma, chronic obstructive pulmonary disease (COPD), obstructive sleep apnea, and obesity-hypoventilation syndrome, as well as postoperative respiratory complications, such as atelectasis and venous thromboembolism.[43]

The prevalence of COPD increases with aging, and an age of older than 65 years predicts a poor survival in this patient group.[26] In persons with COPD, body weight and lean body mass significantly influences pulmonary function and respiratory muscle strength, with some increased

mortality in those who are underweight. In addition, current smokers with COPD tend to have lower BMI than persons without COPD, and BMI decreases further with progression of the disease.[44] Nevertheless, obesity can worsen exercise tolerance in persons with COPD; limited exercise capacity and a sedentary lifestyle can, in turn, contribute to further weight gain and decrease in muscle mass.

EFFECTS OF WEIGHT LOSS ON PULMONARY FUNCTION

Optimal weight management may be particularly important for obese older adults who have concurrent medical disorders or functional impairments that would benefit from weight reduction. However, it is essential that weight reduction programs target excess body fat while, at the same time, minimizing loss of lean muscle and bone.[45]

Weight management and exercise has been shown to improve peak oxygen consumption in obese older adults. In one study, 27 frail older adults (age ≥ 65 years; BMI ≥ 30) were randomized to a 6-month weight loss program or control. The former consisted of weekly weight loss behavioral therapy designed to achieve an energy deficit of about 750 kcal per day and thrice-weekly group exercise training. In contrast to the control group whose weight did not change, the treatment group lost 8.2 ± 5.7 kg (8.4% ± 5.6%) of body weight ($P < .001$), with a reduction in body fat but not fat-free mass. This was accompanied by an increase in VO2max (1.7 ± 1.6 versus 0.3 ± 1.1 mL/min/kg) compared with control subjects.[46]

Weight loss appears to be superior to exercise in improving pulmonary function in obese older adults, with greater changes in static lung volumes compared with dynamic pulmonary parameters. Researchers compared the effect of weight reduction or aerobic exercise in pulmonary function in 140 obese, sedentary, middle-aged and older men (46–80 years). Subjects who underwent the weight loss regimen decreased their weight (−11% compared with baseline values), % body fat (−21%), waist circumference (−8%), waist-hip ratio (−2%) and fat-free mass (−3%). These changes were accompanied by increases in FVC (+ 3%; 4.08 ± 0.71 L versus 4.21 ± 0.76 L), TLC (+ 5%; 6.62 ± 0.99 L versus 6.94 ± 0.99 L), FRC (+ 18%; 3.09 ± 0.58 L versus 3.66 ± 0.79 L), and RV (+ 8%; 2.20 ± 0.44 L versus 2.37 ± 0.52 L). Change in body weight correlated with the change in FVC, but changes in % body fat, waist-hip ratio, waist circumference, and fat-free mass did not correlate with changes in any other measure of pulmonary function. No significant changes were observed for FEV1, FEV1/FVC, DLCO, arterial blood gases, or VO2max in the weight-loss group. Although exercise resulted in a reduction in % body fat (−3%) and improved VO2max (+ 14%; $P < .0001$), pulmonary function, waist circumference, and waist-hip ratio did not change in the exercise or control groups.[47]

SUMMARY

The prevalence of obesity among the elderly in the United States is expected to increase and poses unique challenges to both the general health of older adults and more specifically to respiratory function and pulmonary disorders.

REFERENCES

1. Social Security Administration. The 2002 Annual Report of the Board of Trustees of the Federal Old-Age and Survivors Insurance and Disability Insurance Trust Funds, March 26, 2002.
2. Ogden CL, Yanovski SZ, Carroll MD, et al. The epidemiology of obesity. Gastroenterology 2007; 132:2087–102.
3. Arterburn DE, Crane PK, Sullivan SD. The coming epidemic of obesity in elderly Americans. J Am Geriatr Soc 2004;52(11):1907–12.
4. Ogden CL, Carroll MD, Curtin LR, et al. Prevalence of overweight and obesity in the United States, 1999–2004. JAMA 2006;295(13):1549–55.
5. Li F, Fisher KJ, Harmer P. Prevalence of overweight and obesity in older U.S. adults: estimates from the 2003 Behavioral Risk Factor Surveillance System survey. J Am Geriatr Soc 2005;53(4):737–9.
6. Lapane KL, Resnik L. Obesity in nursing homes: an escalating problem. J Am Geriatr Soc 2005;53(8): 1386–91.
7. Zamboni M, Mazzali G, Zoico E, et al. Health consequences of obesity in the elderly: a review of four unresolved questions. Int J Obes (Lond) 2005; 29(9):1011–29.
8. Yan LL, Daviglus ML, Liu K, et al. Midlife body mass index and hospitalization and mortality in older age. JAMA 2006;295(2):190–8.
9. Patterson RE, Frank LL, Kristal AR, et al. A comprehensive examination of health conditions associated with obesity in older adults. Am J Prev Med 2004; 27(5):385–90.
10. Wright NC, Riggs GK, Lisse JR, et al. Women's Health Initiative. Self-reported osteoarthritis, ethnicity, body mass index, and other associated risk factors in postmenopausal women-results from the Women's Health Initiative. J Am Geriatr Soc 2008;56(9):1736–43 [Epub 2008 Jul 17].

11. McCarthy LH, Bigal ME, Katz M, et al. Chronic pain and obesity in elderly people: results from the Einstein aging study. J Am Geriatr Soc 2009;57(1): 115–9 [Epub 2008 Nov 19].
12. Blaum CS, Xue QL, Michelon E, et al. The association between obesity and the frailty syndrome in older women: the women's health and aging studies. J Am Geriatr Soc 2005;53(6):927–34.
13. Jensen GL, Friedmann JM. Obesity is associated with functional decline in community-dwelling rural older persons. J Am Geriatr Soc 2002;50(5):918–23.
14. Davison KK, Ford ES, Cogswell ME, et al. Percentage of body fat and body mass index are associated with mobility limitations in people aged 70 and older from NHANES III. J Am Geriatr Soc 2002;50(11):1802–9.
15. Friedmann JM, Elasy T, Jensen GL. The relationship between body mass index and self-reported functional limitation among older adults: a gender difference. J Am Geriatr Soc 2001;49(4):398–403.
16. Chen H, Guo X. Obesity and functional disability in elderly Americans. J Am Geriatr Soc 2008;56(4): 689–94 [Epub 2008 Feb 11].
17. Lang IA, Llewellyn DJ, Alexander K, et al. Obesity, physical function, and mortality in older adults. J Am Geriatr Soc 2008;56(8):1474–8 [Epub 2008 Jul 24].
18. Grabowski DC, Ellis JE. High body mass index does not predict mortality in older people: analysis of the Longitudinal Study of Aging. J Am Geriatr Soc 2001; 49(7):968–79.
19. Grabowski DC, Campbell CM, Ellis JE. Obesity and mortality in elderly nursing home residents. J Gerontol A Biol Sci Med Sci 2005;60(9):1184–9.
20. Janssen I, Katzmarzyk PT, Ross R. Body mass index is inversely related to mortality in older people after adjustment for waist circumference. J Am Geriatr Soc 2005;53(12):2112–8.
21. Heiat A, Vaccarino V, Krumholz HM. An evidence-based assessment of federal guidelines for overweight and obesity as they apply to elderly persons. Arch Intern Med 2001;161(9):1194–203.
22. Maurer MS, Luchsinger JA, Wellner R, et al. The effect of body mass index on complications from cardiac surgery in the oldest old. J Am Geriatr Soc 2002;50(6):988–94.
23. Batsis JA, Huddleston JM, Melton LJ 4th, et al. Body mass index and risk of adverse cardiac events in elderly patients with hip fracture: a population-based study. J Am Geriatr Soc 2009;57(3): 419–26.
24. Luchsinger JA, Lee WN, Carrasquillo O, et al. Body mass index and hospitalization in the elderly. J Am Geriatr Soc 2003;51(11):1615–20.
25. Teramoto S, Ouchi Y. Aging lung and possible animal models. Chest 1999;116:1145–6.
26. Chan ED, Welsh CH. Geriatric respiratory medicine. Chest 1998;114:1704–33.

27. Turner JM, Mead J, Wohl ME. Elasticity of human lungs in relation to age. J Appl Physiol 1968;25: 664–71.

28. Fitzgerald MD, Tanaka H, Tran ZV, et al. Age-related declines in maximal aerobic capacity in regularly exercising vs. sedentary women: a meta-analysis. J Appl Physiol 1997;83(1):160–5.

29. Hagberg JM. Effect of training on the decline of VO2max with aging. FASEB J 1987;46:1830–3.

30. Heath GW, Hagberg JM, Ehsani AA, et al. A physiological comparison of young and older endurance athletes. J Appl Physiol 1981;51:634–40.

31. Fleg JL, Morrell CH, Bos AG, et al. Accelerated longitudinal decline of aerobic capacity in healthy older adults. Circulation 2005;112:674–82.

32. Villareal DT, Banks M, Siener C, et al. Physical frailty and body composition in obese elderly men and women. Obes Res 2004;12:913–20.

33. Stathokostas L, Jacob-Johnson S, Petrella RJ, et al. Longitudinal changes in aerobic power in older men and women. J Appl Physiol 2004;97:784–9.

34. Rubinstein I, Zamel N, DuBarry L, et al. Airflow limitation in morbidly obese, nonsmoking men. Ann Intern Med 1990;112:828–32.

35. Poulain M, Doucet M, Major GC, et al. The effect of obesity on chronic respiratory diseases: pathophysiology and therapeutic strategies. CMAJ 2006; 174(9):1293–9.

36. Jenkins SC, Moxham J. The effects of mild obesity on lung function. Respir Med 1991;85:309–11.

37. Thomas PS, Cowen ERT, Hulands G, et al. Respiratory function in the morbidly obese before and after weight loss. Thorax 1989;44:382–6.

38. Canoy D, Luben R, Welch A, et al. Abdominal obesity and respiratory function in men and women in the EPIC-Norfolk study, United Kingdom. Am J Epidemiol 2004;159:1140–9.

39. Wannamethee SG, Shaper AG, Whincup PH. Body fat distribution, body composition, and respiratory function in elderly men. Am J Clin Nutr 2005;82: 996–1003.

40. Lazarus R, Sparrow D, Weiss ST. Effects of obesity and fat distribution on ventilatory function: the normative aging study. Chest 1997;111:891–8.

41. Santana H, Zoico E, Turcato E, et al. Relation between body composition, fat distribution, and lung function in elderly men. Am J Clin Nutr 2001;73:827–31.

42. Rossi A, Fantin F, Di Francesco V, et al. Body composition and pulmonary function in the elderly: a 7-year longitudinal study. Int J Obes 2008;32: 1423–30.

43. Soderberg M, Thomson D, White T. Respiration, circulation and anaesthetic management in obesity. Investigation before and after jejunoileal bypass. Acta Anaesthesiol Scand 1977;21:55–61.

44. Nishimura Y, Tsutsumi M, Nakata H, et al. Relationship between respiratory muscle strength and lean body mass in men with COPD. Chest 1995;107: 1232–6.

45. Villareal DT, Apovian CM, Kushner RF, et al. Obesity in older adults: technical review and position statement of the American Society for Nutrition and NAASO, The Obesity Society. Am J Clin Nutr 2005; 82:923–34.

46. Villareal DT, Banks M, Sinacore DR, et al. Effect of weight loss and exercise on frailty in obese older adults. Arch Intern Med 2006;166:860–6.

47. Womack CJ, Harris DL, Katzel LI, et al. Weight loss, not aerobic exercise, improves pulmonary function in older obese men. J Gerontol 2000;55A:M453–7.

Index

Note: Page numbers of article titles are in **boldface** type.

chestmed.theclinics.com

Moving?

Make sure your subscription moves with you!

To notify us of your new address, find your **Clinics Account Number** (located on your mailing label above your name), and contact customer service at:

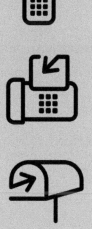

Email: journalscustomerservice-usa@elsevier.com

800-654-2452 (subscribers in the U.S. & Canada)
314-447-8871 (subscribers outside of the U.S. & Canada)

Fax number: 314-447-8029

Elsevier Health Sciences Division
Subscription Customer Service
3251 Riverport Lane
Maryland Heights, MO 63043

ELSEVIER

Moving?

Make sure your subscription moves with you!

To notify us of your new address, find your Clinics Account Number (located on your mailing label above your name), and contact customer service at:

Email: journalscustomerservice-usa@elsevier.com

800-654-2452 (subscribers in the U.S. & Canada)
314-447-8871 (subscribers outside of the U.S. & Canada)

Fax number: 314-447-8029

Elsevier Health Sciences Division
Subscription Customer Service
3251 Riverport Lane
Maryland Heights, MO 63043

To ensure uninterrupted delivery of your subscription, please notify us at least 4 weeks in advance of move.

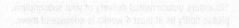

Printed and bound by CPI Group (UK) Ltd, Croydon, CR0 4YY

03/10/2024

01040353-0009